SEX AND SUFFERING

Sex and Suffering

Women's Health and
a Women's Hospital

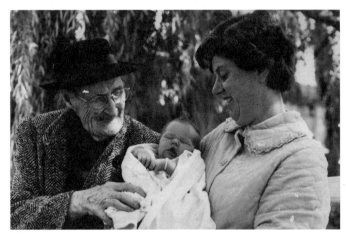

Janet McCalman

THE JOHNS HOPKINS UNIVERSITY PRESS
BALTIMORE AND LONDON

Text © Janet McCalman 1998
Hardcover edition published by Melbourne University Press
All rights reserved

Johns Hopkins Paperbacks edition, 1999
Printed in the United States of America on acid-free paper
9 8 7 6 5 4 3 2 1

The Johns Hopkins University Press
2715 North Charles Street
Baltimore, Maryland 21218-4363
www.press.jhu.edu

Library of Congress Cataloging-in-Publication Data

McCalman, Janet, 1948–
   Sex and suffering : women's health and a women's hospital / Janet
McCalman.
      p.   cm.
   Originally published : Melbourne University Press, 1998.
   Includes bibliographical references and index.
   ISBN 0-8018-6226-4 (pbk. : alk. paper)
   1. Royal Women's Hospital—History. 2. Women's hospitals—
Australia—Melbourne—History—19th century. 3. Women's hospitals—
Australia—Melbourne—History—20th century. 4. Women's health
services—Australia—Melbourne—History—19th century. 5. Women's
health services—Australia—Melbourne—History—20th century.
6. Motherhood—Australia—Melbourne—History—19th century.
7. Motherhood—Australia—Melbourne—History—20th century.
I. Royal Women's Hospital (Melbourne, Vic.) II. Title.
RG501.A8M38   1999
362.1'98'099451—dc21   99-20663
                                                                  CIP

A catalog record for this book is available from the National Library of
Australia.

Contents

VI Human Relations 1945–1970

VII Transformations 1970–1996

Foreword

On 22 January 1866 at two o'clock in the morning, Miss Bridget Kelly, aged twenty-two and born in Ireland, delivered herself of a baby daughter in the Melbourne suburb of Prahran. She knew she needed help and she also knew that somewhere in the city of Melbourne there was a hospital, but the only way to get there was to walk. We don't know how long it took her to walk the four miles to the city. It was dark and the roads unlit, and between Prahran and the river lay bushland and swamps. Once over the river she faced a long, unrelieved climb up Swanston Street, past St Paul's Church and the Town Hall. On the corner of Lonsdale Street she found the Melbourne Hospital, now eighteen years old and the first general hospital in the colony. But it was the wrong place they told her: she needed the Lying-in Hospital, further up the hill in Madeline Street, opposite the university. The hill became steeper and it was a brisk twenty-minute walk for the fit. But this time she was taken in, and when her clothes were drawn aside it was discovered that she 'had the infant in her arms with the *funis* and placenta attached'.

funis: umbilical cord

That is all there is on Bridget Kelly in the Midwifery Book of the Lying-in Hospital and Infirmary for the Diseases Peculiar to Women. She named her baby Ann; the father's name was unknown. If this book is about that Lying-in Hospital which is today Melbourne's Royal Women's Hospital, it is also about all the Bridget Kellys, married and unmarried, who have passed through its wards and clinics in the past one hundred and forty years. Their case histories and the hospital's varying treatments of their childbed and diseases are a window into the private lives and reproductive health of poor women over the past century and a half. The hospital's history is also, therefore, the history of women — as mothers, as lovers, as citizens, as victims, as nurses and medical staff, even as prostitutes and drug addicts. This history is not significant because of where it happened, but because of when it did.

The hospital was born in 1856, in the dawn of anaesthesia, before the antiseptic and aseptic revolutions, and its story will conclude with AIDS and In-Vitro Fertilisation in our own time. Although the Female Convict

Factory and the Sydney Benevolent Asylum had instituted lying-in wards, it was the first of its kind in the Australian and New Zealand colonies, and remains one of the oldest surviving women's hospitals in the world. When the Medical Faculty opened at the University of Melbourne in 1862, it became the Antipodean colonies' first specialist teaching hospital. It has always been a 'charity' or 'public' hospital, serving the poor and the awkward, but in providing the compliant pudenda for clinical teaching, it ensured that in return the poor women of south-eastern Australia often received the best care that contemporary medicine could offer. Its history has its dark times and not all patients were treated well, but a hospital is a product of its society and its time, as much as being a shaper.

This history is about a hospital at work, about its staff and their practices and values, and about the patients themselves. A hospital is a complex web of human relationships — a small stage upon which the wider dramas of life and society are enacted. Moreover, the reproductive health of both men and women is critically affected by their behaviour and their environment, and it is thus a contest between impulse and calculation, nature and society, biology and history. It is here, more than in any other area of health, that beliefs, desires, fears and knowledge impinge on biologically driven behaviour. Consciousness enables us to love and therefore to grieve, to nurture or to neglect, to lust after and to reject, and our libido and our biological reproductive imperative can be locked in mortal conflict. We can want and conceive a baby without wanting sex and we can want sex but not a baby, and human reproduction is riven with such paradoxes. It is a natural process and yet it is also part of nature that it can go tragically wrong. It belongs to the great biological struggle between the fit and the sick, the strong and the weak, yet we resist that and men grieve for their dead wives, and children mourn their lost mothers. Our reproductive efficiency is dependent on social structures and environmental conditions, so that even now the majority of childbearing women in the world are undernourished and overworked, and the best medicine is feeble in the face of poverty and political indifference. Perhaps most difficult of all is the fact that our need for sexual pleasure exceeds the capacity of our bodies to bear safely all the babies that unrestrained sexual passion can conceive: inducing some to wonder whether 'nature's' own method of birth control was the sickness of women.

The story of the medicalisation of childbirth and the treatment of the diseases peculiar to women, as they described them in the 1850s, is the story of human intervention in that biological dilemma. It is not a story of unalloyed progress or of unambiguous benefits, but sex, unmitigated by medical science and contraception, can bring suffering to women. It can burden them with pregnancies which break their health and shorten their lives; it can transmit diseases which disfigure, kill and afflict the next generation; it can even bring pain and suffering to those who remain celibate or infertile. And the rich archives of this old hospital document tens of thousands of lives blighted by the sufferings of sex. They are a vast repository of private female misery: of difficult lives of pain, disablement and sickness. But they also reveal the transformations in the life experience of women brought about by the most dramatic interventions in human biology ever seen in history: the conquest of bacterial infection

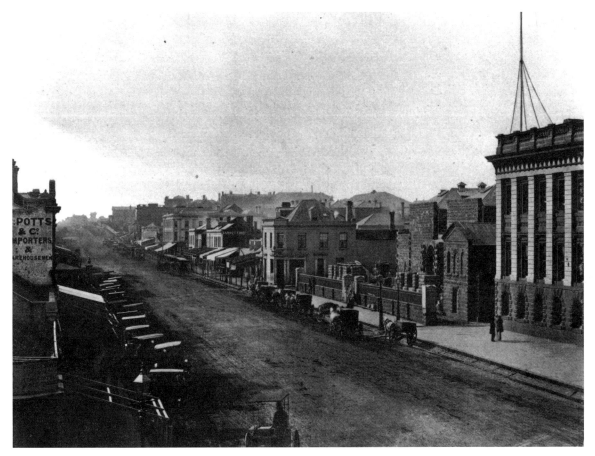

**Swanston Street,
Melbourne, 1858,**
*La Trobe Picture Collection,
State Library of Victoria*

and the safe control of conception. At an ecological level these have been monumental changes for us as a species — changes with which, perhaps, we have scarcely begun to cope.

Inevitably, these are partial rather than complete victories over both biology and human needs. New diseases emerge and old defences weaken, while people continue to act on impulse, to make mistakes, to be unlucky, to be too poor to avail themselves of the benefits of science and technology. Women still become pregnant when they don't want to, or long for babies denied them, or catch dire infections, or do things which endanger their unborn. Their sexual health still depends on their emotions, ideas, behaviour, social condition and economic situation; and on the values and moral health of the society they inhabit. In other words, their health will only be as good as their society permits it to be. And a vital measure of a society's delivery of medical knowledge and care to those in need of it are its public hospitals.

Some readers may find what follows too graphic for comfort. The use of detailed case histories is not gratuitous, however, but carefully considered. This is a history of medical and surgical practice, of nursing techniques and of medical culture; that is, of a hospital at work, and we need to see clearly what that work was and what its consequences were. But most of all, we dishonour people of the past if we shrink from comprehending their pain and the difficulties they faced.

Abbreviations

Sources for Marginalia

AMA	Australian Medical Association
AMG	*Australian Medical Gazette*
AMJ	*Australian Medical Journal*
B of M	Board of Management
BMA	British Medical Association
C of M	Committee of Management
CH	Children's Hospital
IMJ	*Intercolonial Medical Journal*
LIH	Lying-in Hospital
MJA	*Medical Journal of Australia*
MH	Melbourne Hospital
QVH	Queen Victoria Hospital
RCH	Royal Children's Hospital
RMH	Royal Melbourne Hospital
RMO	Resident Medical Officer
RWH	Royal Women's Hospital
RWHA	Royal Women's Hospital Archives
WH	Women's Hospital

Allen & Hanburys: *Catalogue* (London, 1924)

AMD: *The American Illustrated Medical Dictionary* (Philadelphia, 1906)

Black: *Black's Medical Dictionary,* seventeenth edition (London, 1942)

Burbidge: G. N. Burbidge, *Lectures for Nurses* (Sydney, 1949)

OMD: *Oxford Concise Medical Dictionary*, third edition (Oxford, 1990)

Playfair: W. S. Playfair, *A Treatise on the Science and Practice of Midwifery* Vol. II (London, 1882)

Townsend (G): Lance Townsend, *Gynaecology for Students* (Sydney, 1974)

Townsend (O): Lance Townsend, *Obstetrics for Students* (Sydney, 1978)

Acknowledgements

The first to thank are the members of the former Board of Management and of the Archives Committee who, in planning a history of Melbourne's Royal Women's Hospital, decided that it should be a social history of women's health as well as a history of a hospital: the last two presidents, Mary Murdoch and Dr Gytha Betheras, and with them Elizabeth Chernov, Dr John Colebatch, Dr James Evans, Dr Cliff Flower, Alison Leslie and Margaret Mabbitt. In addition, Professor Patricia Grimshaw, Ian Ness and Professor John Poynter served on the advisory committee. They have been part of the project for more than seven years and their support and inspiration have been unfailing. No historian could hope for a better reference group.

Second, an Australian Research Council Fellowship and a large research grant made the project possible in the History Department of the University of Melbourne. Among my colleagues there I thank in particular the two succeeding heads of department, Professors Patricia Grimshaw and Peter McPhee; also Associate Professor Warwick Anderson and my new colleagues at the Centre for the Study of Health and Society at the University of Melbourne.

Third, there have been my day-to-day colleagues who have shared more of this project than anyone else: Robyn Waymouth, the Archivist of the Royal Women's Hospital, Margaret Mabbitt, and my research assistants, Jane Beer and Dr Cecile Trioli. They have been a joy to work with, unfailingly patient and wise. Liliana Ferrara, Madonna Grehan, Catherine Hallam (Dedman), Helen Johnstone, Marlene Kavanagh and Margaret Mabbitt conducted the oral history survey as well as providing constant support and advice. Among the many past and present members of staff of the hospital I single out Gary Henry, Netta McArthur, Margaret Peters, Jo Raw and her staff, the library staff and the many people who talked over lunch and morning tea and slowly taught me the ways of the Women's. I also thank the staff at the Educational Resource Centre of the Women's and Children's Healthcare Network who scanned most of the illustrations.

Dr James Evans, Dr Robin Bell, Dr James Smibert, Mr A. G. Bond and the late Dr Frank Forster all read case histories and interpreted them for me. Robin Bell gave much of her time to the analysis of the birth weight data. Emeritus Professor Harold Attwood provided wise counsel from beginning to end.

I am deeply grateful to all those who read a long and complicated manuscript either in part or from end to end: Emeritus Professor Harold Attwood, Jane Beer, Dr Robin Bell, Dr Gytha Betheras, Professor Shaun Brennecke, Dr Ian Britain, Dr James Evans, Dr Suzanne Garland, Dr Robin Haines, Dr Caroline Hannaway, Dr Bill Kitchen, Margaret Mabbitt, Mary Murdoch, Dr Ralph Shlomowitz, Professor F. B. Smith, Dr Cecile Trioli and Robyn Waymouth. Remaining flaws are my responsibility alone.

Finally, many friends and colleagues have helped along what has been a long and difficult road. I thank them all. But I thank most of all my family, Al Knight and our children, Nicholas and Imogen, who help far more than they can ever know.

I

Tracy's Hospital
1856–1874

Founding a Hospital 1

Dr Tracy, Dr Maund and Mrs Perry

Melbourne clung to the southern rim of the inhabited world and, when the hospital was founded in 1856, it was a raw, new city just twenty-one years old as a European settlement and in the midst of a gold rush. It was a frontier society, blending English, Scots, Irish, American, European and Chinese with the released 'old lags' and their Currency lads and lasses of the Australian penal settlements. But the vigour and wealth of the colony concealed tragedy, because the Koori people, whose land the Europeans had stolen, were already pushed to the margin, their population cut by 90 per cent by murder, disease and despair.[1]

Victoria was one of the last settled colonies after the First Fleet landed in Sydney Cove in 1788 — Van Diemen's Land, or Tasmania, had been the first southern settlement and a harsher penal colony than Sydney. In 1803 a party of soldiers and convicts had attempted a settlement at Sorrento in Victoria, until discord and a shortage of water drove them away. Whalers and sealers worked from the Victorian coast, but it was not until the 1830s that the push into Victoria began, first in the west at Portland and then in 1835 at Port Phillip Bay at the mouth of the Yarra River. The best sheep-grazing land in New South Wales and in the midlands of Tasmania had all been claimed, and the Vandemonians became interested in the lands across Bass Strait. In 1836 Major Mitchell returned from his inland explorations extolling an 'Australia Felix' of rolling plains and good soils, and the squatters and their flocks streamed into the western district. The Melbourne, Portland and Geelong settlements became firmly established and the society built by the colonists was soon very different from the older colonies. About two thousand former convicts (Derwenters) came of their own accord from Tasmania, and since they were willing to go to the bush as shepherds, where they could live out a life of uninterrupted alcoholism, they formed the rural labouring class. By 1851 about 15 per cent of the adult population were convicts or discharged convicts. There were assisted immigrants, but the long voyage to Australia was beyond the means of the destitute, so that even the Irish who came during the famine years had something behind them. Only 1300 Irish orphan girls from the workhouses and the Gaelic-speaking Scots brought out by the Highland and Island Emigration Society who arrived in Victoria in the 1850s were truly survivors of the potato famine. It is scarcely surprising, therefore, that only 15 per cent of the assisted immigrants from 1839 to 1850 were illiterate. Those who came to Victoria and paid their own way in the 1830s and 1840s were a relatively skilled and educated class, so that for a time the colony was the most literate society in the British Empire.[2] There were enough with capital and 'breeding' to establish a polite society of calls and clubs, balls and duelling and, for some, duties of public spiritedness.[3] Andrew and Georgiana McCrae were 'quality', even though she was illegitimate and he was improvident, yet they both were prominent in society, and Andrew was a participant in numerous societies and networks which bound the new community together in chains of mutual obligation and social responsibility.[4] The philanthropic impulse was integral to the workings of gentility.

The philanthropic impulse was also integral to the workings of evangelical Christianity, and among the cultural baggage brought to the new colony was a practical Christian charity which was voluntarist. In England by 1700 concern for the sick poor had displaced the respect for poverty as an ascetic holy state: poverty was now seen to be the just burden of the lazy and improvident, whereas sickness could be blameless. Moreover, unwillingness to provide became a masculine failing, so that charity was gendered. The sick poor, along with dependent women and children, were thus deserving of charity, and groups of Protestants had formed voluntary hospitals which, in the words of K. S. Inglis, were 'like the new joint-stock companies, from whose profits much of the revenue for philanthropy was drawn, they owed their strength not to the work and wealth of one man, but to association. They invited all who could afford it to become subscribers, with rights analogous to shareholders'.[5] In constructing a new society, the genteel classes of the colony of Victoria established an impressive network of asylums for the indigent, the deaf and blind and the immigrant, all without a Poor Law which criminalised poverty.[6] In 1848 the philanthropically-minded supported with subscriptions the founding of the Melbourne Hospital. It had all the hallmarks of a charity hospital: its medical staff were honoraries and it was governed by an unpaid committee elected by the subscribers. The government, however, considered it had no direct financial responsibility for the hospital, thus Melbourne's first hospital was a voluntary institution because the government forced it to be.

In 1851 Victoria was made a separate colony from New South Wales, but barely had the celebrations ceased before the news burst that gold had been discovered. In the next ten years more than half a million men, women and children flooded the colony, and among them were a quarter of a million permanent settlers from the United Kingdom. By the time most of them arrived, however, the alluvial gold had been found and there was little opportunity for the adventurer digger. There were riches deep in the ground, but that mining required capital and machinery and management. For all those hoping for Eldorado on the track to the gold-fields, there were just as many disappointed diggers trailing their way back to Melbourne.

Among those disillusioned goldseekers was a young Irish doctor, Richard Tracy. Tracy was born in Limerick in 1826, to a Protestant professional family. At sixteen he determined to be a doctor and not enter the Church as his mother had hoped. In preparation, he worked for a time as a wardsman and dresser in the County Limerick Infirmary — a medical apprenticeship he later much valued — and at the age of nineteen began his proper medical studies in Dublin. It was the time of the famine, and during each of the three succeeding summer vacations Tracy volunteered for service with the Irish Board of Health. Typhus broke out and at Celbridge, near Dublin, Tracy himself contracted it and very nearly died. In 1848 he received his Licentiate of the Royal College of Surgeons of Ireland and immediately afterwards went to Paris 'where he saw a good deal of useful surgical practice during that epoch of revolutions'.[7] At the end of the year he moved to Glasgow where, during an epidemic, he was in charge of the City Cholera Hospital of seven hundred beds, and in May 1849 he took his MD from the University of Glasgow. He returned to Ireland but, finding it difficult to establish himself, tried practice in England. He was on the point of starting a military career when he suddenly became engaged to his cousin, Fanny. News came from Australia and from Canada of opportunities for practice, and one evening in his brother's rooms in Lincoln's Inn in 1851, Tracy tossed a coin and Adelaide was the winner. The cousins married and on 16 May set sail for Australia. Tracy was a not untypical colonial immigrant: talented, energetic and ambitious, but lacking in the capital which could build a leading practice in his native land.

The Tracys settled in Adelaide, but by February 1852 it seemed as though nearly every able-bodied male in South Australia had left for the Victorian diggings. Tracy, despite the birth of his first daughter, could not resist temptation either, and in the company of the future historian James Bonwick, tried his luck in Bendigo and on the Loddon. It was soon clear that medical practice was more predictable, and after a quick return to Adelaide, the Tracys moved to Melbourne where he set up in Brunswick Street, Fitzroy. The house was tiny, with four rooms, and the rent was an exorbitant seven guineas a week — more money was being made out of the goldseekers than by them. Tracy, a founder of the Australian Medical Society in 1852, hosted meetings where his colleagues sat on the piano and on the cupboards. In 1854 he had made enough to build a two-storeyed house on the west side of Brunswick Street, and the Irish aspirant was well established. But he was also widely loved, for in two years that unpretentious house had become 'as well known as any public building in Victoria'.[8]

One of Tracy's Melbourne friends, Dr John Maund, was another not untypical immigrant. He was born in Bromsgrove, Worcestershire, and his father, Benjamin Maund, Fellow of the Linnean Society, was a world famous botanist. John Maund was the eldest of three sons and, despite a delicate constitution, he wanted to study medicine. He served an apprenticeship under a surgeon in Lancashire before going on to the University of Glasgow where he won many prizes. At the age of twenty-one he

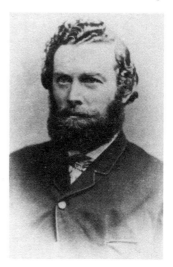

Dr Richard Tracy, 1874
RWHA

became assistant surgeon at the St Pancras Infirmary in London while studying at the Royal College of Surgeons. He received his Diploma in 1845 and then spent a year attending hospitals and lectures in Paris, achieving membership of the Parisian Medical Society. In June 1847 he qualified for the Diploma of the Apothecaries' Society, and then the MD at St Andrews. He began private practice in Harlow.

However, it was soon clear that he had contracted tuberculosis. It seemed advisable to emigrate to a warmer climate in Australia and to pursue a less taxing career as an analytical chemist. He sold his practice in 1851 and, before leaving, took out the certificates of the Royal College of Chemistry, London, and of the Polytechnic Chemical School. Dr Maund, with one of his three sisters, arrived in Melbourne in the *Janet Mitchell* on 3 January 1853, and his fellow passengers presented him with a silver tankard in gratitude for his services to them during the voyage. Some continued to consult him in Melbourne, and he eventually decided to stay in medical practice. His first rooms were in a small, cramped house in Lonsdale Street East in the city, and he practised there until May 1857 when he moved into a new house in Latrobe Street East. The poor lived close by, down the lanes and alleys of the growing town. He was Victoria's first Government Analyst, making investigations into the quality of Melbourne's new piped water supply from the Yan Yean Reservoir. Maund quickly developed a large practice, especially in the newer suburbs. If his friend Tracy was vital, generous and brave, Maund was a sweet man, thoughtful and reflective. They were both young doctors of exceptional promise and complementary gifts.[9]

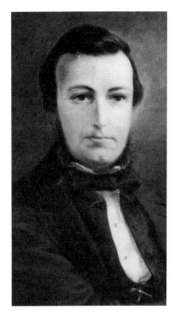

Dr John Maund *RWHA*

Tracy was thirty and Maund thirty-three years old when they began talking to each other about a lying-in hospital for destitute women in Melbourne. They saw the need for a place to confine the numerous homeless and friendless women in gold-rush Melbourne, but they were also subject to very real medical ambition. Both had studied French clinical science in Paris, and they wanted a modern hospital, on the scale of the Edinburgh Maternity — a hospital where health and disease could be studied, where a man could specialise and develop a reputation not merely with his patients, but also with his peers, where medical practice left the private bedchamber and went on public view. Richard Tracy wanted to be an Antipodean James Young Simpson.

But there was another group in Melbourne also thinking about a lying-in hospital. Prominent among them was Mrs Frances Perry, the wife of the Bishop of Melbourne. The Perrys had arrived in Melbourne in 1848, when Port Phillip was still just the mercantile centre for a pastoralist society. Charles Perry was an Evangelical, highly intelligent, outwardly stern and inwardly affectionate. Theirs was a childless but devoted marriage, and Fanny accompanied her husband on horseback as he set about visiting his vast diocese, journeys she wrote about with a sharp and compassionate eye. Her philanthropic instincts were strong, if condescending, and she viewed the moral and social pandemonium of the gold rush with amusement and alarm. On 2 September 1852 she wrote:

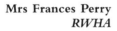

Mrs Frances Perry
RWHA

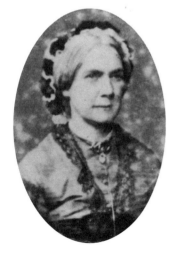

I was all but mobbed today in the street, but happily contrived to rush into Mrs — 's just in time . . . After the mob came a carriage with four dashing past, full of white veils and white satins. It is most amusing to see how completely the tables are turned. There is now a stand of some eighteen or twenty carriages in Collins Street; and these may be seen careering about all day long in all parts of the town and suburbs, full of diggers, varied occasionally, as I have said, by the white veils. Fancy some of these inexpressibly awkward-looking, fat, firm, red-faced Irish girls from the unions [workhouses], dressed out in the best satin, lace and flowers which Melbourne can produce! It is indeed an everyday occurrence; and they are not unfrequently to be seen waiting in front of a public-house, the 'gentlemen' having gone in for a 'nobbler' (did you ever hear such a word before) and I fear it is only the apprehension of spoiling the finery which prevents the bride and her bridesmaids from following them. It is not only on occasion of a wedding that these people drive about, but it seems an every-day's amusement, just as persons in London go out to drive in the Park. You may imagine what a state the carriages get into, with their dirty and often drunken occupants; for the men go driving about in their working dresses.[10]

Most diggers and Irish girls were not so lucky. The colony's resources were stretched to breaking point, and thousands found themselves living in cramped cottages or tents on swampy, low-lying ground. Prices for everything soared and savings were often exhausted before diggers even made it to the goldfields. It may have been 'Australia Felix', but the land itself took getting used to. The winters were bearable for northern Europeans, for if there was rain and cold, it did not snow and only inland on the gold fields were frosts severe. What they were not prepared for was the summer heat. For three months of the year the heat came in three- and four-day waves, brought by savage winds from the dry centre of the continent. The mercury climbed over 100°F, and the only relief was to be found shut away from the wind and in shade; modesty forbade that men and women should strip to barest clothing on dry land, as many had done on board ship while sailing through the tropics. As Isabella Wyly, an Irish immigrant wrote home in 1857:

> You say I told you nothing about the Climate, but what with <u>dust, &</u> <u>Heat</u> & <u>hot</u> <u>winds</u> & <u>Flys</u> & <u>an Insect that the[y] call Moskitoes</u> we do not know what to do with ourselves just now . . . It makes me quite cold to think of [?] winter yet for just now we are all just <u>Melted with heat.</u>[11]

Australia was a land of flies that delighted in the human and animal waste the European invasion now daily dumped on the earth and in the waterways. Food left out soon became black with flies; flies crawled over children's sticky faces and colonised open wounds. With summer came drought and water shortages so that drinking water itself became an expensive commodity. In 1857 piped water was brought to Melbourne, but the supply was insufficient and the low pressure often saw it fail on the hottest days. All creeks and rivers soon became open sewers wherever they were close to dense human settlement. Thus on the goldfields, in the small towns, in the city and suburbs, and in the canvas town of the immigrants, while gastro-enteritis carried off babies and children, 'colonial fever' struck down adults. It would be another twenty years before doctors would reliably recognise it as typhoid.[12]

The hopes dashed were not just for instant wealth. The bid for a new life prompted many to marry quickly before boarding ship, only to find the marriage sour amidst the tedium and tensions of a long sea voyage. Single women, hoping for employment and a husband, succumbed to the promises of strange men and found themselves pregnant and alone. Married women were suddenly deserted or widowed, or left wandering alone in Melbourne while their men tried their luck 'up-country'. By 1854 the colony was plunged into economic depression as thousands of failed diggers struggled to find work in an economy too small to accommodate the surge of population. And drink and gold, dislocation and waywardness led to moral ruin. There were desperate women at risk of falling.

Or so it looked to the evangelical conscience in 1856. Bishop Perry had already burnt his fingers at the Melbourne Hospital. In 1853 he had attempted to evangelise the hospital with daily readings of prayers and the preaching of sermons in the wards — the Catholics objected to being subjected to Protestant services and the doctors objected because soon all denominations would be doing it, 'leading the helpless congregation in continuous worship'.[13] This time the Evangelicals would be more

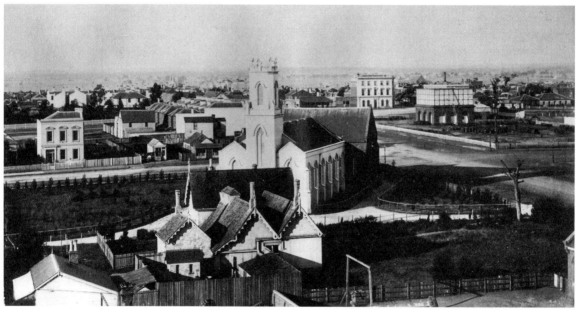

Eastern Hill, 1866, photograph by Charles Nettleton: original Lying-in Hospital in Albert Street at left of St Peter's Church *RWHA*

careful. In the first week of August 1856, under the advice of the Dean of Melbourne, Frances Perry and her committee first approached the Melbourne Hospital to see if twenty beds for lying-in and four to six beds for delivery could be provided for 'destitute women in their confinements'.[14] The Melbourne Hospital declined and the Treasurer of the Colony made it known that the government could not be expected to support such a venture until it was demonstrated to be both needed and feasible. The committee then heard that Dr Maund and Dr Tracy were in the process of establishing a lying-in hospital in Albert Street, East Melbourne. The ladies approached the doctors, and despite differences, they quickly decided to join forces. The property was a nine-roomed stone house capable of accommodating seventeen patients, a matron and two resident servants. On 19 August 1856 the first patient, Mrs Hingston, born in Ireland and expecting her first baby, was admitted. Three weeks later, after an exhausting twenty-seven hour labour, she was delivered by Dr Maund of a stillborn son.

A Simpson Hospital

The doctors and the Ladies' Committee were not entirely united in their ideas on the form the institution should take. The Ladies took charge of the lay running of the hospital and the admission of patients: theirs was to be a committee of Protestants only, but women of all faiths were to be admitted.[15] To their mind the hospital would need public good will if it were to prosper, and respectable people of means were unlikely to become subscribers to a hospital full of diseased prostitutes and wayward single mothers. As it was, the English lying-in establishments, aside from Queen Charlotte's in London, admitted only the married. Moreover lying-in hospitals were notorious for their high death rates, especially from puerperal fever, so Melbourne's Lying-in Hospital would be best served by admitting only the respectable and clean down on their luck. The doctors saw it differently, however. They wanted to admit on both medical and social need, and to have the discretion to admit emergency cases: a sick woman, however abandoned, they believed, still had a right to treatment. The doctors had wide support among the medical profession and Tracy's friend Dr Motherwell reminded them that the great Rotunda Hospital in Dublin — 'perhaps the noblest institution in the world for lying-in women' — made no such discriminations. Motherwell, a Scot and political radical, then threatened to speak ill of the hospital in the town if he heard that single women were being kept out.[16] It was a conflict that would continue to fester.

The Ladies' Committee had much to do. The providing committee ran the financial side of the household, and discussions were under way to persuade the government to support the establishment of a proper hospital: the East Melbourne property was merely a staging post. Neither was it welcome in a genteel suburb, where owners of neighbouring properties soon complained of the screams from the labour room.[17] The doctors also wanted a purpose-built hospital because they had advanced ideas about the way hospitals needed to be organised if puerperal fever were to be prevented and their professional ambitions realised. In April 1857 the government granted them two acres of land in 'Madeline Street, North Melbourne' — later known as Swanston Street, Carlton. In the meantime the East Melbourne establishment concentrated on midwifery, with only a few admissions for 'diseases peculiar to women' such as one woman who was tapped of seventeen pints of ascitic fluid, but the out-patients service was keenly sought. The medical officers were required to attend alternately every Monday, Wednesday, Thursday and Saturday between the hours of two and three o'clock for the outpatients. The Matron, a divorced but remarried woman known by her first married

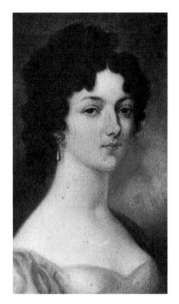

Mrs Sarah Gillbee, matron 1856–1857 *RWHA*

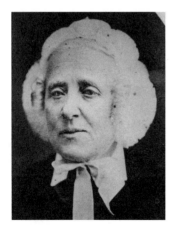

Mrs Elizabeth Tripp, first secretary *RWHA*

name of Gillbee, ran the household with two servants. The names of the first midwives and nurses were never recorded.

The Ladies' Committee supplied the household, visited the hospital three times a week, and reviewed applications for tickets of admission.[18] An applicant would come with a reference, preferably from a subscriber, which would attest to her need and her respectability. Sometimes she stood before the committee for forty minutes to be questioned: was she married, and if so, where were her marriage lines; was her income less than 30 shillings a week; did she have friends who could take her in for her confinement; was she suitably repentant for her sins if she was pregnant and single; would the child's father marry her in time; was there hope of salvation? If they looked for remorse from the fallen, they also took it upon themselves to force the putative fathers to accept their responsibilities. Ellen, 'an ignorant Irish girl', had been impregnated by her master, Mr Delaney in Dandenong, and was now so 'absolutely destitute' that the local police officer was 'at a loss as what to do with her'. The committee's response was to reject her and recommend that the police take action against Mr Delaney.[19] Two months later Eliza G. did better. For nine months she had worked for the wife of Edward Cotton, Registrar of the County Court of Bourke, and then moved on. Two months ago she returned to the Cotton household, pregnant and 'needing help'. Her other employer testified that she had been a 'nursemaid and [servant] for eleven months and in both situations she behaved in the most trustworthy, honest and sober manner'. Mrs Cotton felt 'much interested in her' and took her in, but it would not be 'convenient' for her to be confined in the home. And so, with the generous references of respectable people, Eliza G., aged twenty-three and born in England, on 18 January 1857 gave birth after a three-hour labour to an 8-pound son, 24 inches long.[20] Eliza G.'s story was a common one. Many of the single women were cared for by employers or neighbours, past and present, and were given lodging — perhaps nothing more than a corner with some straw for a bed — but it was still an intimate, face-to-face society.

The Ladies' Committee, most of them wives of clergymen, visited huts and tents, public houses and boarding houses — down back lanes and across paddocks — asking after the applicants. They saw a lot of raw colonial life and could be moved to genuine charity. Mrs M. F. was in an awful state: 'Her case, if true, is very sad, and needs such prompt assistance that I hardly know what is best to be done'. Quickly, however, Mrs F.'s daughters were taken into the Immigrants' Home and she into the Lying-in Hospital two weeks before her baby was due. After a ten hour labour, she produced a son of nine and a half pounds.[21] Mrs R. M.'s husband had left her and returned to England, and she was taken in as a servant by Dr Florance of Collingwood. She was thirty-six and her first baby was stillborn, having died *in utero* two days before labour began.[22] Another who lost her baby was Mrs M. K., Scottish and known in Emerald Hill as 'a decent well-doing woman' whose wharf-labourer husband had been 'a good deal out of work lately'.[23] The Ladies' Committee did not always detect vice when it was there. They did not realise that A. E., nineteen and Irish, was diseased. She was admitted in labour, and her small baby died five days later from 'secondary syphilis'. The doctors kept her in hospital for ten weeks afterwards, perhaps for mercury treatment, and no one on the committee either objected or knew of her real condition. Tracy was well informed on syphilis. He used a translated French text on the health of children and the *Australian Medical Journal* published the latest research on syphilis.[24]

John Maund and Richard Tracy had each undergone medical training in Scotland and they brought to Melbourne the Simpson legacy of 'obstetrical science'.[25] They believed that isolation was the best preventative against infection — Tracy had considerable experience in fever hospitals — so the terrace house was far from ideal for a lying-in establishment and they were determined to build an institution on scientific principles. They saw themselves as men of science: they were among the founders of the Medical Society and its journal, the *Australian Medical Journal*. They shared the excitement of building a colony, which being made afresh could be better; and they were tantalised by the scientific challenge of observing disease and death in a new world. In the Scots tradition of medical topography, the Medical Society had its members recording the weather and studying the new social and geographical characteristics of the colony. Surely disease would behave differently here in so novel an environment, and already Dr Kilgour had declared phthisis less dangerous in Victoria, but miscarriages more common, even among women who were not engaged in heavy physical work.[26] The Medical Society was also much concerned with medical reform by the obtaining of an Act to regulate entry to the profession and eliminate quacks. For Tracy and Maund, a lying-in hospital like James Young Simpson's in Edinburgh would not only provide care for destitute women, it would advance the quality and the standing of their practice and profession.

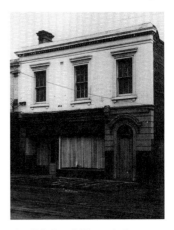

Dr Richard Tracy's house in Brunswick Street, Fitzroy, photographed in 1964 *RWHA*

Simpson's astonishing success depended not just on scrupulous care but also on clinical scientific method. He had measured everything from length of labour to the length of umbilical cords, and by careful evaluation of practice he was able to create standards for improvement.[27] The charity hospital made possible the practice of clinical science: doctors could observe, measure, compare and the patients could neither object nor demand therapies and nostrums. In the charity hospital the doctor exercised a control denied him in the private medical relationship. Moreover, the concentration of cases made comparison and analysis easier. The statistical enumeration of conditions and treatments elevated medical analysis from the particular and anecdotal, to the general and scientific. It was an empirical clinical science that the two young doctors had also studied in Paris.[28]

By the beginning of December Tracy and Maund had a Simpson's Midwifery Book and they began their system of full record taking. Recorded were the patient's name, place of birth, age, marital status and parity — the number of her confinements, including the impending one. Labour time was recorded, but with less precision than later and this seemed to cover the time the labouring woman needed to go to bed. The baby's presentation was noted, its condition, its sex, its weight and length. Lastly the time of discharge was meant to be entered. Any complications were to be briefly described, but it seems that the doctors were not consistent in recording whether a baby died during the mother's time in hospital. They were scrupulous about noting any interventions by instruments or the hand, but not whether a woman suffered a postnatal infection. The record taking improved, but not until 1857 was the system in place and fully functioning.[29]

In the founding year, Tracy and Maund delivered twenty-five women, of whom seven were unmarried. Twelve came from Ireland, ten from England, and one apiece from Scotland and Wales. The one Australian was eighteen-year-old Mrs T. from Tasmania, and she had the only instrumental delivery after an agonising labour of sixty-two hours with the baby's head 'face-to-pubis'. Her son was a giant — 11 pounds and 23 inches long — and her exhausted uterus haemorrhaged 'for want of contraction'. Maund delivered her with forceps under chloroform 'without difficulty' and she was discharged only sixteen days later. Mrs H., aged twenty-seven and from England, was not so lucky. She also had a difficult labour but her 10-pound son was stillborn and she was in hospital for nine weeks after, presumably recovering from infection and weakness.

Attitudes of the foetus A. Vertex presentation: the head is fully flexed and the sub-occipito-bregmatic diameter presents. B. Face presentation: the head is fully extended and the cervico-bregmatic diameter presents. C. Brow presentation: the head is partially extended and the supra-occipito-mental diameter presents. *Townsend (O), p. 123*

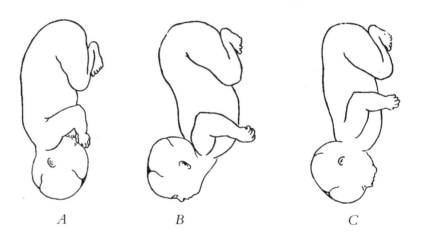

A   *B*   *C*

In the October issue of the *Australian Medical Journal* Maund published his analysis of the first hundred confinements in the hospital. The mothers had comprised 52 Irish, 36 English and 12 born elsewhere. Only 16 were unmarried. Sixty-five were having their first baby, and there were 99 head presentations and one footling. The average labour time was nine hours, the shortest just one hour and the longest lasted sixty-two hours. As for the babies, there was one set of twins and six babies were stillborn. Of the live babies there were 45 male and 40 female, average weight 7 pounds — the smallest weighing 5 pounds, the biggest 11 pounds. The forceps were applied only three times, with two live babies resulting. And there was no death or severe injury to a mother. Dr Maund was proud of the record and announced that such statistical work was essential if they were to discover whether 'any or what differences exist in parturition in this and other countries'. It was also a way in which the doctors could measure whether the mortality in a lying-in hospital was better or worse than in home deliveries.[30] These were the beginnings of a clinical school.

The building of the new hospital in Madeline Street proceeded rapidly and it was opened by the Governor, Sir Henry Barkly, on 22 October

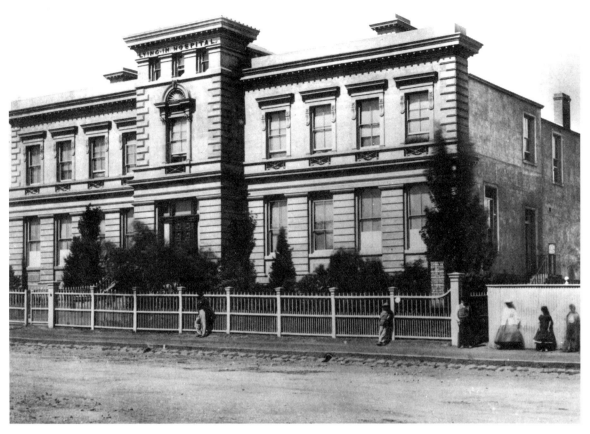

Melbourne Lying-in Hospital, Madeline Street, photographed by Charles Nettleton *RWHA*

1858, just eighteen months after the grant of land. The doctors had had their way with the committee and Tracy was to be deeply proud of his hospital for the rest of his life: it had cost to this stage £6190 10s. The outside world was impressed: the façade was pleasant and beautifully situated on a hill opposite the University's gardens. It had handsome stone steps leading up to a spacious vestibule, which was to be 'panelled and supported by pilasters and entablatures with columns of the Ionic order': a dignified setting for the unfortunate few who, rushing to the hospital in labour, made it only so far as the vestibule and delivered their babies on the floor. On the ground floor were the boardroom, the dispensary, the house surgeon's apartments, and 'two large wards for married women expecting their accouchement'. Beneath there was extensive cellarage.[31] Upstairs in the two-storeyed front building were the matron's apartment, the linen room, an operating room, three gynaecological wards and 'a very fine corridor for the patients to promenade in'.

The hospital's distinctiveness lay in its midwifery wards. These were adjoining the front building and ranged on the side of a central courtyard. They were each twelve feet square, twelve feet high, with a fireplace, a window ventilator in the wall and movable fanlight over the door; the walls were painted for about five feet from the floor, the remainder lime-washed. An eight-feet wide veranda along the entire range of wards made it possible to move patients in their beds from one part of the hospital to another. On the other side of the courtyard, which was to be planted with shrubs, there was a matching wing containing the servants' rooms, the kitchen, storeroom, bathroom and water closets. The laundryroom was large enough for the fumigation of mattresses. The water supply was not reticulated to individual wards, nor were there toilets in the main building. Water was collected from the roof and stored in four large zinc tanks. The refuse water was conveyed underground to two large filtration tanks outside the building, where, 'after undergoing a self-acting deodorising process, it passes into the street in a comparatively pure state'.[32] Tracy designed the waste filtration system himself, and in 1860, when the hospital was connected to the reticulated water from the Yan Yean reservoir, the system was complete.[33] (Not until 1869 did the filter system fail and the Melbourne City Council take action against solid sewage matter being discharged by both the Lying-in Hospital and the Melbourne Hospital into the open street drains.)[34] This was to be a hospital where fever and inflammation were to be blown away with fresh air, sluiced away by clean water and soap, and expelled by limewashing and fumigation. Above all, the diseased were to keep their illnesses to themselves by isolation: each woman was to be accouched alone in a single ward, and kept thus isolated for nine days after delivery; if by then she was free of any 'bad symptom', as they wrote in the medical records, she could rejoin the other mothers recuperating in the large ward. Tracy was later to admit that the women found their sanitary isolation very lonely and would beg for a companion.[35]

While the deliveries were shared between Tracy and Maund in the first year, Tracy was performing the majority by 1858. Maund was ailing, and just as the new hospital on Madeline Street was nearing completion, his body, weakened by consumption and selfless work, succumbed to typhoid. Tracy was with him as he died, and he was widely and deeply mourned both as a doctor and as a man. His colleagues in the Medical Society remembered him as the outstanding doctor of his time in the colony.[36] John Maund's private practice and place in the hospital as honorary physician were taken over by William Mackie Turnbull, an Edinburgh-trained and therefore a Simpson man.[37] And like Maund, he was a consumptive.

Lying-in 2

The new hospital was more than just a new building. It was a pre-meditated medical system, designed to regulate a natural and passionate event, childbirth, and impose an order which was believed would prevent or ameliorate the unexpected and the dangerous. It was also making public in a new way a life experience which was normally private. Even traditional home births attended by flocks of female relatives and friends were essentially private because they were domestic.[38] The parturient woman in a lying-in hospital was delivering her child among strangers. The new building in Madeline Street was constructed to the doctors' orders; it represented a system to prevent infection and to maintain control over the inmates, both patients and their attendants. If the hospital was disorderly, it would quickly become a hive of infection, and if it did it would incur public wrath and be judged a failure. And if the hospital failed, then so did its honorary and resident medical staff, conferring on them an odium that would harm their private as well as their public medical practice. If Tracy and Turnbull's lying-in hospital fell short, then so would they.

The hospital also gave the doctor a new authority over the patient. In private practice, the doctor was invited into the patient's home, and while he could request water, cloths and other necessities as well as assistance, it was not his own place, adapted to his ideas of a suitable setting for a medical procedure. He had to negotiate his way to controlling the birth scene. In the hospital, the rules were set for the patients, and if they refused to comply they could be dismissed, and so they were for 'impertinence', 'drunkenness', or if they 'complained of their food' or 'refused to help themselves when they were able to do so'.[39] It was possible to discipline patients in a way that was different from private practice; it was easier to enforce procedures that a patient might fear or resist; patients could be washed and reclothed more readily than in a private setting; and they could be physically restricted to the bed and their allotted space. Above all, the charity patient could not demand a therapy — a curative intervention — and the doctor was free to deny therapies which were deemed useless or irrelevant.

The hospital was a site of medical authority and power, but it was not necessarily perceived by patients as oppressive. Within a year of opening, the new building could not meet the demand for beds either for midwifery or in the infirmary. The desperate and the shameless tricked and bullied their way into admission, taking advantage of the doctors' willingness to admit on medical need irrespective of moral character. Some, like Mrs O. of 7 Rathdowne Terrace, regarded admission as a right, not a privilege, and when refused a ticket because she would not tender character testimonials, simply presented herself in labour and was admitted.[40] Many exhausted and undernourished women sank thankfully into warm, dry, clean beds; ate heartily of the meals and imbibed in imposed moderation the hospital stimulants. They complained, nearly always about the food, but their complaints were not appreciated and the Ladies' Committee instituted a formal inquiry before discharge as to their satisfaction or otherwise with their treatment in the hospital. This forced final roll-call before the committee succeeded admirably in stifling criticism and arming the hospital with public testimony of its patients' content and acquiescence. The one complaint the hospital was proud to make public was that of the loneliness of the women lying-in alone in the labour wards for the first nine days after delivery.

The unrespectable were a problem. They were often dirty, drunken and diseased. If the hospital admitted too many, then the respectable would stay away and the public-spirited would withdraw their financial support. The Lying-in Hospital was to be a hospital not a moral reformatory, and while the Ladies' Committee was compassionate towards those whose fall was not really their own fault, it had to be realistic about the unregenerate. They refused Mrs M. B. a ticket in June 1860, because she was 'of indifferent character', but she threatened that she would 'come in anyway' and she did on 30 July, while in labour and with a doctor's letter. She was thirty-two, Irish and this was her sixth confinement and she was delivered of an eight-pound daughter after a long labour. The hospital had no alternative but to allow her to stay, but she was kept in a room by herself to the end to protect the other patients.[41]

The issue was more profound than this. The problem of the unrespectable had festered between the committee and the doctors from the hospital's first days. Tracy, warmly supported by his friend Dr Motherwell of South Yarra, believed that all women were entitled to medical care, whatever the state of their morals. He disagreed with his fellow honorary surgeon, Dr Turnbull, that the hospital should admit more medically interesting cases rather than keep an open door, and in 1860 matters came to a head. Rumours began circulating in January that the hospital had recently admitted 'six or seven women from Brown's Lane' in the notorious north-western end of the city. The House Surgeon was questioned and the midwifery book checked for emergency admissions. Only eight were found since July 1859 and just two were from the lane in question.[42] The issue finally exploded in a public debate in the Town Hall a fortnight before the hospital's Annual General Meeting. Sir James Palmer, president of the Legislative Council and vice-president of the Melbourne Hospital, declared that single women should not be admitted at all; Tracy vigorously defended his hospital, insisting that few women of low char-

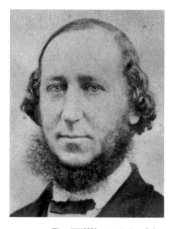

Dr William Mackie Turnbull *RWHA*

acter had found their way into the hospital as emergency admissions. Anyway, 'really debased and abandoned women were not likely to apply, as they could not bear the restrictions of the place'. If the doctors' discretion to admit emergency cases were abolished, then the hospital would 'lose sight of one of the objects of doing good' and he would 'cease to have anything to do with the hospital'.[43] The doctors won the debate and it was a crucial victory.

Tracy had a high sense of calling to obstetrics, and in defending the place of the male physician in the lying-in room, argued that only the trained practitioner, educated in the surgical science of anatomy as well as physical medicine, knew when to allow nature to take its course and when to intervene. In his inaugural lecture on obstetrics to the students of the infant University of Melbourne Medical School in 1865 he argued:

> Nor is it any sufficient argument against the utility of obstetrics to assert that the great proportion of all labours, even in the most civilised form of existence, are natural, and that they do better without any interference whatever. For the truth is, it is this very simplicity of treatment and non-interference at which the accomplished accoucheur constantly aims. Every practitioner knows from sad experience that some of the very worst complications of labour he is called to treat, are directly brought on by the mischievous meddlesomeness of ignorant midwives. The fact is that these women are never content to let well alone, and you will hereafter find the solicitations of the patient and her friends, to, as they term it, 'help her'.[44]

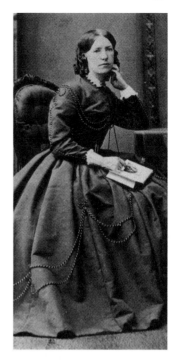

Mrs Sarah Ellen Fetherston, matron 1860–1864 *RWHA*

There were qualified medical practitioners who also did not know what they were doing, and legal action against them was almost as frequent as that against midwives.[45] As the hospital became established, more and more emergency cases arrived where midwives or doctors had not known what to do. The journey to the hospital must have sometimes been almost as appalling as the travails that led up to it. There was no form of ambulance service: those who could afford it hired a cab; those who were destitute walked or were carried. On 29 May 1864 Mrs M. B., aged thirty, Irish and having twins for her tenth confinement, arrived:

> This patient was confined of first child nine hours previous to coming to hospital. Arm of second child presenting four hours before arrival at hospital. Membranes ruptured all that time and the funis of the first child had not been tied. A good deal of haemorrhage must have occurred. Mother drunk. Second child delivered by version but was dead. Chloroform given.[46]

The living child weighed seven and a half pounds, the stillborn eight. Mrs B. did well and was discharged twelve days later.

The admission of emergency cases, particularly of women with complications, ensured the hospital's transition from a lying-in refuge to a specialist hospital. In time, women who expected complications — such as those who had an abnormal pelvis and had already lost babies — sought the hospital's services for medical rather than social reasons. Turnbull, more narrowly ambitious than Tracy, wanted the hospital to be a specialist one, while Tracy was determined to keep the normal midwifery.[47] Tracy, like many of his medical successors in the hospital's long history, had a strong emotional commitment to women. He felt for them, and held medical service to them in their reproductive role in the highest sense of duty. Within the Lying-in Hospital this same devotion to women was to be extended to even the most debased. Few of the patients would have passed a present-day test of cleanliness. In the mid-century personal hygiene and daily washing with soap and water were still a comparative novelty. The poor notoriously washed only the exposed parts of their bodies, and slept and worked in the same clothes for weeks on end. Women were only just beginning to wear underwear and some still menstruated into their clothes. In the United Kingdom the excise on soap had only just been lifted in 1853, and it was not until the 1840s, as F. B. Smith has shown, that doctors began to complain about the odour of their patients, presumably because doctors themselves had begun to wash.[48] And yet it is significant how rarely the hospital records display distaste at the physical state of patients: one of the few recorded was Mrs A. McC., Irish, twenty-four and delivered of her first baby outside five days before, who was admitted on 5 December 1861 in 'a very deplorable state of filth'.[49] They cleaned her up and kept her in for eleven days to recover her strength.

After 1857 the committee gradually became more lenient and for the next eight years the proportion of single mothers admitted ranged between 25 and 39 per cent. And while married women made up the majority of patients, it was those without partners who engaged most of the committee's attention. Of those who did have husbands able and willing to support them, many were temporarily destitute because of unemployment or sickness. Mrs J. E.'s husband was a surgical instrument maker and had found no work. They were in service in Warrnambool but not receiving wages until another party brought them to Melbourne for two months work. Mrs E. was only twenty-one, and after a dreadful thirty-six-hour labour had a stillborn child.[50] Another young woman's husband had gone 'up country to find work' and left her with nothing. The committee organised for her to be admitted to the Immigrants' Home on her discharge from hospital, made her a subscription so that she could redeem some baby clothes that she had pawned, and gave her five shillings.[51]

More striking than marital status was national origin. The patients were disproportionately Irish, but they were also less likely than the English, Scots or locally born to be unmarried. While some Irish may have been drawn to the hospital by Tracy's reputation in the local Irish community, there is evidence that Irish women found it harder to survive in the new colony. Most came as young single women, and more Irish proportionately than of the English or Scots have been identified among the destitute, vagrant, alcoholic or criminal.[52] The Ladies' Committee sometimes betrayed disdain for 'ignorant Irish', so perhaps pregnant, single Irish girls had even less chance of obtaining a ticket. It was the Scots single mothers who got the best hearing, but their representation also reflected the strong family networks of Scottish immigration, and the casting out of women who 'fell'. M. E.'s mother, on being interviewed by the committee, 'appeared deeply sensible of the disgrace into which

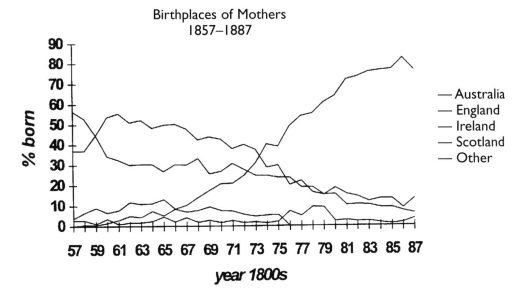

Birthplaces of Mothers 1857–1887

Birthplaces of Mothers (per cent)

Birthplace	1857	1887
Australia	0	76.9
England	37	13.5
Ireland	56.5	6.1
Scotland	3.7	0
Other	2.8	3.5

her daughter had fallen' and, as a widow, could not afford to pay for a home confinement; and G. B., also Scottish and single, was entirely dependent on the kindness of her former employer.[53] As the number of native born grew, they too were mostly unmarried, again alienated from their family networks by shame or family breakdown. Some girls who 'got into trouble' spoke of drunken fathers and flights from unhappy homes; one refused to marry the father of her child because of his drinking and his debts.[54]

The Ladies' Committee's selection procedures also had obstetric consequences. The age and marital structure of the colony determined that more than half of the women confined were *primigravidae*, that is women having their first pregnancy. They were therefore predominantly young, more than two-thirds being between the ages of twenty-one and thirty, while another 16 per cent were even younger. They were therefore in their obstetric prime, and few were weakened by frequent childbearing and lactation. In fact in these early years the number with five or more confinements (*grand multiparae*) averaged under 10 per cent. The most fertile was Mrs E. K. from England, who was forty-eight when she was delivered of her nineteenth child — an eight-pound breech on 24 April 1863. On 18 January 1863 Mrs R. S. from Ireland had identical twins, each eight pounds, for her twelfth confinement. She was forty-four, and her exhausted and over-distended uterus could not contract properly in the third stage so that her life was nearly lost to post-partum haemor-rhage. The usual treatment was compression, cold packs and sometimes the baby was put to the breast to strengthen the contractions. She went home after just six days.

Extract from Midwifery Book

accoucheur: one skilled in midwifery

Most women were admitted the day they deliv-ered. Many walked to the hospital while in labour, and those who were brought in a hurry in cabs sometimes did not make it because horse-drawn transport was slow. It is not clear whether they were washed and changed into hospital clothing, but a form of culotte was put on to cover their legs, with a hole for the birth passage. The delivery was under the control of the house surgeon who had to be in residence. It is unclear how many of the nurses were competent midwives in their own right, but the nurse training that began in 1862 produced 'ladies' monthly nurses' who were qualified as midwives after observing one hundred cases of labour and delivering babies under supervision. Thus Melbourne's Lying-in Hospital was the first in Australia to train nurses and award certificates, and it began nurse training in the same year that Florence Nightingale opened a maternity ward at King's College Hospital, London. (The Nightingale Ward was closed by puerperal fever five years later.) The nurses were also trained in general nursing and it was an intensive three months for the £8 2s 6d fee. In the first decade thirty-four women com-pleted the course, twenty-one of them married or widowed. The matron's position was an adminis-trative and housekeeping, not a nursing, one, and Mrs Gillbee was suc-ceeded by the pretty Miss Harvey who married Dr Gerald Fetherston. Their son 'Bertie' (Richard Herbert) was born while Dr and Mrs Fetherston were resident surgeon and matron respectively, and the fam-ily was to be associated with the hospital for sixty years.[55] The women who sought nursing training were often widows who saw midwifery as a means of supporting their families, and a number of former patients returned for training. It was exhausting work. The nurses were required to stay on duty until each patient who had been under their particular care was discharged.

The women were delivered in the classic British obstetric position, lying on their left side. This position gave the accoucheur clear access and was good for teaching, but the most important reason for the left lateral position was the control it gave the accoucheur over the speed of the birth. One of the dreads of childbirth was a major tear of the perin-eum. If the rent was big enough, a woman would lose the anal sphincter muscle and forever after have no control over her bowels. Her uterus could also prolapse. If left to heal without suturing and care, she would finish with a perineum that was nothing but scar tissue — if it healed at all and did not become chronically infected. The inevitable faecal incon-tinence was every bit as devastating to her life as the dreaded fistulae or holes that could form between the vagina and the bladder or the vagina and the rectum. Women so afflicted suffered the stench of the endlessly unclean and the skin excoriation from constant wetness and fouling with urine and excreta. A moment's accident could destroy a woman's life. Therefore control over the perineum was everything in responsible midwifery, and the technique was to support the perineum from below and thereby to slow down the birth of the head and the aftercoming shoulders. If a woman stood or used a birth chair, the accoucheur could both see and do less, and the assistance of gravity might accelerate the delivery dangerously.[56] The births were delayed, and at times this was a risk to the child, but in 1859 and 1860 only nine women suffered a ruptured perineum — that is one in about forty deliveries. The technique was not foolproof, for in one case the Midwifery Book recorded, 'Was present and supporting the perineum when the accident happened'. These were not the nicks to the perineum which were inevitable and best left alone; these were full ruptures and the women were not discharged until they were healed. Healing often took six or more weeks, though one woman stayed in eight. From 1860 silver wire sutures were inserted and the patient spent her convalescence lying on her side in the obstetric position, with her bowels confined with opium — faecal contamination was known to produce infection and thereby prevent healing. All those in 1859 and 1860 were primiparas; one unfortunate, having her second child in 1862, had her perineum rupture again in the old scar.

It is difficult from this distance to evaluate the quality of the labours. The timing of labour for the Midwifery Book appears to have changed, for why else did 53 per cent of the women in 1860 labour for more than ten hours and just 11 per cent in 1861? Presumably a judgement was made about strong labour and the point at which the labouring woman was forced to take to her bed. There was no pain relief other than chloroform and that was used sparingly only for forceps deliveries and version. Women traditionally used alcohol and certainly some, again like Mrs

version: the act of turning, especially the manual turning of the foetus in delivery. Abdominal v., version performed by external manipulation. Anopelvic v., that which is accomplished by manipulating the pelvis of the foetus by means of a finger passed into the rectum of the mother. Bipolar v., that which is effected by manipulating both poles of the foetus. Cephalic v., version which causes the foetal head to present. Combined v., a combination of external and internal version. External v., that which is performed by outside manipulation. Internal v., version produced by the hand introduced into the uterus. Pelvic v., that which is performed by manipulating the breech. Podalic v., version which causes the feet to present. Spontaneous v., version which occurs without artificial interference. (AMD)

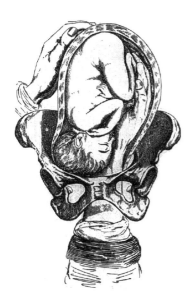 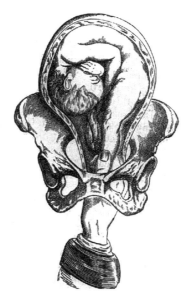

**Podalic version
Seizure of the feet when the hand is introduced into the uterus**

Drawing down the feet and completion of version
Playfair, pp. 172–3

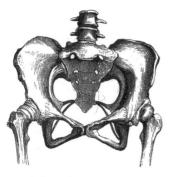

Adult pelvis retaining its infantile type

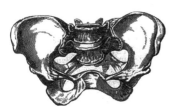

Rickety pelvis, with backward depression of the symphysis pubis

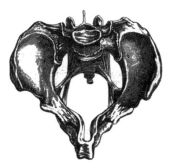

Osteo-malacic pelvis

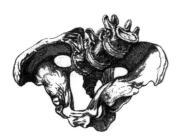

Extreme degree of osteo-malacic deformity

M. B. who had her first twin outside the hospital, were intoxicated by the time they were admitted. Many women screamed and screamed so that the young ladies' school next door to the East Melbourne house had reason to object to having a lying-in hospital as a neighbour. But many too would have suffered in grim, stoic silence. And some underwent a purgatory of pain.

One problem was the size of the babies. Between 1859 and 1865 around half weighed eight or more pounds — an indication of the physical well-being of the mothers. The women themselves, however, were not big in the skeleton, and one guide to this was the proportion of women with contracted or deformed pelves. Contracted pelvis and the consequent difficulties in delivering a baby consumed more intellectual energy in nineteenth-century obstetrics than any other topic. It had underwritten the man-midwife's entry into the birthing chamber, for it had been the Chamberlens' invention of the obstetrical forceps which gave men a specialty with which to stake their claim against traditional female midwifery. The problem itself of the pelvis being too small or misshapen for the baby to pass through the birth passage was appalling and sufficiently common to justify the European obsession with it.[57] If there was no room, then the baby had to be removed by a destructive operation, most often a craniotomy where the baby's skull was perforated and collapsed, or the child was taken apart in the uterus and extracted in pieces. These were dreaded procedures which involved religious as well as ethical dilemmas. A destructive operation could be seen as an act of murder on a non-baptised soul, but any sort of invasive abdominal operation which removed the child from the uterus meant certain death for the mother. Until anaesthesia, such an operation had to be performed on a conscious patient who was probably already far gone physically and mentally. But if she survived that, it was almost impossible to ensure that the uterus healed — the first successful caesarean sections were still a quarter of a century away.

By the 1850s the measurement and classification of deformed or narrow pelves was well advanced, and the skill in delivering either with forceps or by turning the baby was high among the best accoucheurs. The destructive operations also were well done, but doctors were also fully sensible that the more often forceps were resorted to, the more complications seemed to arise, and in particular, the more susceptible the woman became to infection. The standards set by Simpson were very conservative indeed. In 1404 deliveries associated with the Edinburgh Maternity Hospital between 1844 and 1846, there was intervention in one in 107 cases, and forceps were used only in one in every 472 deliveries. Yet there was immense variation within the United Kingdom and in Europe. Siebold in Berlin used forceps in one in seven cases, and Busch in one in eleven, with a craniotomy rate of one in 342.[58] In cases where the child's head had become fixed in the brim of the pelvis, Simpson advised craniotomy in preference to forceps delivery if the child was certainly dead; but he also recommended the use of long forceps.[59]

The causes of contracted or deformed pelvis could be congenital or environmental, the most frequent cause being varying degrees of malnutrition both in the woman herself and possibly even in her own mother during pregnancy. The effects of malnutrition are complex and not always plainly obvious. The easiest to diagnose was rickets (later understood to be caused by a shortage of vitamin D in the diet exacerbated by lack of sunlight on the skin) which softened and bent the bones as the growing child stood, walked and developed. Typically, the lower part of the spine — the sacrum — pushed forward into the pelvis, narrowing the diameter from back to front and elongating the pelvis from left to right. This produced contraction at the inlet of the pelvic brim. Less obvious was subclinical rickets, other disease and poor bone development which left a flatter, or smaller, masculine or heart-shaped pelvis which still made childbirth difficult. It was reckoned that an anterior/posterior diameter of three and a quarter inches was the minimum size where a child could be delivered. Diseases such as spinal tuberculosis and osteomyelitis could damage the pelvis, and conditions such as congenital hip and spinal deformity twist it. To be afflicted with gross pelvic deformity doomed every pregnancy to end in tragedy, with death at least for the baby, and possibly for the woman herself. Pregnancy could be a death sentence. On 1 March 1863 Mrs M. C. lost a baby for the third time because of her narrow pelvis. Twice before she had been delivered with forceps; this time it was by version; and on 15 January 1864 Mrs M. O'C. was delivered of her sixth stillborn child; her pelvis was deformed and heart-shaped. Both these women were born in Ireland and of an age to be entering adolescence as the potato blight brought starvation. And such victims of early malnutrition presented Tracy and Turnbull with their most frequent obstetric complications. At its worst, in 1860, one in fifteen of the patients born in Ireland had a contracted or deformed pelvis and all of them were of an age to be children during the famine. H. C., aged nineteen and utterly destitute, endured a thirty-hour labour, but her baby was dead, delivered by the forceps through her inadequate pelvis. The only English-born woman that year with a narrow pelvis was just fifteen and had barely stopped growing.

The true incidence of rachitic and deformed pelvis is problematic. Loudon, after reviewing hospital statistics for Ireland, England, Scotland, Paris and Vienna, estimates that the true incidence of rachitic pelvic deformity was around one per cent, and reminds us that hospital statistics are plumped out by the fact that problem cases were referred to them.[60] The Melbourne Lying-in Hospital records reveal a specific and quite short-lived problem, as a particular generation of Irish and Scottish immigrants passed through its doors between 1856 and the late 1860s. Also these figures include contracted pelves which were sub-clinical manifestations of the same deficiency diseases, but they were none the less a terrible disability in childbirth. Rickets soon disappeared from medical prominence in Australia, to reappear only in subdued form with another group of immigrants after World War II.

Sometimes tumours of various kinds blocked the birth passage. Mrs A. L. had 'a large tumour growing from upper part of sacrum which had so filled the cavity of the pelvis that the antero-posterior diameter was only one and a quarter inches'. Craniotomy had to be performed with her first child for that reason. B. Q., aged twenty-three and having her first child, had a narrow pelvis; after a nine-hour labour, forceps failed

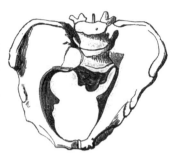

Obliquely contracted pelvis

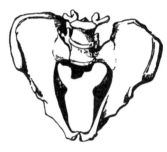

Robert's or double obliquely contracted pelvis *Playfair, pp. 191–5*

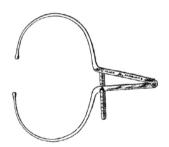

Mathews Duncan's pelvimeter, external

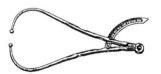

Martin's pelvimeter, external *Allen & Hanburys, p. 498*

Applying the forceps according to Playfair (1882)
1. Position of patient for forceps delivery and mode of introducing lower blade
2. Introduction of the upper blade
3. Forceps in position: traction of the axis of the brim, downwards and backwards
4. Last stage of extraction: the handles of the forceps are being gradually turned upwards towards the mother's abdomen.
Playfair, pp. 191–5

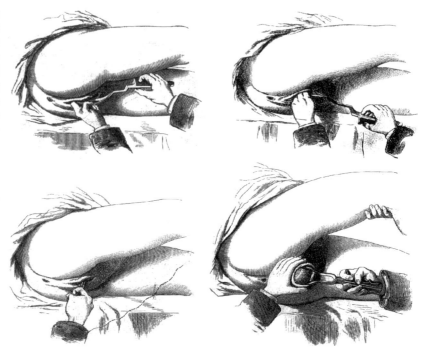

ergot: fungus that grows on rye, used to stimulate contractions of the uterus. An alkaloid derivative *ergometrine* replaced it after World War II, and was usually administered by injection to enhance labour and control bleeding. (*OMD*).

Barnes bags: for artificial dilatation of the cervix—a series of india-rubber bags of various sizes, with a tube attached through which water can be injected by an ordinary Higginson's syringe (Playfair, p. 153)

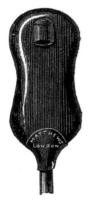

Barnes bag for dilating the cervix *Playfair, p. 153*

and the baby was delivered by turning but not without the cord ceasing to pulsate so that the child did not breathe for thirty minutes after birth. Tracy experimented with the premature induction of labour 'to avoid the revolting operation of craniotomy' in cases of pelvic deformity. At the seventh month of gestation he would use the stethoscope to find the position of the placenta, and then 'using Simpson's sound, and taking the greatest care *not* to rupture the membranes and if possible pass it between them and the anterior wall for around 4 inches, and move it from side to side to ensure separation of the membranes'. He then withdrew the sound and waited for labour. If it did not begin in five to six hours, he would inject a few ounces of tepid water into the uterus by use of Higginson's elastic syringe. And sometimes he had to give ergot to strengthen contractions. If he needed to bring labour on quickly, as in a case of eclampsia, he used Barnes bags to dilate the cervix.[61] (In that pre-bacteriological age Tracy had not the least idea of how dangerous this was, for it was tantamount to introducing infection into the sterile uterus.) Mrs M. F. was another Irish famine victim with a deformed pelvis and was in hospital for three weeks before she gave birth. She survived an appalling forty-eight-hour labour but her daughter did not. Delivery was by craniotomy.

O. A. was also admitted before her time in 1863, and after eleven weeks of rest, produced a ten-pound daughter after eighteen hours labour. The forceps were on for twenty-three minutes, slowly compressing the head so that it could pass through the brim. That was the other side of the story. These stunted survivors of famine and poverty, when they had plentiful food and rest produced babies which were far too big for their once starved skeletons. Australia might potentially have been a land of plenty, but in the 1850s and 1860s the diet of the poor was limited and monotonous. Melbourne was growing rapidly, but the food supply infrastructure lagged well behind. The poor lived on damper (unleavened bread), salt beef or underdone mutton, beer and endless cups of very sweet tea. Their diet was deficient in fresh foods, especially fruit and vegetables: scurvy ('Barcoo rot' in the bush) was to remain a problem for the very poor and the isolated into the twentieth century. The shortage of fresh meat as well as green vegetables exposed menstruating and parturient women and girls to anaemia. The strengthening diet recommended for pregnant women included much farinaceous food and milk which, combined with rest in a warm, dry bed and no work to do, made women put on condition quickly in hospital. And the beer drinkers were accommodated, even if in moderation.

Despite all these impeded deliveries, forceps were used as little as possible, and only by the honorary surgeons. But at least by 1856 the doctors had chloroform. Tracy, like many, on reading Simpson's first paper on chloroform, immediately thought 'Oh, I will give chloroform in every case I attend'. He tried it and soon observed that it delayed and suppressed labour, and that the after-effects were so unpleasant that women declared that they wished they had never had it. 'Every accoucheur knows how readily and speedily the feeling of perfect ease takes possession of a patient as soon as delivery is accomplished, and how soon the pangs of the previous hour are forgotten', and chloroform denied them that. However, he saw its great benefit in obstructed and tedious, exhausting labours: 'although you can positively assert to anxious friends that "all is right", still there is much apparent cause for uneasiness, and the poor sufferer has almost lost hope; the inhalation of a little chloroform causes a deep and refreshing sleep'. But above all chloroform made forceps deliveries safer:

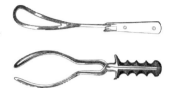

Simpson's forceps

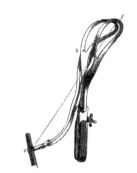

Simpson's axis traction forceps
Playfair, p. 186

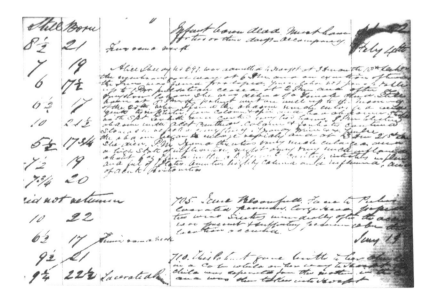

Extract from Midwifery Book

**Various destructive
instruments**

Crochets

Perforators

**Simpson's cranioclast
and craniotomy forceps**
Playfair, pp. 204–6

we all know the natural horror of 'instruments' entertained by all women, the state of wild excitement often induced, when their use is hinted at, the valuable time lost in trying to persuade a patient to submit, and last, not least, the injuries that have been caused by the struggles of the patient during such operations.

Tracy, in his vivid and feeling way, went on to relate the case of A. C., admitted in labour to the Lying-in Hospital on 19 September 1857:

> She was a domestic servant, and at the time of admission had been forty-eight hours in labour; she was below the middle stature, frame altogether stunted and pelvis narrow. On examination, the os uteri was found dilated to the size of a crown piece, the head presenting naturally, the strait of the pelvis and outlet both being under the average capacity; pains were strong and at short intervals. She progressed pretty favourably for some hours, but though the pains increased in violence and frequency, still there was not corresponding progress. My patient now lost all control of herself, her shrieks were terrific and caused no little commotion in the hospital and neighbourhood; she would not allow herself to be touched, and I had great difficulty in making an examination, the poor creature dashed herself about in a state of frenzy, and became quite unmanageable. The head of the child was at this time free of the uterus, firmly impacted in the strait of the pelvis. With the approval of my colleague, Dr Maund, chloroform was now administered, and the woman was speedily under its influence; then our troubles ceased, or rather, we got fair play to grapple with them. After waiting a sufficient time, it was evident that delivery by the natural powers unassisted, was impossible. I applied the forceps and exerted all my strength in the use of them; I was relieved by Dr Maund, and he in turn by my friend Dr Black, who happened to be with him when sent for; and the amount of patient, steady force required to complete the delivery, was greater than in any case I have attended.
>
> She was delivered of a male child, which had to all appearances died during the early stages of labour, when the head was so many hours in entering the brim of the pelvis. The child weighed nine pounds and was 21 inches in length. There was not the least injury to the perineum, the parts having relaxed considerably under the influence of the chloroform. Our patient soon awoke, and said she had been dreaming about home; great was her surprise when she found her trouble was over. She recovered speedily, without a single bad symptom. The struggles which this woman would (if conscious) undoubtedly have made while the forceps were being used, must have caused lacerations, and the shock of her morbidly excited nervous system, would have been terrible.[62]

Tracy gave chloroform on a handkerchief, which he acknowledged made the simultaneous administration of anaesthesia and delivery or operation difficult for the lone practitioner. He does not seem to have given anaesthesia for agonising labours in the hospital, but then Simpson had recommended it primarily for 'ladies' because they were more sensitive to pain than the poor, but where Tracy did use it with some success was in eclampsia.

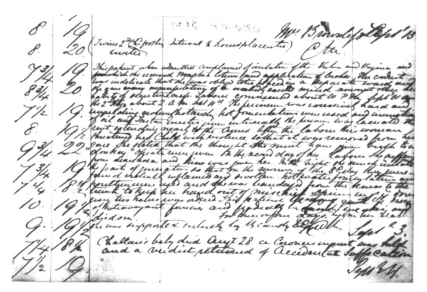

Extract from Midwifery Book

Eclampsia, or 'kidney fits', has been one of the most reluctant complications of human parturition to yield up its secrets. It is generally preceded by 'pre-eclampsia' or 'toxaemia of pregnancy', with a rise in blood pressure, fluid retention, oedema of the legs, and albumin in the urine. If the condition advances, a woman can go into convulsions and even suffer a cerebral haemorrhage. Only delivery of the baby stops the convulsions, and severe eclampsia often resulted in the death of both mother and child. The accoucheur had to bring labour on and deliver the child as quickly as possible; but it had also become popular to practise venesection — opening a vein — and bleeding the patient until her blood pressure went down. This was an empirical not a scientific finding, as blood pressure was not understood. Tracy, along with a handful of other practitioners, tried chloroform. In 1858 he bled a convulsing woman of ten ounces of blood and then administered chloroform. She struggled so he gave her more and she slept for three hours. He then watched her for twelve hours, giving her chloroform four times of two minutes inhalation. She survived.[63] His first eclampsia case in the Lying-in Hospital came in April 1859: B. B., 'a young healthy woman, in labour with her first child — margins of the os hard — convulsions came on severely as soon as child's head began to press on the os — during the convulsions the patient's face was much congested — quite livid, breathing loudly stertorous'. He administered chloroform during one of the convulsions, her symptoms ceased and her face cleared. To soften the os — the opening of the cervix at the neck of the womb — he ordered tartrate of antimony in half-grain doses every hour. After the second dose, vomiting occurred and 'the bowels freely relaxed' after which the patient slept calmly for three hours. When she awoke, labour pains came on, the os dilated rapidly and the labour was over in ninety minutes. Mother and child did well.[64]

tartrate of antimony: (tartar) a toxic and irritating salt of antimony, used as an emetic as 'constitutional treatment' (*OMD*)

This was courageous medicine, even if with scientific hindsight we can be alarmed at recourse to treatments which were almost as dangerous as the condition itself. Also we need to remember that more than 80 per cent of the deliveries in the Lying-in Hospital were normal and concluded with mothers and babies 'doing well'. But obstetric hospitals are judged not only on the quantity and quality of normal deliveries, but also on the manner in which they cope with the complicated and the life threatening. Ultimately a hospital stands or falls by its record of deaths in childbirth.

When the new building opened in October 1858, not one woman had died in childbirth, then on 26 April 1859 Maria Chick, aged twenty-five and born in England, was admitted at midnight as an emergency case. She was reported to be 'an unhealthy woman'. She had already been in labour for forty hours. Her 'vaginal discharges were most offensive' and 'a large caput succedaneum had formed — no foetal pulse could be heard. A warm enema was given and the vagina was well syringed with tepid water. The physician of the week was sent for, but before the messenger had been gone five minutes, a sudden pain caused the head to pass into the vagina, and another which quickly followed completed the delivery; the child was dead'.[65] The midwifery record continued:

> Lochia after labour most offensive and required frequent injection of chloromate [sic] of soda. On 28 complained of slight pain in abdomen which was relieved by an opiate. Bowels opened freely on 29 but pain came on Friday night with much tenderness on pressure. Warm turpentine fomentations and opiates with Calomel given and urine drawn off about 6 ounces. Tongue furred and she complained of thirst, pulse soft, about 90. 30th she was better and free from pain in the morning, but at 10 am it returned and the tenderness became excessive, her pulse reached 120. Already thirst extreme & anxiety of countenance well marked, her abdomen which had already been enlarged was quite tympanic. Leeches 24 were applied and bled freely. Cal & opium cont'd. Sickness came on about midday . . . water fluid constantly rejected. She became worse & sickness increased. Chloroform in 10 drop doses given every hour during the night and brandy & lemonade freely. At times her pulse was scarcely perceptible in the evening. She died at 9.30 am on 1st May.[66]

Maria Chick thus became the first woman to die in childbirth in the Lying-in Hospital. Peritonitis was a horrible way to die; the pain was unendurable yet the victim remained conscious to the end. The post-mortem revealed the peritoneum to be 'extremely congested. Adherent to bowels'. The uterus contained 'remnants of dark brown membranes which had escaped attention when the placenta had to be removed manually. And the os of the cervix was lacerated'. Tracy's comment on the post-mortem was that this wound allowed 'absorption of unhealthy matter to take place'. The injury to the os had been caused by the rapid passage of the child's head.[67]

Maria Chick was reported to be 'an unhealthy woman' which suggests venereal disease. Her waters had broken long before, during her prolonged labour before she arrived at the hospital, and a malodorous anaerobic infection was present; existing venereal disease was often the pre-condition and trigger to grave puerperal infection. The syringing of the vagina may have unwittingly introduced vaginal flora into the normally sterile uterus, resulting in an ascending infection, but Tracy was quite right to regard

---

caput succedaneum: a temporary swelling of the soft parts of the head of a newly born infant that occurs during birth, due to compression by the muscles of the neck of the womb (*OMD*)

lochia: the material eliminated from the uterus after the completion of labour

chloromate of soda: ?sodium chlorate, 'detergent and alterant' (*AMD*)

opiates: given for inflammatory conditions such as peritonitis, as well as to treat diarrhoea, cough, and pain (Black)

calomel: subchloride of mercury, given as a purgative (Black)

os uteri: the orifice of the canal of the cervix or neck of the womb

anaerobe: a microbe able to live and grow in the absence of free oxygen the laceration in the cervix as a possible entry point to further infection. Then as her peritonitis advanced, the hospital tried everything it knew in its struggle to save her life, from ancient bleeding of bad humours with leeches to the modern marvel of chloroform — revealing the eclecticism of practitioners in the midst of what Charles Rosenberg has called the 'therapeutic revolution'.[68]

Then on 5 September another Englishwoman, Rebecca Catchlow, aged twenty-seven, was admitted:

> This patient when admitted complained of irritation of the Vulva and Vagina for which she received morphia lotions and applications of leeches. Her conduct was so indelicate that she was obliged to be placed in a separate ward and she gave many manifestations of a morbidly excited mind, amongst other habits [of a disagreeable nature].
>
> Labour commenced about 10 pm Sept 10 and the second stage about 2 am Sept 11. The perineum was extremely hard and unyielding notwithstanding hot fomentations and [applications] of oil of Tartar. Emetic given internally. The perineum was lacerated the rent extending nearly to the anus.

She had a daughter weighing a healthy seven and three-quarter pounds:

> After the labour the woman threatened her child with violence so that it was removed from her care. She stated that she had given birth to a 'donkey'. Opiates were given her on the second day after labour. She suffered from diarrhoea & wine was given her. In the night she much irritated her parts of generation so that on the morning of the 3rd day they were found to be violently inflamed and swollen. Hot water fomentations & poultices were used & and she was bandaged from knees to trunk to keep her hands out of mischief. Opium of 7 dcms every 2 hours was ordered. This patient became quite free of... and fancies & gradually became weaker & died. For 3 or 4 days before her death she was supported entirely on brandy and egg.[69]

So did poor deranged Rebecca Catchlow depart this world, but the hospital forgot to record her date of death and a post-mortem was deemed unnecessary.

The last to die that year was Mrs Cross, English also and aged twenty-five. She was admitted on 1 December and went into labour three days later. She had premonitions of death:

> Mrs Cross when admitted was in a very distressed state of mind on account of her [numerous] afflictions. She also stated that after her first labour she was unconscious and very ill for many days and was also ill after her second labour. Two days after labour [this] her lochia ceased and her breasts became very painful and distended. Next day she complained of violent pain in the head across the eyebrows and afterwards at its summit. Next day her pulse was very rapid and soft but the pain in her head was as bad as ever. She vomited many times and had no sleep in the night. Next day she appeared to be a little better, but in the evening she became unconscious

valerian: is the root of *Valeriana officinalis,* a European plant. Used 'chiefly in form of tincture of valerian to quiet nervousness, insomnia and hysterical attacks'. Also 'useful in doses of two or three drops on sugar for the relief of dyspepsia associated with spasm of the stomach'. (Black)

hyoscyamus, or henbane: preparations made from leaves 'have an effect of quieting pain and relieving spasm. In large quantities it is a narcotic poison'. Used for 'all spasmodic and painful conditions, particularly in colic and irritable states of the bladder'. Hyoscine, an alkaloid obtained from it, was later used in very small doses to control mania and, with morphine, for the production of 'twilight sleep' in childbirth. (Black)

arachnoid: one of the membranes covering the brain and the spinal cord (*OMD*)

secondary post-partum haemorrhage: bleeding occurring twenty-four hours or longer after delivery, most commonly caused by the retention of pieces of placenta or membranes; less often by infection (Townsend (O), p. 479)

stupe: a hot fomentation sprinkled with turpentine, applied over the abdomen for distension

and her pulse was very rapid and compressible. She rallied in the day until the day before her death, at times rational and then unconscious. The day before she died she was considerably better and drank nourishing broth, but in the evening she was seized with rigor and from the collapse did not rally but died about 1 am on 12 December. She was treated with Valerian & Ammonia & Hyoscyamus, Beef tea and wine & when she could not swallow, beef tea was administered by injection.

At P[ost] M[ortem]. several patches of lymph were found in the surface of the brain and the arachnoid was opaque. The uterus contained a large clot (there had been a discharge from the vagina for 3 days before her death) the brain was congested and full of bloody points from which blood exuded when the brain was sliced with the knife.

This tragic threesome were the first of twenty-three women to die in the hospital during the first nine years of its history. Considering the class of women the hospital served, it was a creditable performance although Tracy later tended to be over-sanguine in public.[70] In 1860, however, there were five maternal deaths out of 197 confinements. Included among them were two mothers of large families and three were cases of women bearing babies too big for them, requiring traumatic forceps deliveries. Mrs D. B. was one of the one in fifteen Irishwomen that year whose pelvis was too small. She was twenty-five, and in her five previous deliveries either forceps or version had to be used. After sixteen hours she delivered a stillborn daughter and nine days later died from a secondary post-partum haemorrhage. S. P. had a similar problem but a very different story. She was fifteen and English. She had been in Dr Tracy's service as a nursemaid and had been admitted formerly to the hospital 'suffering from disease'. Now she was pregnant and infected with venereal disease and 'the circumstances of her reduction were most painful'. Dr Tracy had pitied her and 'had taken her into his family' and her sister was still in his service. Her mother 'only lived in a tent and could not have room for her [daughter] during her confinement'. She was given a ticket without demur.[71] She was admitted on 12 October and ten days later went into labour. Her pelvis was narrow, and after sixteen hours of agony she was delivered of a nine-pound son by forceps under chloroform. Her perineum was lacerated.

On second day complained of tenderness of the abdomen. Had twenty-four leeches applied. Had Hy of Sup Emetic opium. Third day stuped . . . Mania with high fever set in on the fourth day which terminated fatally on the 6th. Discharge very foetid. No [tympanic] was perceptible on the abdomen foreshadow to death. Tongue clean and moist.

Death from puerperal mania remains an unexplained phenomenon which disappeared early this century. To the modern clinical microbiologist it looks like an acute toxic state.[72]

Of the twenty-three deaths, while many were multi-factorial and diagnosis from this distance is difficult, eight began with cases of contracted or deformed pelvis. There were nine cases of operative intervention: two of version, three of forceps and four of craniotomy. Two of the craniotomy deaths occurred within two hours of the delivery. Eleven cases involved severe infection: nine cases of peritonitis and two of pyaemia. Two women suffered from *Phlegmasia alba dolens* or 'white leg'; one of debility after diarrhoea; two were clear cases of eclampsia including a seventeen-year-old married Afro-American who died after giving birth to twins. There were two deaths from 'puerperal mania', with another couple which may have been eclamptic, and finally one from 'obstetric shock'. Many were unavoidable deaths and their causes both social and medical. The hospital in fact had started well.

Over the next nine years the patterns began to change. The Australian-born grew in numbers until by 1874 they comprised 40 per cent of the midwifery population; and the proportion of single mothers rapidly increased with them, because 73 per cent of the Australians in that year were unmarried. For the first time, the unmarried accounted for more than half the midwifery patients, and ten years later, in 1884, 76 per cent of all mothers were Australian-born and 61 per cent were single. But as the Ladies' Committee became more tolerant of the unmarried, the hospital population became less healthy. Venereal disease was more often noticed: usually syphilis and only on those with syphilitic lesions at the time of the confinement. In later years it would be understood that perhaps most syphilitic babies would not reveal their condition until some months after birth. More alcoholic women were brought in after giving birth in public places. As Melbourne expanded to absorb the massive immigration of the 1850s, the society settled and while many prospered and built a cottage in the suburbs, in the inner city others sank to form a residuum of casual employment, alcoholism and sexual promiscuity. By the early 1870s the hopefuls of the 1850s had either risen or failed, and those who failed now lived in the crowded cottages and terraces of the city, working as sweated labour in homes and tiny workplaces, where tuberculosis and typhoid fever began to take their toll.

But the most telling measure of the increasing poverty and deprivation of the midwifery patients was the steady fall in mean birth weight as the Ladies' Committee relaxed their moral standards. The fall in mean birth weight by the mid 1870s of about one pound (~0.45 kg) which is more than the decrease in the mean birth weight seen during the much studied Dutch famine of World War II. To achieve a fall of this magnitude, many

pyaemia: 'pus in the blood', now understood as blood poisoning by pus-forming bacteria released from an abscess. Abscesses may appear in various parts of the body, often with fatal results. (*OMD*)

phlegmasia alba dolens: ('white leg') inflammation of wall of a vein with a secondary thrombosis occurring within the affected segment of a vein, resulting in an 'enlarged, white and painful leg'. May come during convalescence from an acute febrile disease such as pneumonia or typhoid, but most commonly occurred after childbirth as an accompaniment of puerperal fever. (Black, *OMD*)

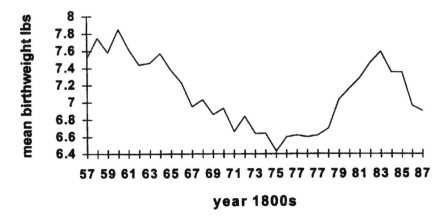

Mean birth weight 1857–1887

pregnant women delivering in the hospital after 1870 had to be severely underweight before they became pregnant and then be subsisting on less than 1500 calories a day — in the Dutch famine, the ration was 800 calories. Therefore despite the macro-economic evidence which points to substantial growth during this period of Australia's development, those members of the poor trapped in the casual labour market in the inner city were being left behind.[73]

As the hospital's reputation grew, more undelivered women suffering grave obstetric complications were admitted as emergency cases. Between 1866 and 1874 nearly a quarter of the fifty-six women who died in the midwifery wards had eclampsia, a figure far above the actual incidence of eclampsia in the community. Three died from tuberculosis and a mother of six aged forty from chronic alcoholism; three suffered a ruptured uterus after forceps or craniotomy, and three others died after traumatic instrumental deliveries. Five died from haemorrhage. Mrs M. B., who had suckled her six children 'for long periods', 'sank from exhaustion induced by the extreme heat of the weather' during a heat-wave in January 1872. And Mrs E. E., having been 'previously exhausted by phthisis' and haemorrhage, expired on a day when it was '104 degrees in the shade' the following summer. Infection was, of course, still the major killer, and adding to the death list of the hospital by the end of Tracy's years was the first genuine outbreak of puerperal fever.

Death from peritonitis and pyaemia, while infection deaths, were not the same as puerperal fever. Most commonly they were infections caused by bacteria already within the mother's genital tract; they were anaerobic infections which thrived in the absence of oxygen. These infections smelt and doctors believed they sprang from the absorption of unhealthy matter. Puerperal fever, the dread of lying-in hospitals, was different. It came in epidemics; it was obviously contagious; it struck down perfectly healthy lying-in mothers who had not necessarily had long and exhausting labours and birth injuries. Puerperal fever seemed 'to come out of the air' as one great doctor of the hospital would say sixty years later, and it assumed a terror in the public and medical mind almost as great as the cholera. Doctors dreaded it because it could ruin their practice for ever; lying-in hospitals feared it because it could close them down.

As cholera became 'the greatest of sanitary reformers', so also did puerperal fever and post-partum infection lead the way in the understanding of all wound infection. The very first advances in cell pathology were in response to puerperal infection, and while it is customary to invoke the names of Semmelweis and Oliver Wendell Holmes, there was also a Scot, Alexander Gordon, who published in 1795 a treatise on an outbreak of puerperal fever which had occurred in Aberdeen. He comprehended that it was contagious, and anticipated Semmelweis's exposure of hospital filth and contamination by fifty years. He missed only the role of the examining finger of the doctor or medical student, fresh from the decomposing cadavers of the dissecting room that Semmelweis was to implicate.[74] As soon as the first medical students were admitted to the Melbourne Lying-in Hospital in 1865 they were prohibited from entering the wards while they were doing anatomy and dissection. And the hospital maintained good standards of cleanliness from doctors. There had been a small outbreak of puerperal fever in Melbourne in 1868, coinciding

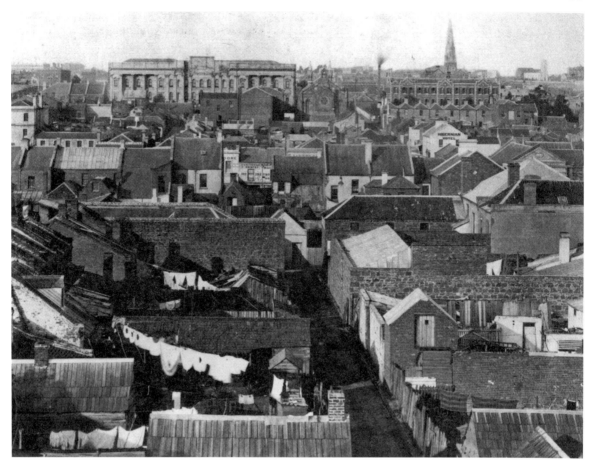

with an epidemic of scarlatina, but the hospital was untouched and the Annual Report noted with a certain smugness that the Nightingale Ward at King's College Hospital, London, had registered a death rate of one in thirteen.[75] In 1873, however, the hospital's time had come.

Dr L. J. Martin was now an honorary, along with the ailing Tracy (Turnbull had finally died of tuberculosis in 1868), and the intellectual armoury he brought to the emergency was an interesting mixture. He knew that the best authorities believed that puerperal fever, 'especially in its putrid malignant form' was contagious and that birth attendants could carry it from patient to patient. Yet in his own experience in this later epidemic, he could not see that he had carried anything from patient to patient. It was a conundrum which would not be understood until the middle of the 1920s, but while he was attending puerperal fever cases in other men's practices and in the hospital, none of his private patients fell ill. Similarly in the Lying-in Hospital, even though the wards were unusually full, and though forty-one women were accouched, and though most were attended by the same nurses, yet only four were attacked and the wards were now free of the disease, although a few cases were 'still occurring throughout the city'.[76] The four died within a week of each other in what was to be the hospital's worst year with sixteen maternal deaths out of four hundred and forty-four confinements. Martin knew the latest literature, even if he did not agree with it, but he did accept

View of Melbourne looking east, *circa* 1860 by Charles Nettleton: the lanes and cottages of the inner city
La Trobe Picture Collection, State Library of Victoria

erysipelas: ('the Rose', 'St Anthony's fire') is a disease characterised by diffuse inflammation of the skin or of subcutaneous cellular tissue, attended with fever. In the Middle Ages this disease was confused with ergot poisoning. (Black) It was also known as surgical fever and was gradually being linked with puerperal fever by the 1870s. It is now known to be caused by *streptococcus pyogenes* and is treated with antibiotics. (*OMD*)

that erysipelas and this dangerous form of puerperal fever were closely linked. The discussion that followed his paper to the Medical Society was revealing. Dr Gerald Fetherston, now a young honorary at the hospital, was anxious that the Lying-in Hospital not be seen as the source of the outbreak. The first patient to succumb had not been attended by either Dr Martin or himself; rather the midwife alone had delivered the baby and the patient 'had no bad symptoms for some days after delivery'. He was convinced that erysipelas and scarlatina were more likely to spread puerperal fever than other puerperal cases. He reminded all present of the peculiarly foggy and damp weather that June and of the fact that all the surgical cases had done badly in those same weeks.[77] The dissident voice as to the contagiousness of puerperal fever itself was Dr Gillbee, the son of the first matron of the Lying-in Hospital and in 1868 the first champion of Listerism in the Melbourne Hospital.[78] He had no doubt that it was contagious and that medical attendants had to quarantine themselves if any of their patients succumbed; but his was a lone voice in 1873.

The Lying-in Hospital honoraries were sensitive to any imputation on the healthiness of their model hospital, but they also had to be realistic about the condition of the women confined there. As Dr Addison reminded them, 'In hospital women suffered much more from mental anxiety, single women, for example, so that they were much more susceptible to the poison' — many believed it was the shame of unmarried motherhood that predisposed them to fatal infection. But if the rising maternal death rate confirmed this, a more telling statistic was again the falling mean weights of the babies. And the mothers most at risk were either young Australian-born single women (in particular Tasmanians), and older immigrant women with large families. But there were also more older women with bad obstetric histories, who sought the hospital's care in case of repeated or worse complications. Between 1869 and 1872 about a quarter of all deliveries registered some form of complication, ranging from death of the mother and stillbirth of the child, to forceps delivery or a baby under five pounds. Among those women who had had six or more children, the complication rate was 10 per cent higher. In 1872 39 per cent of these women had a complication, 24 per cent resulting in death either of the mother, the baby or both. Interventions such as forceps deliveries remained conservative: in 1870 it was still under 2 per cent. However, as birth weights fell dramatically after 1871, forceps rates rose, largely for young single women delivering small babies: in 1875 when mean weights were lowest, the forceps rate was one in nineteen deliveries. As for the babies, vigorous efforts of up to an hour or more were made to resuscitate babies at birth, but the records neglected to note all neonatal deaths. From 1856 to 1874 stillbirths fluctuated between 4 per cent and 11 per cent, and usually little was said about them. All that was recorded was whether the death of the foetus was recent or a pre-labour death *in utero*, a proportion which fluctuated wildly. The substantial number each year of putrefying foetuses delivered suggests a higher incidence of venereal disease than the hospital ever suspected. But the statistics also suggested that the hospital was not operating quite to the standard Tracy had first set. The records were no longer as fulsome and the rate of accidents a little higher, but then in the 1860s Tracy's greatest intellectual energies were being expended in the Infirmary.

The Diseases Peculiar to Women

3

The hospital was also dedicated to treating the diseases peculiar to women and children, but this was a discreet, secretive world that did things that could not be spoken about except in the privacy of the medical meeting or the medical journal. Medical men enjoyed a freedom denied all other respectable people of speaking and thinking frankly about human sexuality. During a century when it became increasingly difficult to discuss sexual relationships and contraception, medical men alone were free to speculate and philosophise. They were responsible for some of the appalling notions that deformed nineteenth-century society's fear and fascination with sex; but for all those who blamed madness on masturbation, there were others who observed that shameless masturbation was merely a symptom of madness and that sexual desire in women was as normal as it was in men. If Dr William Acton proclaimed that sexual anaesthesia was normal in respectable women and that only prostitutes experienced desire, and Mr Isaac Baker Brown implicated excessive uterine sexual excitation in sterility, there were others who still shared the folk belief that conception was only possible with female orgasm.[79]

This is not to deny that the nineteenth century was not an age of sexual anxiety. Human sexual desire produced both pleasure and pain, because uncontrolled fertility could inflict physical and mental suffering on women. And it was in the wards of the infirmary that the female casualties of desire and poverty were to be seen. Mrs MacF. was to be admitted to the infirmary in 1887, but she had only just reached puberty and was already a mother when the Lying-in Hospital was founded. She had been born in Waterford, Ireland, and brought to Victoria at the age of ten. At twelve years and three months of age she was married off; at fourteen she began menstruating. In the next twenty-seven years she had seventeen babies, the last at the age of forty-two. She was remarkably well, except for a vast varicose ulcer on her leg; and that had only started eight years before when she fell into a cellar. She worked as a cook and a laundress around the genteel slopes of the Melbourne suburb of Kew. Three weeks bed rest, with the leg raised, good food, poultices and aperients

35

saw it healed over again.[80] Mrs M. S. did not fare so well. Born in 1823, she was also of the Irish poor, so low in body weight that she did not menstruate until the age of eighteen. She married late, but between the ages of twenty-eight and forty-three she bore eight children. Now aged sixty, she had been sick for a year after a severe cold and 'a fall which seemed to strain her'. She had a foetid discharge and a lump in the neck. Dr Stephen Burke operated and 'drew off "three barrels" of thick, greenish, coffee-coloured fluid'. During the operation she began to gasp for breath so he thought it unwise to continue. Three weeks after the operation the tumour in her neck began to discharge. Dr Burke diagnosed a cancer of the uterus and after six weeks in hospital she went home to die.[81]

'The diseases peculiar to women' afflicted both the fecund and the barren. Miss E. C. was born in Perthshire in 1834 and came to Victoria with her family at the age of twenty-seven. Her family had not prospered in Australia. Only her mother was well. Her father had tuberculosis and two sisters and one brother had already died of it. One sister and one brother had both died of heart disease and a sister had died of general paralysis of the insane, due to syphilis. Miss E. C. had reached puberty at fifteen and worked all her life. She had a responsible job as a postmistress, but now, at the age of fifty-three, she was dying of ovarian and abdominal cancer: the Resident Medical Officer saw her as 'rather pale, wan, worn, cachectic appearance, emaciated. Abdomen distended with ascitic fluid'. Dr Fetherston drew off seventeen pints of fluid, but within five days her abdomen was filling again. She was discharged as 'relieved'.[82] Mrs P. G. of Richmond had been 'so frightened at herself being poorly' — that is menstruating — for the first time at the age of fifteen in 1850, that she sat in cold water. Her period had stopped and she remained in bed for six weeks. Ever since her periods had been irregular and caused 'great pain'. She married at forty-six, had never been pregnant, and she was beset with difficulty in passing urine, haemorrhoids, 'bearing-down pain' and pain over her left ovary. The doctor found her 'fairly nourished' but she was 'dark and undersize'. Dr Balls-Headley operated without anaesthetic to enlarge the os of the cervix to relieve her menstrual pain, but he suspected that she had an old infection of the ovary and fallopian

cachexia: a condition of abnormally low weight, weakness, and general bodily decline associated with chronic disease. It occurs in such conditions as cancer, pulmonary tuberculosis and malaria;

ascites: the accumulation of fluid in the peritoneal cavity, causing abdominal swelling. Causes include infections (such as tuberculosis), heart failure, portal hypertension, cirrhosis and various cancers (particularly of the ovary and liver). (*OMD*)

Madeline Street photographed from the chimney of Carlton Brewery, with the university gardens and the Lying-in Hospital in the distance. Carte de visite by Charles Nettleton, 1870 *La Trobe Picture Collection, State Library of Victoria*

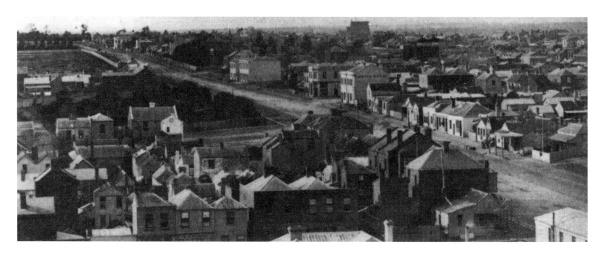

tube. One night in hospital she had a 'severe hysterical fit' and at 1 a.m. the RMO had to use the 'battery' to shock her into her senses. Hers was a life made miserable by her sex.[83]

Those doctors who were drawn to specialise in the diseases of women often had a particular emotional, or sublimated sexual commitment to women. No doctor could afford to ignore obstetrics in his professional armoury. In general practice it was the most frequent and lucrative of all family medical work, and a well-conducted first confinement was often the beginning of a family's lifetime attachment to a particular doctor. But specialisation in women's diseases was not to the taste of all medical practitioners. For one, it had only recently become a reputable specialty. As Tracy himself said, physicians and surgeons had long disdained the specialist in midwifery and the diseases of women as 'a timid surgeon, a very mild physician, with a dash of the old woman, or, in other words — a ladies' doctor'. It had been elevated to the front rank, however, by the rise of gynaecological surgery, made possible not just by new instruments and anaesthesia, but essentially by the careful application of anatomical study and clinical observation. The new surgical techniques could be applied because of the growing understanding of the mechanics of labour. The rediscovery of the speculum by the pioneering American gynaecologist J. Marion Sims brought the vagina into clear view and Simpson's sound made internal exploration of the uterus easier. Tracy listed his heroes of 'obstetrical science': Simpson, Wells, Baker Brown, Sims, West, Tilt, Meigs, Bouchet, Kiwisch, Clay, Montgomery, Barnes, Churchill, Henry Bennett, McClintock. These were men from Great Britain, America and Europe. It was a professional college of print that Tracy could now only consult by reading and correspondence. He had left England too soon to see the great men operate and he would not see them again until 1873, but he was deeply proud of what his profession was achieving and was determined to emulate them as best he could:

> As a result of the labours of men such as these, we can now point to cases that were regarded for ages as positively incurable, now everyday restored to health; and I think that I may be allowed to state, without fear of contradiction, that the modern operations for removal of diseased ovary, and for the cure of vesico-vaginal fistula may rank with the greatest triumphs of the healing art.[84]

Even though Tracy emphasised that 'surgical measures and appropriate constitutional had to go hand in hand', it was increasingly a surgical specialty and not all doctors were deft surgeons. Moreover, it required a particular tact, a 'way with women', a balance between professional distance and social charm. The doctor had to persuade the most modest of women to permit him to a physical intimacy society otherwise only granted to their lawful husbands.[85] One of the debatable benefits of chloroform was that it enabled doctors to perform intimate examinations on the terrified and the refined.[86] Ornella Moscucci argues that the availability of chloroform after 1850 increased the speculum's popularity with doctors, and that at the Chelsea Hospital for Women, most *per vaginam* examinations were performed under anaesthesia.[87] This was not quite

battery: electricity was being experimented with in the treatment of fibroids, menorrhagia and chronic pelvic infections. The Australian experience was disappointment with a technique much vaunted in France. The battery was rarely used at the Women's Hospital, and usually only for nervous or cardiac stimulation as in this case. (Intercolonial Medical Congress of Australasia, 1889, Discussion between Drs Foreman, Rowan and Balls-Headley, pp. 717–20.)

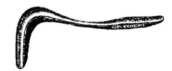

Sims's vaginal speculum
Allen & Hanburys, p. 460

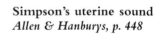

Simpson's uterine sound
Allen & Hanburys, p. 448

per vaginam: an internal pelvic examination

the case in the Melbourne institution, however, where only the virginal
or resistant were examined under chloroform. The right to use the speculum became the dividing line between the legitimate medical practitioner
and the quack and the midwife. Tracy gave evidence in 1871 in the trial
of a herbalist, William Frith of Brunswick, who had used a speculum and
treated a Mrs Evans for 'ulceration of the womb'. Tracy diagnosed a fibroid
and declared that Mrs Evans was lucky not to lose her life: even some
doctors refused to use a speculum because of the special training necessary,
he declared.[88]

In 1858 the English gynaecologist Charles West in his *Lectures on the
Diseases of Women* reminded his fellow practitioners when they undertook a vaginal examination:

> This examination must be extremely painful to a woman's feelings, since
> she is not now, as in the time of labour, impelled by the extremity of her
> sufferings to submit to anything for the sake of relief. She seems indeed
> to be now particularly alive to every painful impression; and while she
> feels almost overwhelmed by a sense of humiliation at having to undergo
> an examination, of the necessity for which she may yet feel fully con-
> vinced, she will judge with painful minuteness each act of yours, any care-
> less exposure of her person, any apparent want of delicacy, or consideration.
> With the greatest care, indeed, you will not always escape from undeserved
> blame. Without it, you will perpetually wound your patient's feelings, and
> if you did not injure your own prospects, you will yet fail to support the
> dignity of your Profession.

It was a different matter when treating the poor, however, and hospital
practice among charity patients 'whose sensibilities are not always as keen,
as those of persons in a higher class of life . . . leads but too often to
carelessness in these respects, on the part of men who would yet shrink
from the idea of inflicting a moment's unnecessary suffering upon
anyone'. West concluded with a lesson well taken by his Australian medical
readers:

> I am, therefore, all the more anxious to impress upon you that the delicacy
> with which you ought to conduct all your investigations into the diseases
> of women, is not a thing which can be assumed for the nonce, but that
> it must be the habit of mind, must therefore have been acquired now
> during your pupillage, and in the midst of your intercourse with the
> poor.[89]

It was probably Tracy who selected this quotation for the January issue
of the *Australian Medical Journal* for 1858, and it accorded with his own
principles and practice. No infirmary case books survive from the hospital
before 1879, and so we do not have the narratives for Tracy's time which
take us directly into the private world of poor women in the 1860s and
1870s, but we do have Tracy's own published cases, and his scientific papers
reveal much of the relationship between doctor and patient. We also have
two of his lectures: one an address to the Medical Society on 2 September
1863 and the other his inaugural lecture to the first class of fourth-year

medical students in 1865, in which he reflected on his specialty and revealed something of his therapeutic understanding.[90]

The 1860s was an exciting decade for Tracy and his hospital.[91] With Australia's first medical course under way in the infant University of Melbourne, his was the first specialist teaching hospital in the land for midwifery and the diseases of women. He was conscious of the historical moment and very proud of the hospital he had at his disposal for teaching: 'The student will here find every facility afforded him for study, a noble anatomical room, chemical laboratory, and an excellent library'.[92] The student was to master medical science, for how else could he 'follow and understand the advancing researches of learned workers in every branch of medical science'; and he must learn at the bedside: 'become learned in the daily practical details of hospital, medical and surgical practice'. Tracy was an eclectic physician and a 'scientific' surgeon, trained in both the older therapies of constitutional regulation — the resort to bleeding, purgatives, blistering — interventions to produce changes and secretions which could be monitored as signs of recovery or deterioration; and in the clinical science of anatomical analysis, which by the 1850s was underwriting the dramatic new interventions of surgery. He advised his students that they had to combine theoretical knowledge with empirical learning: theoretical knowledge was useless without clinical experience, but without theoretical competence and scientific method, they would be left behind in the march of medical advance. His own teaching, however, would be 'practical instruction; to show you what is to be done and how to do it'. The 'exhaustive scientific treatises' of 'eminent men' were for the students' private study. Medical education had in the past been 'too much lecturing and too little study or real clinical teaching'. The lecturer had to be a guide, but above all

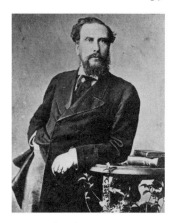

Dr Richard Tracy
RWHA

> . . . he should be the counsellor and friend of every member of his class, and by teaching at the bed-side, seek to fix indelibly on the plastic unprejudiced mind of the painstaking intelligent student, the true rules of practice, so as to stir up and keep alive a constant spirit of enquiry, showing his class that he their teacher is daily learning himself; for happily, and to the credit of our noble profession be it spoken, a man must be a student, in the truest sense of the word every day, to keep pace with modern research and improvement in practice.[93]

Tracy regarded the treatment of women as the hallmark of a society's state of moral culture, and the new scientific midwifery, 'as yet almost entirely limited to the more polished communities of Europe, America and Australia', as 'evidence of our advancement'. But if he was gratified by the relief good practice of the obstetric art could bring to women in childbed, he was even more moved by the relief surgery offered women for their gynaecological problems. However, his theory of disease was mechanical rather than constitutional, and he was sceptical of those who explained the reproductive diseases of women as the inevitable consequence of 'higher civilisation', of the 'artificial life' over the state of nature. Even if 'civilised' women appeared more prone to puerperal complications, the comparisons with 'savage women' were often ill informed.

He told his students that 'savage tribes' destroyed 'all very weakly or deformed children' so that most women who survived were fit for healthy childbearing. Furthermore, close observers of parturition among indigenous peoples around the world had less sanguine reports: 'and those who have had the opportunity of observing the aborigines of this continent have found that parturition is often followed by great and dangerous exhaustion [haemorrhage]'.[94] Simple environmental and moral explanations were insufficient. Gynaecological disease had its aetiology in mechanical failure, or constitutional disease, or injury, or improper management of the processes of reproduction, therefore its correction, more often than not, needed to be mechanical, that is surgical. In passing, in a paper in 1862, Tracy noted that the bulk of the hospital gynaecologist's work came from the mischief caused 'by the want of care and rest after miscarriages — the most inveterate forms of leucorrhoea may as a general rule be traced back to this cause'. He conducted a survey of 'women in the humble classes' and discovered that they generally returned to work and housekeeping 'about the third day' after. He was diagnosing 'congestion and ulceration of the cervix' — a condition which would be reframed dramatically by the end of the century and which would dominate the work of the infirmary until the discovery of antibiotics. But Tracy had no surgical remedy, so in fact he scarcely wrote about it, as neither did he comment on induced abortion, even though it was widely practised.[95]

Tracy concentrated on what he could mechanically change, and rather than being oppressed by how little doctors could do for sick women, he was overwhelmed with how much they could now do. The experience of medical advance had been so rapid and dramatic in a mere decade and a bit, that it seemed that for the first time in human history, medical knowledge could intervene effectively in the age-old diseases of women. These could begin well before a woman's child bearing career. A doctor known to be interested in 'women's problems' soon drew a clientele of patients afflicted with misery every month from their periods. Sympathetic doctors took great interest in menstrual disorders, including the crushing discomforts of dysmenorrhoea. West wrote of women writhing in agony on the floor, and identified three forms of the condition: 'neuralgic' dysmenorrhoea which resulted in pain both in the head and in the pelvis; 'congestive' which would approximate to premenstrual tension and finally 'mechanical' dysmenorrhoea resulting from a contracted or pinhole os, which was too small to permit an easy passage of menstrual blood and clots from the uterus.[96] In a mechanical age the last was a logical explanation, for if the natural release of a bodily fluid caused pain, then there must be a blockage. In such cases Simpson advised the incision of the os of the cervix by a device known variously as a hysterotome, metrotome or uterotome.[97] In 1861 Tracy reported the successful treatment of a private patient for a stricture of the cervix and the case was remarkable for the intimate and co-operative relationship between doctor and patient. Mrs L. was thirty-four:

> This lady resides in the bush. She is very tall and slight, of exceedingly active habits, and highly intellectual. I at once found I was called to treat

leucorrhoea: white or yellowish mucous discharge from the vagina. An abnormally large discharge may indicate infection of the lower reproductive tract. (*OMD*)

dysmenorrhoea: painful menstruation. Primary (spasmodic) dysmenorrhoea usually begins with the first period and is heralded by cramping lower abdominal pains starting just before or with the menstrual flow and continuing during menstruation. It is often associated wth nausea, vomiting, headache, faintness and symptoms of peripheral vasodilatation. The cause is thought to be related to excessive prostoglandin production. *Secondary dysmenorrhoea* usually affects older patients who complain of a congested ache with lower abdominal cramps, which usually start from a few days up to a few weeks before menstruation. Causes include pelvic inflammatory disease, endometriosis, fibroids and the presence of an intra uterine contraceptive device. (*OMD*)

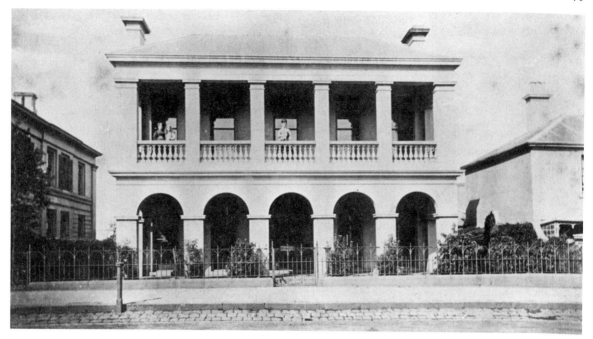

a patient who, from having suffered long and severely, had been led to endeavour to ascertain for herself, if possible, the cause of her sufferings, and having some facilities for obtaining a perusal of medical works, had read up on the subject, and had formed, from an exact comparison of her own symptoms with those related in some of the cases she had read, an opinion that she was suffering from mechanical obstruction in the canal of the cervix uteri.[98]

Dr Tracy's house, 190 Collins Street, Melbourne, 1874: Mrs Tracy and daughter Blanche on balcony
RWHA

Tracy welcomed this feminine intellectual achievement and invited her to write up the case notes herself and thus they became joint authors of the paper. The treatment was exactly that recommended by Simpson, where the uterotome was introduced, without anaesthetic, and incisions made in the os. But after two weeks the symptoms returned, so Tracy asked his patient to insert metal pessaries, shaped like mushrooms, of graduating sizes for a fortnight. Her condition improved, but it remained necessary for her to have 'the instrument regularly inserted to prevent stricture recurring'.

pessaries: instruments designed to support a displaced or prolapsed uterus

It was never a satisfactory treatment but it was to prove one of the most frequent surgical procedures in the hospital for the next thirty years, and if it worked at all it was because dilatation of the cervix can momentarily bring relief or because it severed nerve endings. At worst damage to nerves and tissue could cause cervical incompetence. The forced dilatations of the cervix also made the procedure excruciatingly painful, especially for those whose cervix had never been dilated by labour. Many would have fainted at the pain. Tracy found Simpson's instrument difficult to use because it required turning, and to do that it needed to be extracted and re-inserted. He designed instead an instrument with extra blades and a screw device to open them out, and it thus became the first surgical instrument wholly developed in Australia.[99] Tracy's new procedure had

cervical incompetence: may cause a miscarriage in the second trimester. Now often averted with a stitch. (Townsend (O), pp. 579–80) sponge tent: a piece of dried vegetable material, usually a seaweed stem, shaped to fit into an orifice such as the cervical canal. As it absorbs moisture it expands, providing a slow but forceful means of expanding the orifice (*OMD*). Slippery elm bark was commonly used in this way to induce abortion.

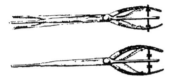

Tracy's hysterotome
Australian Medical
Journal, *1863*

fibroid: a benign tumour of fibrous and muscular tissue, one or more of which may develop in the muscular wall of the uterus (*OMD*)

anaemia: reduction of oxygen-carrying pigment (haemoglobin) in the blood (*OMD*)

Liquor Secalis Cornuti: ergot of rye

the patient lying in a recumbent position for eighteen to twenty-four hours, and the sponge tent, inserted into the cervix to keep it open and reduce bleeding, would be removed so that the vagina could be syringed with tepid water. Every day he would insert his index finger, 'well greased', into the incisions 'so as to counteract any tendency to adhesion of the cut surfaces'. On the fourth day he would cautiously insert the sound.[100]

Tracy's relationship with private patients crossed the divide from an older age where the doctor was a practitioner of healing arts to the age of the scientific doctor practising with scrupulous clinical detachment. In 1863 he reported on another private patient whom he treated for years for an infantile uterus, and who year after year painfully inserted sponge tents and pessaries in graduating sizes. In the middle of the treatment Tracy sent her to Scotland 'to consult Professor Simpson' which led to a fruitful correspondence between the specialists in women's troubles. Tracy lost hope that the treatment could work, but 'I was exceedingly fortunate in having a thoroughly intelligent lady to deal with, who not only bore the irksomeness of the appliances well, but often urged me to persevere in the treatment when I was very much inclined to be discouraged at the apparent hopelessness of my efforts'. Finally 'in September 1861 to her great delight a well-marked coloured discharge appeared for two days'. (There was no record if this was a genuine menstrual flow which returned.)[101]

This was not the only surgery performed through the vagina. Tracy and his fellow surgeons were also confident enough of their skills to be excising uterine fibroids via the vagina. Fibroids were not only painful, they were life-threatening if they resulted in prolonged bleeding. They could grow as big as a football, filling the entire pelvis: an obese woman at the Melbourne Hospital in 1871 yielded at autopsy a tumour weighing forty-six pounds.[102] In 1865 two women were operated on in the infirmary to have fibroids removed. Elizabeth K. was thirty-three and had had two stillborn children, the last ten years before. For nine months she had suffered bearing-down pain and flooding, leaving her weak and anaemic. Tracy ordered rest and a 'supporting diet', and began to insert tents to dilate the cervix while she was prescribed ten drops of *Liquor Secalis Cornuti* (BP) three times a day. Next he incised the os and the cervix to equalise the pressure of the uterine fibres on the tumour and to lessen its vascular supply. Inside the uterus the tumour, deprived of a proper blood supply, began to slough, that is become gangrenous. Nature was now allowed to take its course, but the patient became very sick before the uterus, with the assistance of ergot, finally expelled the fibroid as a 'foreign body'. Once rid of it, the patient became quickly better. The second patient was forty-five and had never been pregnant: 'She was a largely built, masculine-looking woman, but presented a most anaemic appearance; the skin was of greenish-white colour, exactly like the appearance presented by a patient suffering from a malignant disease'. Again *Liquor Secalis* was administered to aid the uterus in bringing down the fibroid 'within the range of the os'. After two weeks she haemorrhaged violently and 'ergot was given in large doses to good effect'. He continued with the ergot, awaiting a second haemorrhage to justify operative interference. The patient within days was in great pain, 'as in childbirth', and with the aid of forceps Tracy 'delivered the tumour' which was 'the size of a coconut'. Four weeks later she was 'discharged well'.[103]

These operations—the incisions of the cervix and the removal of fibroids—were all conducted without anaesthetic, and surgical interference was used only as a last resort. The risks of post-operative infection were so high that there had to be no other humane alternative. Chloroform offered the surgeon-gynaecologist new opportunities for considered abdominal operations, but every major intervention Tracy took in these years was after great heart-searching. None the less, it was his surgery which gave him the greatest personal satisfaction and which brought him widest recognition. And perhaps the most gratifying of all were the first plastic operations to close vaginal fistulae. Fistulae or holes between the bladder and the vagina and the rectum and the vagina were easily come by when long labours could not be averted by caesarean section. Prolonged pressure of the baby's head on soft tissues could bring about bruising, leading to the death of tissue and the formation of holes. Fistulae were also a common consequence of pelvic abscesses of gynaecological or tubercular origin. Urine or faeces perpetually leaked through this hole. Tracy described the condition of one patient:

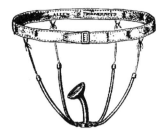

Barnes pessary, cup and stem
Allen & Hanburys, p. 474

> Mrs H., residing at Sandridge, aged twenty-six years, was admitted to the infirmary wards of the Melbourne Lying-in-Hospital, December 7th 1864. She stated that she was taken in labour of her first child on the 14th of October; that she was attended by a woman; that the head of the child was born four hours before the body was extracted; that much force was used, the ears being torn off the child's head; that she had not passed water for more than twelve hours before delivery, and that she was never able to retain it after.
>
> All the usual miserable symptoms of urinary fistula were well marked in the case on admission. The labia and thighs were much excoriated. On examination, the vagina was found to be much contracted by bands of adhesion, the result of what must have been very acute inflammatory action. The fistulous opening was rather close down and about three-quarters of an inch from the urethral orifice. It was about an inch long, and from its position and the contracted state of the vagina, extended quite across the bladder. The mucous coat was protruding considerably, and the parts were altogether in a most filthy and irritable state, the patient moreover being in a very bad condition and weak. She was put on good diet, cleanliness strictly observed, and the state of the bowels attended to.[104]

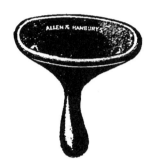

Simpson's pessary, cup and stem
Allen & Hanburys, p. 475

excoriation: the destruction and removal of the surface of the skin or covering of an organ by scraping, the application of a chemical or other means (*OMD*)

After nearly seven weeks care she was strong enough for surgery. The operation was performed without anaesthesia, with the patient on hands and knees—just as J. Marion Sims, the father of American gynaecological surgery, had first experimented on his slaves.[105] The edges of the fistula were pared and 'four iron wire sutures introduced'. Tracy decided not to leave in a catheter 'as the patient was a most irritable woman and the stitches were so near the urethra', so the young Resident Medical Officer, Dr Gerald Fetherston, was instructed to insert a catheter each time she needed to pass water. On the tenth day the sutures were removed and 'perfect union was found to have occurred'. A week later she was allowed to pass urine herself and she was able to retain it for six or eight hours so that 'shortly afterwards she left the hospital quite well'.

Mrs C. G. was not so fortunate. She was twenty-nine, 'a very slight, unhealthy-looking woman' who spoke only Gaelic. Another patient did her best to interpret for her, and although it was not clear what had really happened, it seemed that three months before she had been two days in labour with her third child:

> Her health never seems to have recovered — she is exceedingly thin and anaemic. On making a vaginal examination a rent fully two inches long was found extending across the floor of the bladder, about half an inch from the orifice of the urethra. It was very irregular in its outline, the edges hard, and in many places bound down by adhesions, resulting from the attempts at healing set up after inflammatory action. The cavity of the bladder was almost obliterated. A catheter introduced through the urethra, after traversing the fistulous opening, could only be made to pass a short distance, and that only towards the right side. This cavity was full of phosphatic deposit, which also covered the vagina all round the margins of the fistula. The vulva was much excoriated. Altogether the case presented a most unpromising appearance. A liberal and nutritious diet, the internal administration of bark, and scrupulous attention to cleanliness, and suitable injections to free the bladder from the thick layer of phosphates, were the means used for many weeks.[106]

Ten weeks later she was fit for surgery. Nine doctors attended, but there was still a small leakage a month later, so she was operated on again. Five weeks later she was operated on a third time, but there was still pus. Six months after her admission Mrs G. was 'very restless and in a low and weak state — cramps in the legs', a fourth operation would be needed but she was sent to the country to recover her strength first. She disappeared and was never heard of again.

These two victims of what Tracy called 'that most distressing lesion' were still fortunate to receive surgical relief within months of their fistulae forming. Mrs H. S. was denied Tracy's surgical skills when she needed them in 1872. She had married at the age of twenty-three and borne five children. Two decades later only two were alive: two sons had died and another was stillborn. She had been well twenty-three years before when her dead child was delivered by forceps. She was certain that her bladder was torn and Dr Henry 'foretold that it would be'. Four months later she was admitted to the Infirmary where she waited for five months and endured six vaginal examinations until she was told that Dr Tracy was too ill to operate. For the next twenty-two years she had coped 'pretty well' with being widowed, raising her family and working on her feet as a 'first class cook'. Then as she entered menopause, her symptoms became worse. In 1885 she was operated on at the Melbourne Hospital after trying the Austin Hospital, but she was in great pain and urine still ran out. The doctor offered to try again but she refused and got herself into the Infirmary. By now the pain had stopped 'but the urine still flowed'. Dr Balls-Headley then operated and for the first time in twenty-three years she had relief: she 'was in heaven after that as before she couldn't sit down'.[107]

adhesion: the union of two normally separate surfaces by fibrous connective tissue developing in an inflamed or damaged region (*OMD*)

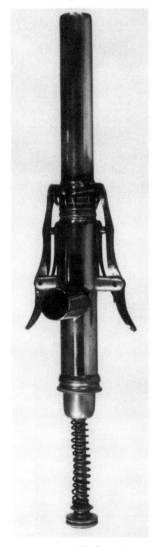

Siphon-trocar (T. Spencer Wells), used for perforating and aspirating an ovarian cyst
RWHA

Tracy and Turnbull's other major successes in plastic surgery were in the repair of torn perinea. Not only were their operations successful, they were a tribute to their skill because neither had seen the surgery performed. Tracy prefaced his proud report on the first three repairs with an extract from Mr Isaac Baker Brown's textbook instructions from *Surgical Diseases of Women*. It was a most complex procedure:

> . . . the new perineum is formed by dissecting off a crescentic portion of the skin (varying in extent as to its upper margin, according to the nature of the case) half an inch in width from the junction of the skin and mucous membrane lining the vagina. A corresponding width of the mucous membrane is removed, and when bleeding has ceased, three deep double-wire sutures are passed by means of a long and very flexible needle. The point of the needle is made to penetrate the skin one inch external to the margin of the denuded surface. Care is taken that there it has sufficient hold of the mucous membrane, as it is made to emerge from the tissues, it is then carried across the vaginal cavity, taking hold of the margin of the mucous membrane, as it penetrates the tissues of the opposite side, and it is brought out an inch from the margin of the incision as at the other side. Those three sutures having been passed into the loops at one side, and the parts being assisted towards coaptation, by bringing the patient's knees together, the free ends of the wires are tied over a corresponding portion of bougie at the other side. The procedure brings the deep or inner margins of the cut surfaces into opposition. The external margins are then united by three ordinary wire sutures, and as soon as it is ascertained, by passing the finger into the vagina, that the deep margins are in thorough opposition, the patient is removed to bed, placed on her side on a water pillow, her knees kept well flexed, and retained in that position by means of a bandage passing from the flexure of the knees to the top rail of the bed. In cases where the rupture extends through the rectum, or where the parts are tense and rigid, the sphincter ani is divided (before passing the sutures) by means of an incision with a straight probe pointed bistoury outwards and backwards on each side of the anus towards the tubera ischii.[108]

bougie: a hollow or solid cylindrical instrument, usually flexible, that is inserted into tubular passages such as the oesophagus, rectum or urethra (*OMD*)

coaptation: the fitting together or adjustment of displaced parts, as of the ends of a fractured bone (*AMD*)

sphincter ani: anal sphincter

bistoury: a long narrow surgical knife, straight or curved (*AMD*)

tubera ischii: thickened ends of the bones forming the lower part of each side of the hip bone

Empirically the doctors knew that the success of the operation depended on the wound not being contaminated, and so tied into this flexed position, the patient was to have her bowels confined by opium for three weeks and for all urine to be drawn off by catheter 'at short intervals' for the first twelve days, and the vagina regularly syringed with tepid water after each use of the catheter.

Mrs S. E. was the first patient to have her perineum repaired in the Infirmary. She had three children and her perineum had been lacerated at the first labour, so that now, 'on the slightest exertion, the womb protrudes to the size of an orange. It is needless to say that her sufferings are severe, and that she is unable to attend to her household duties'. Dr Tracy, assisted by Dr Turnbull and five other colleagues, operated on 18 September 1859. Four days after, the deep sutures had begun to suppurate despite the careful nursing; on the fifth day the deep sutures were removed and there was a strong union. On the eleventh day the catheter was omitted and the patient 'was allowed to pass water after placing her on her hands and knees in the bed'. Opium was given in grain doses at intervals of four, six and eight hours 'as seemed necessary to ensure constipation and allay irritability'. After three weeks the union was complete and five days later the 'patient left her bed and sat up for a few hours, the new perineum being supported by a suitable pad and bandage'. And six days later she left the hospital 'quite cured'.

Tracy's most acclaimed surgical success was in ovariotomy: the removal of all or part of the ovary for malignant, cystic or inflammatory disease. While the history of ovariotomy goes back to the beginning of the nineteenth century, it was one of the abdominal operations to benefit early from the discovery of chloroform. Chloroform was not without its problems: the dosage needed to relax the abdominal muscles was high and the anaesthetist had to maintain a delicate balance between deep insensibility and depressed vital functions. The danger of fatal infection at a time when all operative wounds were expected to become infected was also a deterrent to invasive surgery. To counteract internal infection, the pedicle or stump of the ovarian tumour was brought outside the body so that it could slough and rot in much the same way as the umbilical cord does in newborn babies. The suffering of those with multilocular ovarian cysts was intense: Turnbull reported a case where he had tapped a private patient where at first he drew off sixty-five pints of fluid; three months later it was thirty-three pints and four months after that, thirty-six pints. He believed that injections of iodine were slowing down the accumulation of fluid.[109] Even this had its dangers, for the patient ran the risk of serious infection every time the trocar was inserted. In the 1860s the woman's condition needed to be very serious indeed to justify surgery.

Tracy's first operation was on a private patient in 1864, and he went on to perform the operation seventeen times with only four deaths (two of whom had malignancies), a success rate superior to that of his idol Spencer Wells in England.[110] Again he was self-taught, relying on his correspondence with Spencer Wells, and again the case record brings alive the nursing, the hospital routines and the patient herself.

pedicle: narrow neck of tissue connecting some tumours to the normal tissue from which they have developed

trocar: a sharp-pointed instrument used with a cannula for tapping or piercing a cavity-wall in paracentesis (*AMD*)

> Mrs C., aged forty-six years, residing in Rutherglen, was sent to me by Mr H.B. Wilson of that town, and was admitted to the Infirmary Ward of the Melbourne Lying-in Hospital, on September 24th [1863]. She gave the following history: — In the year 1855, she had first noticed a swelling in the left side, which continued to increase but slowly. Two years after its first appearance she ceased to menstruate. She had been married fourteen years but she had never been pregnant. On the 12th July, 1862, she was first tapped, and the operation did not require to be repeated until 3rd December, 1862. She was again tapped in June, 1863; November, 1863; April 1864; and 3rd August, 1864, seven weeks before her admission; and already she had filled up, and felt that tapping must very soon be resorted to again. In all other respects her health had been good; but since the tumour had begun to fill so rapidly, she had lost flesh, and when admitted she was considerably emaciated.
>
> On examination, the belly was found uniformly enlarged; the measurement round the body at the umbilicus was 37 inches; from the ensiform cartilage to the umbilicus, $8^{1}/_{2}$ inches; from the umbilicus to the pubes,

$9^1/_2$ inches. There were no marked irregularities in the surface of the swelling, and the wave of fluid on palpation was as free from side to side as in ascites. On examination, *per vaginam*, the uterus was found to be drawn up behind the pubes, and it was not possible to introduce the uterine sound more than an inch within the os. There was no evidence of adhesions within the pelvis, nor indeed anywhere else, as the integuments of the abdomen could be freely moved over the surface of the tumour.

Mrs C. was seen in consultation by several medical friends, and all agreed with me that it was a most suitable case for operation, especially as the patient was most anxious to be operated on, after being made fully aware of the danger involved.

The preliminary treatment consisted in the use of the warm bath two or three times a week, nourishing diet, and occasional doses of Ox Gall and Compound Rhubarb Pill, and warm water enemata the day before the operation.

On October 27th, I proceeded to operate in the presence of a large number of the medical men residing in Melbourne and suburbs. Mr. I. B. Brown, jun., of London; Dr Christy, of H.M.S. *Esk* ; and Dr McGrath, of Castlemaine, were also present. I was most kindly and ably assisted by the same gentlemen, as in my first case in March last, chloroform being administered by Dr Motherwell. The catheter having been introduced, the abdomen was opened by an incision between four and five inches long. There was no ascitic fluid. The sac was tapped by means of Mr Spencer Wells' syphon-trocar, and about six or seven pints of a straw-coloured fluid escaped. The point of the trocar was then pushed on into another cyst, and several pints of a clear fluid evacuated. The sac was now gently drawn out, and found to be entirely free from adhesions; and so well were the sides of the wound kept together, by my friends Mr. James and Dr Fetherston, that none of the intestines came into view at any period of the operation. Several small cysts were found developed in the mass, but only four required tapping in the way already described. The pedicle was found to be of good length; it was transfixed by a needle armed with a double hemp ligature tied on each end, and also firmly tied by a double hemp ligature in the ordinary way. The clamp had to be put on before the ligatures were applied. The tumour was not cut away, not a drop of fluid had escaped into the abdomen; so that there was no necessity for sponging-out the cavity. The wound was closed by six silken hare-lip pins, the lowest pin being made to transfix the pedicle. The pins were carefully made to go through the peritoneum at both sides about half an inch from its cut-edge. The superficial edges of the wound were brought together with five wire interrupted sutures; the patient was made thoroughly dry, placed in bed, and a warm linseed-meal poultice applied over the abdomen.

The temperature of the room during the operation was 73 deg. of Fahr., and the time occupied altogether twenty-seven minutes. The amount of fluid contained in the cysts was twenty-one and a-half pints. One small sac was filled with fatty matter.

integuments: 1. the skin. 2. a membrane or layer of tissue covering any organ of the body

ox gall: in a purified and dry condition, used in medicine for the purpose of relieving certain forms of indigestion which depend upon deficient secretion of bile, or which occurs in persons who digest fats badly (Black)

Very little chloroform was given. At 4 p.m., the patient was found to have rallied very well; the pulse was 95. Two grains of opium were given, and she was allowed to suck ice *ad libitum*.

Tracy then added the nursing notes, revealing the Infirmary's routine in post-operative care:

10 p.m. Has once been very slightly sick. Has taken iced soda water. The catheter has been used twice. The pulse is 97. The clamp was removed as it was causing pain, and could be of no use, as in this case I had trans-fixed the pedicle with the pin. A strip of greased lint was passed around the base of the pedicle, and the poultices continued.

28th, 7 a.m. Has slept well; is free from pain; has not been sick; pulse 110. The pedicle was dressed as before, and a small muslin bag of charcoal placed over its decaying surface. The patient wished to have a little dried toast and tea. During this day she also wished for, and was given, a little weak brandy and water. She took barley water and gruel pretty freely.

29th. Feels very well. Did not sleep so well last night as the previous one. Pulse 98. Urine by catheter loaded with lithates. The treatment through this day was continued as before. The pedicle was dressed morning and evening, and one grain of opium was given at bedtime.

30th. Has slept well the past night. The pulse 103. The wound is healed down to the pedicle. Removed the first, third, and fifth pins, and applied two strips of adhesive plaster.

31st. Going on well. Pulse 98. The pins were now all removed except the one through the pedicle. The pedicle is suppurating well. She had some chicken broth for dinner.

Nov. 1st. Has slept well. The pulse 98. Removed the pin from the pedicle, as it was suppurating freely. The poultices were now made much smaller, and only applied over the pedicle. The belly has never been in the least swollen or tender. Flatus has passed freely.

2nd. Going on well. Asked for sponge-cake and a glass of port wine, which were given. Had also chicken broth, maizena, and barley-water. Three of the interrupted sutures were removed.

3rd. Pulse 94. Ordered to have two Ox Gall and Rhubarb pills, and in the evening a warm water enema.

4th. Has had one good night. Ordered a repetition of the warm water enema, which acted freely. Passed urine without aid from catheter.

5th. Going on well.

6th. Tenth day. The pedicle came away this morning. The wound is very small and granulating well.

7th. The two last superficial sutures were removed. The wound is firmly closed. The surface where the pedicle separate, is closing in well. Had a chop for dinner.

Further detailed report is unnecessary. Everything went on favourably. On the twentieth day, the patient was sitting up, and she is now (30th November) making arrangements to return home to Rutherglen. She has gained flesh considerably, and is in excellent health and spirits.

Remarks: I kept this patient a month in hospital before operating on account of her weak state and exhaustion from a journey of 184 miles, which she was obliged to make by easy stages in a waggon.[111]

lithates: a urate (salt of uric acid) (*AMD*)

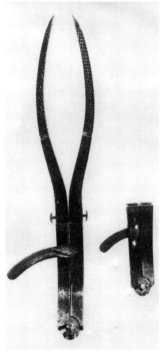

Pedicle clamp (T. Spencer Wells), in three sizes, with detachable handles
RWHA

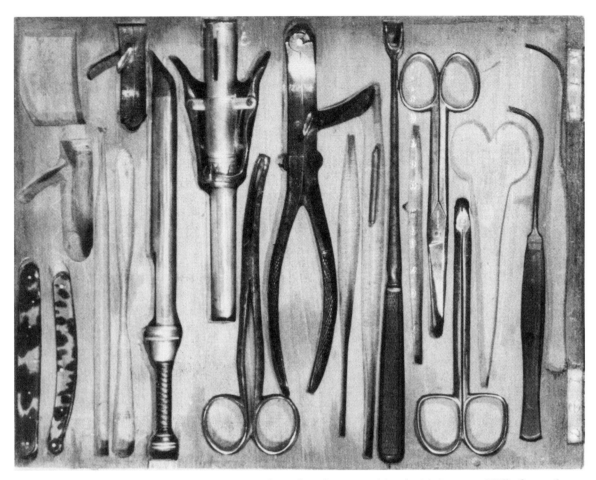

Richard Tracy's ovariotomy instruments, selected and sent to him by T. Spencer Wells from the London instrument maker, Weiss. The case of instruments was presented to the hospital in 1963 by Robert Tracy-Inglis of New Zealand. *RWHA*

Tracy concluded by thanking the RMO Dr Fetherston for his 'unremitting attention' and it was young Dr Fetherston who supervised all the nursing and wrote up the notes.

Tracy had his failures and they devastated him, and he was particularly distressed by two deaths from ovarian cancer in women under twenty-two in the hospital in 1865. One was too sick for surgery; the other, on being opened up, had cancer through to the bladder and Tracy inadvertently perforated the bladder and was publicly criticised.[112] It was his surgery that brought him recognition, however, and in 1871, to his delight, he was elected an honorary fellow of the London Obstetrical Society. But at this moment of triumph he was already mortally ill. The 'great days' of Richard Tracy's hospital were over. In 1871 his health began to deteriorate, and a trip to England in 1873, financed by £600 public subscription raised by his Melbourne friends and admirers, failed to arrest his physical and mental decline. In his last year of life the Melbourne medical fraternity recorded his sufferings in detail. His colleague Dr Martin published his case notes:

May 14 — Had a little more than $\frac{1}{2}$ gr. morphia injected last night, and suffered horribly the whole night from a return of the nervous disorder, the same as after the atropine; dryness of fauces; choking; contracted pupils and great excitement and alarm. Very low and depressed today; refused the morphia, and would prefer any pain to the horror of last night.[113]

Tracy's obituary concluded with the report of the post-mortem conducted by his dear friend Dr Motherwell. He had died of cancer of the bowel and was only forty–six years old. His funeral was the biggest so far in the history of the colony.

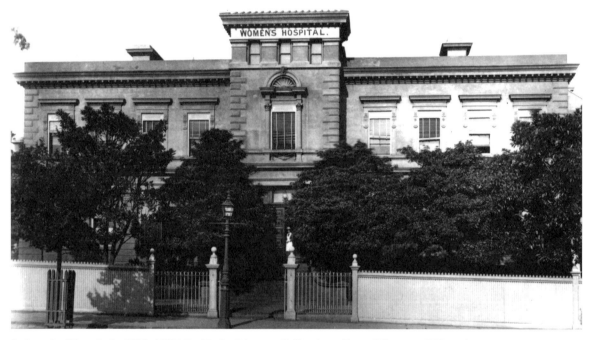

Lying-in Hospital, 1886–1887 *La Trobe Picture Collection, State Library of Victoria*

II

Sepsis and Antisepsis
1875–1902

Fever House
1875–1889

4

Tracy had gone and in 1875 so too had Mrs Perry, and a new generation of doctors and ladies were in control of the hospital. Tracy's immediate replacements, Drs Martin and Black, did not last long, and only Dr Gerald Fetherston and his sister-in-law Miss Emily Harvey, the matron, were left from the Tracy days. The new generation of honoraries were to dominate the hospital into the 1890s and beyond, and they were a volatile mix. The Fetherstons were Protestant Irish, and so was Dr Thomas Rowan, just twenty-four when elected an honorary in 1876; Dr Stephen Burke, elected three years later, was Irish also, and a Roman Catholic. He had already built a large practice from his elegant house in Victoria Street, West Melbourne, and was revered among the poor of North Melbourne for his kindness. The fourth, Dr Walter Balls-Headley, was the lone Englishman. A graduate of Cambridge University and linked to the Cambridge intellectual aristocracy, he had claims to gentility and was listed in Burke's *Colonial Gentry*.[1] He seemed destined for better things than the colonies when he contracted pulmonary tuberculosis as private physician to the Marquess of Bute during a journey through Palestine and Syria. Thus he emigrated to Queensland for the sake of his health in 1869 and in 1875 moved to Melbourne. Three years later he was honorary physician at both the Alfred and the Lying-in hospitals. As a gentleman and Cambridge scholar, he at once assumed the role of leading honorary, so antagonising the young black-bearded Rowan in 1880 that they once nearly came to blows. That year also he was publicly attacked for 'butchering' a Mrs Atkins in a series of unsuccessful operations for a septic fibroid. The Committee stood by him, but Balls-Headley reminded them that for as long as midwifery patients were within earshot of surgical operations which were conducted in the wards shut off by only a movable screen, it was very likely that 'a woman in ordinary labour might be reported to them as being murdered'. It was a professional embarrassment that he converted into a plea for small wards and a separate operating room for surgical patients.[2]

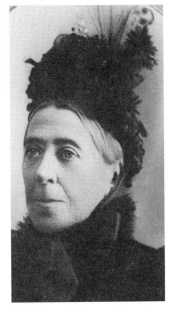

Mrs Turnbull, president
RWHA

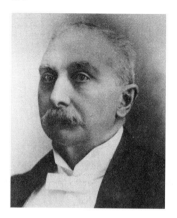

Dr Walter Balls-Headley
RWHA

Balls-Headley also succeeded in antagonising another leading player in Melbourne medical life, Dr James Jamieson, the newly appointed lecturer in obstetrics and the diseases of women at the University of Melbourne. Jamieson was a Scot, trained in Glasgow, and was a spirited medical controversialist. As Health Officer to the City of Melbourne from 1877, he did much to educate the community about typhoid fever and he lectured at the university first in obstetrics and later in medicine until 1907. He lacked the social prestige and private practice to be elected as an honorary in his own right, but he had every right to feel offended when Balls-Headley commenced clinical lectures in the hospital on placenta praevia; and he was outraged when in those lectures Balls-Headley revealed that he did not know what he was talking about. Between May and June 1879 the two of them sparred: Dr Balls-Headley making assured pronouncements; Dr Jamieson correcting his misunderstandings and illusions in the interests of medical students.[3]

This conflict had consequences which went beyond the management of placenta praevia, because Jamieson's most urgent campaign in the late 1870s was on behalf of germ theory and the aetiology and contagiousness of 'hospitalism', among them erysipelas and puerperal infection. The progress of germ theory after Pasteur's discoveries and Lister's antiseptic reforms was tortuous in Melbourne, as it was almost everywhere else. Furthermore, the constantly clinically observed relationship between infection and the retention of decidua after both childbirth and abortion confirmed the belief that infection arose from contact with putrefying matter. In the case of the Lying-in Hospital, if the patients could be kept physically isolated when infected, if basic cleanliness and good care were practised, and if sickly, diseased and undesirable patients could be kept out, then infection might be kept at bay. And that was what had appeared to have happened. Still by 1875 there had been only one outbreak of puerperal fever in Melbourne which had penetrated the hospital's wards. In October 1876 there was an epidemic of scarlet fever, which was believed to be related to puerperal fever, so the hospital was closed for three months during which it was cleaned and whitewashed.

The problem was that Melbourne was growing very fast as the capital generated by gold now moved into urban and industrial development. The population expanded and new suburbs spread containing houses built for both the poor and the comfortable by building societies and property developers. The pressure on the hospital was acute. In 1864 319 women had been confined there; in 1878 there were 565 confinements but only four more beds. Women stayed for a shorter time after birth and there were fewer prolonged antenatal admissions for complications. There were now refuges and homes for fallen women and unmarried mothers, so they were quickly confined at the hospital then returned to their protectors. The hospital patients were now overwhelmingly native born, going from 64 per cent in 1880 to 76 per cent in 1884. And more than half were single women, with around a third under the age of twenty. Many were sad cases, and doctors like Walter Balls-Headley believed that the hospital would be better off without so many of them, but his motion to that effect received no support from the Board of Management in

October 1880. He did not shrink from treating the respectable suffering poor, but he reminded the committee and the general public that the mortality figures in both the midwifery and infirmary wards would inevitably look worse than those from private practice because the poor and the fallen were sicker.[4] As it was, some medical opinion blamed the higher maternal death rate of the fallen on melancholia and shame.[5] In the circumstances there were all sorts of things to suspect for infection, rather than actual medical procedures.

The first discussion of Listerism in Melbourne had been at a Medical Society of Victoria meeting on 4 December 1867, when Dr William Gillbee of the Melbourne Hospital (and son of the Lying-in Hospital's founding matron) presented a paper 'On the treatment of abscess and compound fracture by Mr Lister's New Method'. In a brilliant study, the late Diana Dyason argued that Gillbee became the first champion of Listerism in Melbourne without ever conceptually quite grasping the germ theory which underpinned it.[6] To be fair, Lister himself was never an aseptic surgeon, operating in street clothes and not being particular about ordinary dirt; also, like Gillbee and the miasmic contagionists, he believed that one major purpose of antiseptic dressings was to keep 'the atmosphere' out of a wound.[7] But he did comprehend and teach that micro organisms were in Bynum's words 'the source of surgical mischief', and it did take many of the most competent and skilful medical practitioners time to be convinced. Tracy had been a non-antiseptic surgeon and Balls-Headley was to remain sceptical into the late 1880s.

Soon after he arrived in Melbourne Jamieson began his campaign with an article on germ theory in the *Australian Medical Journal* in 1877. The next year he followed it with a sensible piece on the prevention of bladder infection in parturient women by the antiseptic use of catheters. Then in January 1879, just as he began his first year as the university lecturer in obstetrics, he published a careful epidemiological study of puerperal fever and its relationship to erysipelas or 'hospitalism'. He compared the death rates from 'metria' (childbed fever), scarlatina, diphtheria and erysipelas in the colony from 1868 to 1877. He showed how the 1874 puerperal fever epidemic started in Melbourne and spread to the country districts, and that it was more common in places of dense population. He concluded with a stinging attack on the Melbourne Hospital for its refusal to practise Listerism consistently and effectively, and its consequently scandalous rate of fatal wound infections contracted in hospital. Lastly Jamieson saw what took so many so long to see, and that was that puerperal infection was a wound infection, in just the same way as erysipelas. Therefore safe midwifery depended on antiseptic principles: on the antiseptic cleanliness of the patient's skin and tissues close to any lesion or with access to the open placental site within the uterus, and on the disinfecting of the examining or intervening hand or instruments. However, he commended to the medical practitioners of Australia the antiseptic midwifery practice advocated by the German Dr H. Fritsch, which Jamieson had translated from No. 107 of *Volkmann's Sammlung*. Most important of all, argued Fritsch, was keeping the tissues surrounding existing or imminent wounds clean by irrigation. He saw that wounds

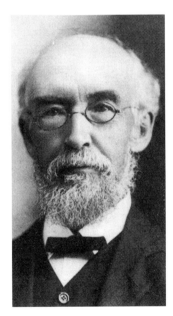

Dr James Jamieson
RWHA

such as tears to the cervix or the perineum were the entry point of infection, therefore postnatal care and prevention of infection required constant antiseptic irrigation of the vagina to promote rapid healing of lesions. And for those who had intra-uterine operations, such as removal of a putrid foetus, or with strongly smelling lochia or fever, the uterus itself should be washed out. Fritsch insisted that involution of the uterus proceeded more quickly with antiseptic irrigations. Jamieson was able to quote figures from Strasbourg that revealed a decline in maternal mortality over five years from 2.4 per cent to 0.6 per cent. Jamieson doubted that such irrigations could be carried out routinely in home deliveries — this was more a procedure for the hospital; but hand washing and the use of carbolised soap and oil and lard should be practised everywhere and no Lying-in hospital could afford to ignore antiseptic midwifery.[8]

involution: shrinking of the womb to its normal size after childbirth

The furore ignited by the paper came mostly from the Melbourne Hospital: from Dr Webb who claimed he did practise Listerism (even though he had just arrived and Jamieson's paper focused on the time he wasn't there), and from Dr (later Professor) Harry Allen, the pathologist, who accused Jamieson of misusing statistics. The row revealed the Melbourne Hospital to have inadequate medical records and no systematic infection control, and Jamieson in the end was vindicated. The debate over surgical fever drowned out that on puerperal fever, however, until late 1880 when Jamieson read a paper before the Social Sciences Congress on 'the Excessive Mortality among Lying-in Women in Victoria'. He showed, again by careful statistics, that Victoria as a whole had a higher maternal death rate than England and Wales and that the Melbourne Lying-in Hospital had a death rate three to four times higher than Guy's Hospital, London, and the Royal Maternity Charity. Balls-Headley gave an answering paper to argue that puerperal fever was a zymotic disease, and related to diphtheria, typhoid, croup, diarrhoea as well as erysipelas, but not related to scarlatina, measles, whooping cough and dysentery. Balls-Headley detected 'an apparent affinity' between typhoid and childbed fever, probably an observation of the increasing number of women already weakened by typhoid giving birth in the Lying-in Hospital. Jamieson had made no impression at all on the conventional wisdom of the honoraries at the hospital.[9]

zymotic disease: old name for a contagious disease which was thought to develop within the body following infection in a process similar to the fermentation and growth of yeast

He was, of course, very critical of it. He blamed the high maternal mortality rate in Victoria on the shortage of doctors and skilled midwives. The Lying-in Hospital was not training enough nurses — just twenty-eight in seven years at the last count. Balls-Headley came to the hospital's defence the following February when he pointed to the differences in the types of patient served by the London hospitals compared to the Melbourne establishment: the Guy's patients were almost always married and the Royal Maternity Charity delivered poor, respectable women in their homes. A hospital like the Melbourne Lying-in took everyone in, including patients 'moribund from convulsions, &c., from sick patients sent from general hospitals, from paupers from immigrants' homes, from fallen-women refuges &c. which contribute largely to the mortality'.[10] Jamieson could not deny that, but within a month the tragedy that had been waiting to happen at the hospital had struck, and Balls-

Headley's blame of the patients was to be scarcely adequate either.

Annie McKay was the first to die — on 6 January, after using 'violent measures towards herself to destroy her infant whose destruction she threatened while in the hospital. She died suddenly from a clot on the heart'. Then in February came three deaths, four in March, only one in April, four in May, one in June, three in July, four in August. The hospital was closed in September and patients boarded out in midwives' own establishments where they were delivered by a midwife and two medical students — even so there were single deaths in both September and October, then three in November and four in December. From the midwifery book there were thirty maternal deaths in 673 deliveries, a death rate of 4.5 per cent or one in 22.5. The Annual Report only accounted for twenty-three deaths, and of that twenty-three, merely seven were ascribed to peritonitis. Three died from 'puerperal mania', two from 'puerperal convulsions', three from placenta praevia, and eight from causes 'not connected with confinement' such as pneumonia, heart disease, lung disease, cancer, typhoid and 'exhaustive diarrhoea'. One even 'fretted herself to death' while 'all the organs were healthy'.[11]

While there were many good reasons for the death toll, the fact was that a fierce Group A streptococcus was back, both in the Melbourne Hospital in the form of erysipelas and at the Lying-in Hospital with fatal puerperal infection.[12] By the end of March maternal deaths began to rise throughout the colony as well as in the hospital. The Resident Surgeon Dr Felix Meyer was in his first year and responsible, as were the honoraries, for both the infirmary and midwifery beds. Meyer was to have a long and illustrious connection to the hospital, being elected to the honorary staff in 1888 and serving until the end of World War I. Meyer or some of the nursing staff or the patients themselves could well have been carriers of the Group A streptococcus, and the overcrowding made infection control more difficult: the hospital depended on isolation and ventilation to maintain the health of the midwifery wards.

There were also administrative problems. Since early 1880 the matron, Miss Harvey, had been going blind, but she refused to resign and was protected by her brother-in-law Dr Fetherston. She argued that it was only the book work which suffered, and with £30 per annum to employ her sister to assist her, she could continue. She assured the committee that there was plenty to occupy her time besides record keeping:

> I have constant demand on my time in the shape of ladies requiring wet nurses, nurses requiring situations, applicants for admission writing for information as to the best means of obtaining tickets, anxious friends looking for near relatives, detectives and policemen looking for 'information', and other inquiries too numerous to mention requiring books to be searched for years back. All this has occupied my spare time so completely for some time past that I have been obliged to defer the writing up of the books till evening and the result is that I must give them up altogether, which I need not say is a very great trial to me. I have written this with some difficulty and feel quite unable to make a fair copy of it, so I must beg the Ladies to excuse all errors, and to believe that if they accede to

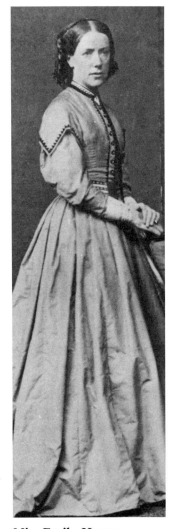

Miss Emily Harvey, matron 1864–1882 *RWHA*

our request, my sister and I will do our best to carry out all their wishes and maintain the efficiency of the hospital.[13]

She was granted £30, but by July 1881, as the new mothers kept dying, the other honoraries, led by Balls-Headley, wanted her to go. Miss Harvey had her loyal defenders on the committee, in Mrs Puckle and Mrs Moorhouse, who had been there from the beginning, so the anti-Harvey party, led by Balls-Headley, convened the meeting before both those ladies arrived and voted to remove her £30 so as to force her resignation. When Mesdames Puckle and Moorhouse arrived at the meeting, they resigned in disgust. Their final sally came in September when they campaigned to reduce the number of single women, especially of 'low character', being admitted as patients. And Miss Harvey stayed.[14]

Mrs Puckle: wife of the Rev. Edward Puckle of St Thomas's, Moonee Ponds, and Mrs Moorhouse, wife of Dr James Moorhouse, Bishop of Melbourne 1877–1886

Balls-Headley was now attending committee meetings and speaking for the honorary staff. The septic crisis in the midwifery wards impelled the honorary staff to insist on new antiseptic rules, but the rules seem to relate only to the changing of straw bedding for each new patient. The doctors had succeeded in persuading the Ladies that a new wing was needed, and in May building commenced on a proper operating room with two small recovery wards and a convalescent ward attached (so that no patients could hear screams suggesting that a woman 'was being murdered'). The new wing also provided better accommodation for medical students and nurses — sitting rooms and bedrooms for two pupil nurses, and at last the nurses would have a dining room and not be compelled to eat their own meals in the wards or service rooms. But before building could begin, the site was found to be contaminated with cesspits and drains, revealing the insanitariness of the hospital grounds and workplaces.[15] Balls-Headley had other proposals also, such as a register of all nurses trained at the hospital, but the honoraries' most bitter dispute with the Ladies' Committee was over the receipt of student university fees. They wanted them shared between the honoraries and the hospital as was practised in England: the hospital wanted the lot.[16]

But there was one final possible cause for the appalling maternal death rate, and for the possible concealment of some deaths, if the discrepancies were not due to the chaotic record keeping under Miss Harvey. If the resident surgeon or some of the honoraries were taking Dr Jamieson and Dr Fritsch's advice and irrigating the vagina after the waters had broken with carbolised water, or the uterus after delivery, especially in cases where septic mischief was feared, then in their eagerness to practise antiseptic medicine, they might well have unwittingly introduced pathogens into the uterus. In the later medical literature, Victorian doctors hinted that they had experimented with such irrigations, only to find that many more women became infected than before. The Boston Lying-in Hospital adopted the practice in 1883 with the best of intentions, and inflicted on its maternity patients an infection rate of 75 per cent and a death rate of one in five.[17] Another unanswerable question involves the clinical teaching of medical students and pupil midwives: if *per vaginam* examinations were routine and increased in clinical teaching, then every examination on a woman whose waters had broken could also introduce infection.

The next two years were much better, with only 1.25 per cent of mothers dying, even though the hospital was under great strain. The committee again attempted to force Miss Harvey to retire and in April she accepted after the committee offered her half a year's salary in recognition of her great service. As it was she stayed until the end of 1882 while her successor was recruited. Patients complained of bad meat; doctors complained of the lack of a proper hot water supply upstairs and of rough nurses (in August 1882 Nurse Jones was dismissed for drunkenness). The septic crisis of 1881 forced the gradual reform of nurse training and practices. The postnatal nursing of midwifery patients both by day and at night was assigned to special nurses, with day and night midwives as accoucheurs only, in the hope that this segregation would reduce contagion. Only the day staff would have pupil nurses. The work of the Infirmary was growing, leading to an increased nursing staff and the 'special wards' for post-operative care being in constant use.[18] In the following twelve months thirteen pupil nurses were trained as midwives and monthly nurses, with lectures weekly from the Resident surgeon and from Dr Jamieson in his capacity as the university lecturer in obstetrics. Meyer was later honoured as one of the founders of nursing education and of *Una,* the first nursing journal in Australia. Jamieson was committed to midwife education because he ascribed Victoria's excessive maternal mortality rate to the shortage of trained birth attendants — both doctors and midwives.[19] As for the advance of germ theory, the public utterances of the Medical Society revealed a growing acceptance among leading Victorian medical practitioners.[20] Even Balls-Headley conceded that various experiments were warranted such as carbolic sprays in the treatment of 'pulmonic disease': 'There was a feeling in the non-professional mind favourable to carbolic acid respirators', yet quite rightly he was 'not satisfied as to their efficiency'. But he is recorded as operating under one in December 1884.[21]

In 1884 the hospital changed its name.[22] With the Infirmary growing, it needed a name which was more modern and representative of its work, and so it became officially 'The Women's Hospital'. And in 1884 it began the worst three years of its history. The summer months passed safely enough with only a death in late January, another in late February and then two within four days in late March. April was worse: five women died within ten days, including Ellen Gollongher who had lingered for fifty-three days, after bearing an 8-lb son. The Ladies' Committee inspected the hospital and found it in chaos. Certainly the wards were clean and comfortable and the patients expressed themselves satisfied with their treatment. The condition of the yard, however, was disgusting; in front of the ventilator to the midwifery wards lay a pile of 'dirt and rubbish'; the straw from the mattress of a woman who had just died of peritonitis had not been burnt and was lying next to the fresh straw, and the toilet close by 'was in a very bad condition'.[23] There seemed to be no alternative but to close the midwifery wards and to arrange for patients to be confined in the homes of reputable midwives. But even then women continued to die: six over the next two months and two of those were extern deliveries, while a third was a woman 'found in the streets by the police, immediately after confinement, at an early hour of a bitterly cold

extern deliveries: deliveries by hospital staff or students in patients' own homes

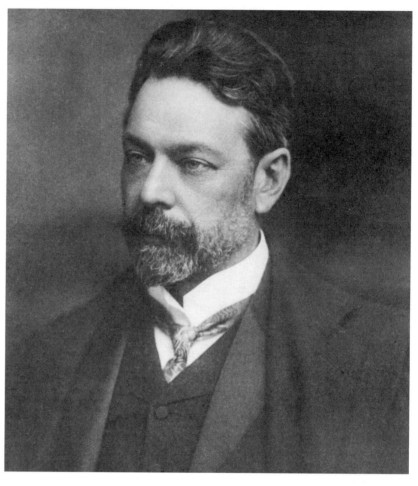

Dr Felix Meyer *RWHA*

morning, suffering on admission from congestion of the lungs and exhaustion from blood loss'.[24]

In the tension of the moment Mrs Puckle, still smarting at her alienation from the Board, brought forth accusations on behalf of an inmate to whom she had given a ticket. The patient accused Felix Meyer the House Surgeon of malpractice, three medical students of levity while she was undergoing an intimate examination, and the nurse of 'rough treatment'.[25] Meyer's version was upheld, but it was an unwelcome distraction as the infection problems in the hospital continued. Then on 20 May the *Age* broke the new 'Contagious Disease' scandal: if the walls of the Melbourne Hospital 'were saturated with erysipelas' as Dr Youl the coroner had proclaimed, then perhaps the walls of the Women's Hospital 'contain all the germs of puerperal fever', and went on to accuse the hospital of concealing deaths from puerperal fever from the public. Certainly the record keeping in the Midwifery Book deteriorated and women did die in the Infirmary who should have been counted in the Midwifery figures. M. P., aged nineteen, for instance, was delivered by forceps after a twenty-four-hour labour on 19 December 1883. She developed peritonitis but 'got on tolerably well' with treatment with leeches and opium. Then on 27 December she developed 'lung symptoms' and she was admitted to the Infirmary. Her condition was 'anaemic, cachectic, dry skin, hot, emaciation — lips dry, herpes, sordes, tongue furred'. She could hardly breathe and there were 'moist sounds all over her chest. By 3 January 1884 she was 'evidently sinking' and the next afternoon she died.[26] There is no record now of the cause of death of the thirty-eight midwifery patients shown to have died in 1884. The hospital spoke only of peritonitis but all Melbourne was calling it puerperal fever. Two days after the *Age* article the Committee of the East Melbourne Refuge wrote asking for an explanation. If the Hospital Board had ordered an 'entire overhauling' while the hospital was empty, 'this would seem to imply that the building contains the germs of fever'.[27] Felix Meyer dealt with the press, and assured them that although some who had died from 'affections somewhat akin', there was no contagious puerperal fever in the hospital.[28] There was also no mention of erysipelas in the Melbourne Hospital, and the deaths were to decline somewhat during the coldest months of that year.

sordes: brownish encrustations that form around the mouth and teeth of patients suffering from fevers (*OMD*)

Then in June the Central Board of Health struck and Dr Youl on inspection found the hospital, while apparently tidy and clean in the wards, was yet an unhealthy place. It had still only twenty-four beds, even though it processed up to six hundred midwifery patients alone in a year. In the midwifery convalescent ward six women and their babies were crammed together. Ventilation was poor and worst of all the earth closets in the infirmary were 'smelling very offensively and empty of earth'. Just as nasty was the hospital's cesspit which was full of blood and decomposing placentae. He inquired into the deaths during the year, and disagreed with Dr Meyer that the hospital could still claim to be free of contagious puerperal fever, for

> Whatever general name may be given to these diseases, there can be no question that they can be conveyed by nurses, by medical attendants, and by clothing to any Lying-in woman; and in addition to that, that a ward, in which any patient suffering from these diseases was, and would become an element of danger to any Lying-in woman who was placed there, unless on each occasion the ward was properly cleansed, disinfected, and left for some space of time empty of patients.

He concluded that it was not safe to have just one Resident surgeon 'who not only has to dress wounds and diseases in the infirmary, but also has to attend Lying-in women, and occasionally to make post-mortem examinations'.[29] The coroner declared there to be puerperal fever on the premises; the hospital medical staff continued to deny it; the *Australian Medical Journal* condemned Felix Meyer and the four honoraries for concealing the gravity of the situation at the Hospital. They were deeply wounded that the Medical Society could turn against them, and continued to insist that there was no actual contagious fever in the hospital.[30] Jamieson had re-entered the fray in June with a timely article in the journal on Puerperal Fever. Death in childbed, especially from 'metria' was higher than it should be in Victoria in general and in Melbourne in particular. Overseas, puerperal infection was being kept at bay with the new antiseptic procedures. It was now clear that it was not a zymotic

metria: infections of the uterus

disease, but was related to erysipelas and it could be prevented. The earlier calls to irrigate the vagina and uterus of all confined women had now been shown in Germany to be highly dangerous, introducing more problems than it washed out. Instead it was the medical attendant who had to be rendered aseptic: 'Let the practitioner cleanse and disinfect himself and everything about him, and see that the same scrupulous cleanliness is observed in the whole of the patient's surroundings'.[31]

Balls-Headley, supported by Rowan, retaliated by using the complaints of a failed medical student to impugn Jamieson's teaching of obstetrics. Their letter of accusations was leaked to the press before it was seen by the Medical Faculty, although neither could understand how anything so improper could have happened. Jamieson defended himself to the satisfaction of the university, and in turn accused the resident medical staff at the Women's of failing to teach practical obstetrics to his students adequately or in time for their examinations. Moreover, he was unable to supervise their clinical training himself because Drs Balls-Headley and Rowan had opposed his election as an honorary. He concluded by calling for the resignation of both those men from the board of examiners.[32]

The Women's Hospital's doctors saw salvation only in a new building, and the press and many of the public agreed. Dr Rowan led a deputation with Dr Balls-Headley to the Premier James Service: they argued that this was Australia's only specialist hospital for women (the Sydney-based *Australian Medical Gazette* was incensed at this slight on the provisions for Lying-in women in other colonies). The hospital needed rebuilding and extending and the government was asked for £5000 towards the cost. The premier was quite uninterested; the sum asked was impossible; married women should be confined at home and wooden cottages would be a more acceptable means to extending accommodation. The premier promised the government could provide some help and would send an inspector to advise, but there could be no £5000.[33]

Felix Meyer, as the lone Resident Surgeon, was under immense strain, and the committee acceded to his request for an assistant; but when his chosen candidate fell ill, Dr Burke helped him out in his ordinary hospital work. The medical staff were firmly united in the crisis. The nursing staff were not always reliable, however (Nurse Plunkett, the night nurse, had to be dismissed for cruelty to patients in November), and the hospital was still dirty. In early July the earth closets for the wards were again empty of earth and foul, and the tank 'smelt very badly'. Over the next months seventy-seven women were confined at midwives' homes, but that was not an unqualified success either. When the visiting committee inspected Mrs Ferguson's house on 19 August they found Mrs Ferguson and her assistant both out, and a servant in charge of eleven patients, one of whom had been confined the night before; 'sheets and pillowcases dirty, room close and unpleasant'. The visitors were not often critical and sometimes too ladylike as in May when they ventured that everything was satisfactory 'except that we would like to suggest that those patients who are recovering in the infirmary should have a little more food'.[34]

In October the death rate began to rise and the hospital was found to be overcrowded again. Boarding out recommenced, then five died in November and seven in December. The clues come now not from the midwifery records but from the Infirmary. On the evening of 12 November Nurse Clara Critchley, aged forty-one, ran a splinter into the forefinger of her left hand; she quickly pulled it out, but she felt sick all night and by next morning her hand was red. By the 14th 'a red line defined the lymphatics up to axilla'. The pain was 'agonising, she says, along the whole of the arm'. She was put to bed in the Infirmary and five days later the finger was 'lanced with deep incisions into the palmar surface of the finger between the joints' to release the pus. It was lanced again next day. Six days later, this time under chloroform, fresh and deeper incisions were made. After a fortnight the finger had greatly improved under daily poultices, there were 'free healthy granulations and fair move-ment in all the phalangeal joints'. Nearly six weeks after she got the splin-ter she was well enough to be sent to the Lady McCulloch Convalescent Home.[35] The pus suggests a staphylococcal infection rather than a strepto-coccal, and she was lucky because if it had been the latter she would have died. Not so lucky was one of Dr Burke's infirmary patients, Mrs A. C., aged 23 from Euroa, who was admitted on 6 December to be treated for a 'contracted os' which was believed to cause her dysmenor-rhoea. The surgery was simple and normally safe, even though it was agon-ising and performed without anaesthesia. This time, however, she also received a streptococcal wound infection and six days later her temper-ature was 103° and 104° in the evening. She was fed champagne and given hypodermic injections of morphine, but eight days after the oper-ation she was dead. Felix Meyer's case notes were ingenuous: 'The rigors were due to a chill which the patient incurred by sitting up in bed tho' warned by Doctor and nurse. This is the first death following metron-omy for 3½ years here'.[36] But there had also been a septic death from a straightforward Emmet operation performed in August by Dr Balls-Headley, only the second ever recorded in the hospital.[37]

The hospital was a fearfully septic environment, and there appeared to be carriers of the two contagious causes of fatal post-partum infection in women: Group A streptococcus and the golden staphylococcus, as well as other members of those bacterial families. Certainly instruments were contaminated. Dr Burke (who had assisted Felix Meyer in the wards in July and August) appears to have passed on staphylococcal infections to an in-patient and an out-patient in December 1884 and January 1885 while using the uterine sound.[38] Felix Meyer and the nursing staff were almost certainly carriers of the staphylococcus, and if it was new in the hospital in November (which is unlikely), perhaps it was introduced by Mrs K. O. who was first examined on 12 November after suffering for five months with a pelvic abscess from her confinement in June. The abscess was discharging, and Dr Meyer found her 'pale, cachectic, emaci-ated, appetite fair, sleep poor'. She was also in an awful emotional state. She had a bad knee but 'resists splint'; she suffered 'outbursts of anger' and was soon 'very discontented — is being made so by other patients in ward'. Finally she could take no more and on 29 January, seven months since she had given birth she discharged herself, with the abscess no better and unlikely ever to get better.[39] These cases are but suggestive clues, but they do explain why Felix Meyer could continue to claim that the prob-lem in the midwifery wards in 1884 was not due to contagious puerperal

Emmet operation: repair of lacerated cervix, developed by the American surgeon and colleague of J. Marion Sims, Thomas Addis Emmet (1828–1919). See: *American Journal of Obstetrics,* New York, 1874, 1875, vii, p. 442.

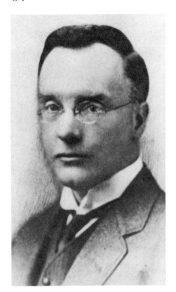

Dr J. W. Dunbar Hooper
RWHA

fever; these were instead 'affections which were akin', and possibly many were staphylococcal. Perhaps for those who died and grieved for them, these were but academic distinctions, but they threw the spotlight of blame not only on the building and its amenities but, more importantly, on the clearly septic state of the medical attendants' hands and instruments. Of the six hundred women confined under the auspices of the hospital in 1884, forty died, a death rate of one in fifteen. Single women had a 2 per cent higher mortality rate; 45 per cent of the dead were aged twenty or younger, compared to 33 per cent overall; whereas 59 per cent of the entire cohort were having their first baby, 82 per cent of the dead were primiparas. Finally, while 56 per cent of the whole cohort had labours of more than ten hours, 72 per cent of the dead laboured for that time, 29 per cent of them for more than 20 hours. Three died after giving birth to large twins. And of the babies, one in thirteen were stillborn; there was no systematic record of neo-natal deaths.

1885 was no better. In February it was decided to appoint two resident surgeons, one for the infirmary and one for midwifery. Felix Meyer resigned to enter private practice where he went on to make a fortune, and in his place were C. J. Shields in midwifery and J. Dunbar Hooper in the Infirmary. Like Meyer, Dunbar Hooper was to have a long association with the hospital. The condition of the patients was not helped by an influenza epidemic during the winter: a Dr Hewlett reported that '70 to 80 per cent of the adult population of Fitzroy and neighbourhood had been attacked', leaving the survivors weak and dispirited.[40] By the winter the wards were so crowded that the committee decided 'that no woman who has a home shall be received for confinement, unless her case has been previously considered or special sanction given by the Admission Committee'.[41] The visiting committee was usually pleased with the condition of the hospital, except for external drains which were still foul at times and for untidiness — the result of the nursing staff reaching the end of their tether on busy days.[42] In the first two weeks of September every midwifery patient bar one 'became feverish' and again the midwifery wards were closed completely for cleansing, disinfecting and whitewashing.[43] The Women's Hospital was both a Victorian and national scandal, and its septic disaster was broadcast nationally through the medical journals. The retiring president of the Medical Society of Victoria called for its rebuilding. The committee and the doctors saw no alternative but to build a new hospital, thus to underwrite the committee's decision to commence large-scale fund-raising with a bazaar, the Annual Report of 1884–1885 provided a detailed analysis of each midwifery death and explained the dangers of overcrowding. With their present accommodation, no more than fifteen to seventeen patients could be safely admitted; instead the numbers sometimes rose to forty and averaged twenty-five. The isolation cottage had to be kept for septic cases, and the hospital could not refuse emergency cases who arrived in a desperate condition. The boarding out of patients was no long-term solution, for it was expensive and not always safe. The midwives' homes were often poorly ventilated and dirty, and another woman had died after being confined by Mrs O'Dwyer without medical assistance.[44]

By 1886 Dr Shields left after not coping with the job, and Dunbar

Hooper was now Senior Resident in charge of both Midwifery and the Infirmary, and he began to show the capacities which were later to take him to the top of the profession. The hospital appointed its first honorary pathologist, Dr F. Dougan Bird, commencing a vital chapter in the hospital's later history. Dr Hooper set about the systematic study of the morbidity of midwifery, and he began to publish. For the first time since Tracy's days, the midwifery patients are vividly portrayed. In July he reported on the death of B. H., aged $18^{1}/_{2}$ and single, who suffered a partial rupture of the uterus and puerperal septicaemia. She was 'admitted June 20th, a very cold and wet day, clad only in one petticoat and a print dress'. Through lack of room, she had to be confined in the cottage, empty after a woman had died there of typhoid ten days before.

Examined at 7.30 p.m. — Child alive; vagina moist; os dilated to size of rim of wine-glass; membranes ruptured; vertex presented at brim in L.O.A. Sacral promontory lying forward, and contracting conjugata vera to $3^{1}/_{2}$ inches; pains feeble; pulse 118; temperature 101°.

11.15 p.m. — Os fully dilated. Chloroform administered by Dr Lynch, and Tarnier's axis traction forceps applied at brim where vertex was impacted. Intermittent traction, without leverage, brought occiput on to perineum in fifteen minutes. Blades removed, and head delivered in five minutes from the rectum. The shoulders and trunk soon followed. Fifteen minutes later the placenta was expelled naturally, but I suspected that some membranes remained, therefore, I inserted the stem of a new Higginson's syringe, charged with diluted Condy's fluid, at 120° F. At the second injection the hot water made the patient give two violent kicks. I removed the tube from the uterus, and found the piece of membrane in the bed. Patient rallied well. The pudenda were thoroughly washed with warm carbolised water, and dusted with iodoform. Perineum found to be untorn,

Condy's fluid: a powerful disinfectant containing permanganate of sodium in water (Black)

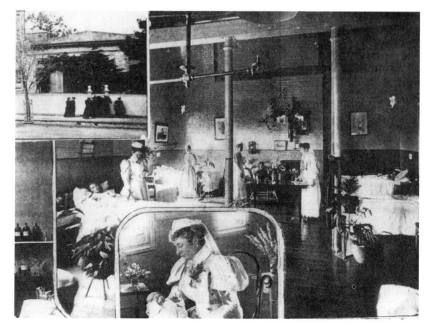

Infirmary ward in 1858 building, Weekly Times, 1897, RWHA

no lacerations inside vulva. The child was alive and exhibited a well-marked depression on the left side of vertico-mesial line, and anterior to left coronal suture.

But within six days she was dead from septicaemia. Professor Allen performed the post-mortem. Cause of death was puerperal septicaemia, but he considered that the small partial rupture of the inside of the uterus was not implicated. B. H. did have a well-marked typhoid ulcer on the large intestine, however. Hooper was not satisfied. The ward cannot have been septic because another girl was confined in the cottage six hours later and was never febrile. There were two small tears to the cervix, but again Hooper had examined 102 women, 44 of whom had cervical tears and none was more than thirteen days in the hospital. He did not think that the traction had caused the tear; it was more likely to have been the baby passing over the projecting sacrum. Finally if the septicaemia were 'autogenetic' then why was the lochia, after being absent for two days, 'sweet'? This surely is 'a curious and instructive fact'. (He did not question his own practice of syringing the uterus.) He concluded by reporting that the hospital's maternal deaths for the past six months comprised two patients who came from the same house, another who came from a very unhealthy neighbourhood, while the fourth died of eclampsia and the fifth of pneumonia.[45]

A month after B. H.'s death Hooper began a detailed record of a hundred consecutive midwifery patients between 2 July and 17 September. Perineal lacerations, actual temperatures and even the slightest complications were all noted. If the hospital was doing better than it had in 1884 and 1885, it was still an appalling record. Just eleven women were discharged as well, six as 'convalescent' and five discharged themselves without permission. Thirty-six had serious infections, from which three died and, as we shall see, one other was to be 'gynaecologically crippled' for life by an infection acquired after leaving hospital. There were seven deaths, that is one in fourteen, but three the hospital would claim were not direct childbed fatalities: Bright's disease, typhoid and pneumonia. The four 'real' puerperal deaths were two from puerperal septicaemia and one post-abortal septicaemia, and the fourth, M. G., from tuberculosis and pyaemia. This last poor soul's temperature reached 106° before death on the seventh day, and one thirty-four year-old mother of eight in the Infirmary was so distressed by the story that she later fled the hospital 'through fright at the death of G.'[46] Forceps were used in but three cases out of the one hundred, and only one of those were long forceps, but a dreadful 35 per cent had lacerated perineums. Lacerations were now routinely sutured if they were more than an inch long, and three unfortunates lacerated through to the anus. Some women left hospital with the rent still unhealed, risking new infection once out of hospital care. Lacerations tended to occur in pairs and on consecutive days. All normal deliveries were now conducted by students, with pupil midwives and medical students taking alternate cases, and the pattern of lacerations suggests that some were better than others. Also it was now realised that protecting the perineum with a finger in the rectum added to the danger of infection.[47] Yet lacerations were not guarantees of post-partum infec-

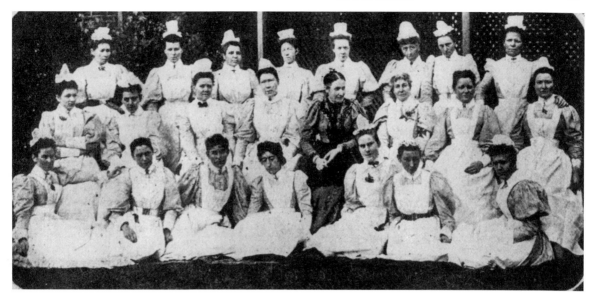

Matron and nurses, Midwifery department, 1897 *RWHA*

tion, for only eight of the thirty-six had both. Perhaps some had gonor-rhoea, but there is no record. Certainly as a group of Australian women, three quarters of whom were under twenty four, they were ill-fed, sickly, neglected and unhappy long before they entered the labour ward.

There was one patient about whom we can know more. Mrs E. S. was one of the 11 per cent discharged well, and she spent nine days in hospital after a six and-a-half hour labour to deliver her third child, Charles, weighing 6 lbs and being only $16\frac{1}{2}$ inches long. She was nineteen, born in England and since marrying at sixteen, had had four pregnancies and three babies. She returned to her home, up one of the dark and dank lanes next to the hospital. She was home for her twentieth birthday, but after a week or so 'she caught cold', and had sharp, shooting pains in the lower back and abdomen. A fortnight later she was admitted to the Infirmary. She had a rigor the first night, and a throbbing headache. Dr Hooper found her 'tongue coated and foul with red tips and edges. Pulse was strong and quick at 120. Temperature 102.4°'. Pains were shooting down her legs, and when she could take nourishment, pain after food. She had 'great weakness and emaciation'. The following week was a fearful struggle against the infection: twice daily warm vaginal douches, hot foments to the abdomen, glycerine plugs in the vagina. The second day she was worse: the douches were increased, her constant vomiting and nausea aggravated her weakness, so she was given nourishing enemas by rectum of strong beef tea and brandy. Each night her temperature rose even higher: 104° on 21 August while her pulse was rapid and feeble at 140. As her temperature fell she was stricken with 'profuse diarrhoea', but after seven days, her temperature was down to 99°. She spent three months in the infirmary before she was fit to go home. The post-partum infection had begun at home: the tubo-ovarian mass and the acute pain suggest gonorrhoea, presumably contracted by her husband during her time in hospital for the confinement.[48]

Fourteen months later she was readmitted to the infirmary under Dr

Rowan. She was an old friend of the hospital by now and the record noted more biographical detail and this time she put down her age at marriage as seventeen, presumably she felt more comfortable about revealing that she had been a pregnant bride. She was nine when her family emigrated. She had been well, she claimed, until that last accouchement and her pelvic inflammation. Ever since she had pains on and off over the left ovary, extending into the lower back, through the hip and down into the thigh. Her bowels were very confined and breath offensive. She got 'vertical headache', and lately much pain on sexual intercourse, so much so that she had been unable 'to stand it for the last six weeks'. There was also a thick, yellow discharge. The doctor saw her as still 'emaciated' and 'losing weight, looks heavy'. He could feel her left ovary to be 'enlarged, adherent and intensely tender', and prolapsed into 'Douglas's space'. The night of her admission she could not sleep for the pain, and was given a morphine suppository, and Dr Rowan operated a day later. The incision was 3 inches. Her pelvic area was a dense, tangled mess of adhesions left over from her infection. With difficulty he separated the enlarged left ovary from the adhesions, brought it to the surface, transfixed and ligatured its pedicle. He found a 'mass of new growth all around the brim of the pelvis and partly into its cavity' and left the right ovary alone. Mrs S. came through, and was taking chicken broth within four days. Next came 'ale, milk and soda, tea and a little bread and butter'. Her chest was very troublesome for a time. The external wound healed well, but a 'disagreeable yellow discharge' indicated that the pelvic infection was still there. A month after admission to hospital, she still weighed a skeletal 6 stone, 4 and a half pounds. But eight days later she had put on two pounds, had a good appetite and was sleeping well.[49] But she would never really be the same again. She would be a 'pelvic cripple' for life, as the infection grumbled away for years, flaring up at times of stress or other illness. The only consolation of pelvic inflammatory disease was that her child bearing was over.

Just after he resigned as senior resident to enter private practice, Dunbar Hooper read a paper before the Medical Society of Victoria. He had analysed all the midwifery cases in the hospital during his two years service. He warned his colleagues that it was not a theoretical exercise, but entirely drawn from 'actual experience'. Finally, and significantly, he insisted that 'the honorary staff are in no measure responsible for the opinions I hold'. Having distanced himself from the senior medical authorities in the Women's Hospital, he presented a painfully honest analysis not just of practices, but also of diagnostic procedures and categories. He confessed that he had 'mistaken puerperal septicaemia for (1) typhoid fever, (2) pneumonia, (3) metritis, (4) puerperal mania, (5) acute rheumatism, (6) tuberculosis, and *vice versa*'. Safe midwifery depended not just on antisepsis, it also needed correct diagnosis and the recognition of the true cause of infection and thereby prevention. By implication, the hospital, in its desire to reduce public fears of puerperal fever, had looked for every other explanation of death in the endeavour to make the 'numbers' look better. He had now come to see puerperal infections as falling into two broad categories — autogenetic and heterogenetic: that is, where infection came from within the woman's system and when it

RULES FOR MIDWIFERY NURSES.

1. The dress, apron, and extra sleeves to be of light-coloured print.

2. In private cases, unless previously prescribed to the patient by the doctor, a small basket is only to contain a 2 oz. bottle of glycerine of perchloride of mercury (six drachms of the perchloride in eleven drachms by weight of glycerine, of which one drachm in half a gallon of water equals 1 in 1000), and a one-drachm measure; or tablets, or powders, each containing 7·3 grs. of hydrarg. perchlor., with 7·7 grs. of ammonium chloride, which dissolved in a pint of water is 1 in 1000; a two-ounce bottle of 1 in 8 carbolic oil, vaselin, a Higginson's syringe with glass tube, a new catheter, a small packet of absorbent cotton wool or tow, thread, scissors, nail-brush, disinfected cloths, and this card.

3. The hands to be thoroughly brushed with soap and warm water, and the nails cleaned with a knife. Before and during labour, and for a week afterwards, on each occasion before touching the neighbourhood of the genital organs, the hands to be dipped in the perchloride solution, and used thus wet during labour, the solution to be kept in a basin at the side of the head of the bed.

4. The edges of all bed-pans, &c., before use, to be wiped with the solution on cotton wool or tow, and similarly, the thread for the cord, and all instruments dipped.

5. Catheters, enema tubes, and other instruments to be smeared with the carbolic oil before use.

6. The bed-pans, &c., to be emptied immediately after use, and washed with the perchloride solution, and nothing put under the bed.

7. All soiled linen, &c., of whatever kind, at once to be removed from the room.

8. If so directed, the vagina night and morning to be injected with a warm red solution of permanganate of potash (Condy's fluid) till it returns of the same colour.

9. The room to be cleared of all hanging clothes, and as far as is conveniently possible, of unnecessary furniture, bed valances being objectionable; and the sun to be freely admitted daily, for one hour at least.

N.B.—These rules being for the purpose of preventing the contamination of the patient, reliance is placed in the nurse that they are carried out.

Dr Balls–Headley's rules for antiseptic midwifery
Collected Pamphlets (Melbourne, 1893) *Brownless
Library Historical Collection, University of Melbourne*

was introduced from outside the environment by the hand, dirty instruments and dressings. Because of these distinctions, prevention was complex. The accoucheur had to ensure that all placental products were removed from the uterus, all lacerations and abrasions treated and made clean, and as little examination and physical intervention in the lying-in period as possible. He recommended extreme caution in the use of syringing, which should never be left to the offices of students or nurses, because syringing succeeded only in making infections worse or setting them off in the first place.

He none the less considered heterogenetic infections to be the greater danger to life. Often all that revealed their presence was a persistent, steady rise of temperature. The lochia after being absent for some days, remained sweet and there might be no abdominal pain. He emphasised the treatment of all ulcers, and implicated vaginal sloughs which he thought were connected with diphtheria. Ventilation and sunlight and removal of wastes were essential. What he had observed but not quite understood were the distinctions between anaerobic and aerobic infections: those that flourished in the absence or presence of oxygen, and that the former, while putrid and obvious and more common, were not as insidious. He also had come to the conclusion that a septicaemic woman was no danger to other patients if contagion were prevented by antiseptic measures. Jamieson opened the discussion and warmly congratulated Hooper. He only added that he believed that few autogenetic infections deserved the title 'puerperal fever' and that they were not so dangerous to life. He also wanted to reiterate that antiseptic irrigations after labour were more apt to cause septicaemia than prevent it. Dr Patrick Moloney declared it was 'refreshing to be told that there really had been puerperal fever in the Lying-in Hospital; and it was honourable to Dr Hooper that he did not hesitate to speak of mistakes as well as of successful diagnoses'.[50]

Hooper's successor was a keen young man called Eugene Anderson. His record keeping was done with a flourish, and he was just as assiduous as Hooper in collecting statistics. A year after he was appointed, he presented his own paper to the Medical Society, analysing the first five hundred confinements that had been conducted under his supervision. It was a triumph of antiseptic midwifery: the maternal death rate was one in 155, the lowest in the history of the hospital since 1858. The hospital played down its change of technique, mentioning it briefly in the Annual Report,[51] but it was a regimen of midwifery that would be recognisable to patients, midwives and doctors for decades to come:

> Every patient on admission is given a warm bath, which many sadly need, her clothes are put aside, and, clad in a hospital wrapper, she is removed to a Delivery Ward, where a simple enema is given to thoroughly empty the lower bowel. An antiseptic injection is then made into the vagina with a Higginson's syringe, with a solution of corrosive sublimate (1 in 1000), and the external parts of generation, the hips, thighs, buttocks, &c, have a similar solution applied to them. An examination book is kept in which is recorded the name of each and every one that examines a patient, to afford facility for tracing any mischief to its proper origin. The urine is drawn from every patient on admission and examined for albumin. The

cases are conducted alternately by students and pupil nurses, but in either case, the student or nurse must have witnessed six cases previously, and the first case conducted must be a multipara. The uterus is followed down by the hand on the abdomen as the birth of the child takes place, and is kept grasped for at least twenty minutes after birth before any effort is made to get rid of the placenta. Expression of the placenta is the rule in every case, being careful to attempt it *only* when acting in conjunction with nature, *i.e.* when a uterine contraction is present. The placenta is received in the hand and given a few turns, when the membranes generally come away, and their digital removal is rarely necessary. The placenta and membranes are examined in every case as to their entirety. A dose of ergot is given directly after the secundines are away. The uterus is still grasped for another ten minutes, while the external genitals, &c., are washed with corrosive solution, and then, if the pulse has fallen to 100 or below, the patient is securely bound and a labor cloth applied. I find the pulse to be an almost perfect guide as to haemorrhage; given a slow pulse, haemorrhage will not occur. The labour cloth is frequently examined for a short time after birth, to see that no undue haemorrhage is taking place, and after the lapse of 12 hours, Tenax pads (wrapped up in muslin) are applied to the vulva instead of labor cloths. A dose of ol ricini is given on the morning of the third day. No vaginal irrigation is resorted to unless the lochia become offensive, or the child born outside, or the liquor amnii was very dirty and disagreeable. A mixture of ergot, quinine, infus. digitalis, is given three times daily for a few days after delivery. For scanty lochia or slight abdominal tenderness, poultices are applied, if there is marked tenderness over or about the uterus, leeches are used, followed by poultices. The patients get up on the 8th day generally, and go out on the 11th or 12th. A solution of corrosive sublimate (1 in 2400) is used to wash the hands before and after every examination by doctors, students and nurses, and the nailbrush well used. All instruments, vaginal pipes, &c., are washed in a solution of corrosive sublimate.[52]

ol ricini: castor oil

quinine: used as a uterine stimulant in labour, to reduce fever, and as a tonic in conditions of debility and exhaustion

digitalis: used as a heart tonic and as a diuretic in dropsy (*AMD*)

In September 1888 midwifery moved into a new wing, built with money first raised by a performance of *Antigone* by the American actress, Mrs Genevieve Ward. The wing was erected not without criticism, particularly from Dr Balls-Headley who declared it unsafe because the ventilation

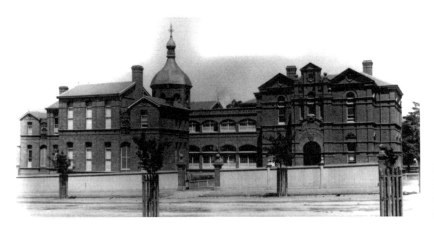

Genevieve Ward Wing, 1886–1887 *La Trobe Picture Collection, State Library of Victoria*

would still permit noxious air to collect. He had become convinced of modern antiseptic midwifery on his recent overseas trip, however, and given it his approval months after it had come into practice. But he also called for an arrangement 'like an incubator for keeping delicate babies warm' and brought back a large collection of medical literature.[53] The new Genevieve Ward wing housed women in large, spacious general wards, even for labour. It had 'antiseptic lavatories' for sterilising the hands, and the wards were separated by covered ways. But new buildings and taps could only achieve so much — the real burden of the fight against infection fell on the staff.

'Servants in the Temple of Purity'

5

In June 1889 Mrs M. S., a housewife of Violet Town in northern Victoria, became pregnant. It must have been a joyous event for she had been married seven years and never conceived before. She appears to have been well nourished as a child for she had reached puberty at the age of twelve, two years earlier than the average for her time; but, like many nineteenth-century girls, her periods had been painful and troublesome. Now at thirty-two, she was finally going to have a baby.

Everything seemed normal at first. In July she began vomiting in the mornings and had some early crampy pains. Before this she had never felt any tumour in her abdomen. At Christmas she felt her child quicken, but at the end of March 1890 the movements ceased. Since Christmas she had lost a little blood four or five times, at intervals of four to six weeks and lasting one to two days. About February she had some slight pains and some water came away from the vagina. Her baby never appeared.

It was now 8 June 1890, a year since she had conceived and she had just been admitted as a patient in the Infirmary. With its twenty-five beds, including only two for post-operative special nursing, the Infirmary's waiting list continued to grow. The back-log was aggravated by the slow recoveries so common still from abdominal surgery; and the longer sick women had to wait, the sicker they were by the time they reached the operating table, and the longer again it took them to be well enough to return to the normal wards. By the end of the year one hundred and eighty women would be awaiting a bed and four years later it would be five hundred.[54] Mrs S. herself had been waiting too long, three months, as it was, since her baby had failed to appear.

She was examined by the Senior Resident Surgeon in the Infirmary, Dr R. H. Fetherston, son of Dr Gerald Fetherston, and he wrote up the case in the case book of her honorary gynaecologist, Dr Walter Balls-Headley. She reported no pain. Her general condition was 'slightly emaciated' and her abdomen was enlarged, containing a tumour of the size and shape of a six and a half months pregnancy. It felt rather hard, but fluctuated in places. Her vagina was discoloured and darkened, and they found a hard rounded mass in the first cul de sac, from which could be distinguished the foetal head. The *cervix uteri* was soft and displaced anteriorly behind the pubes. The condition of the *fundus uteri* could not be determined, but using a Hagar dilator, the cavity of the uterus was explored with the finger and found to be fairly normal. It was a case of abdominal pregnancy — extra-uterine gestation — where the embryo had burst through the fallopian tube and implanted itself within the abdominal cavity.

Twelve days later on 20 June, Dr Balls-Headley, assisted by Dr Rowan, operated. An opening of about five inches was made and there was immediately a lot of bleeding from the incision. The cyst was reached and tapped, releasing some dark brown fluid — *liquor amnii*. Then the opening into the cyst was enlarged and found to be fairly thick — a quarter of an inch and leathery. The child's arm was opposite the opening and the placenta was inserted into the anterior and upper surface of the cyst in its upper portions. With some difficulty a foot was seized and the child thus delivered. It was a male, seeming about eight months at least, quite decomposed in parts but not malodorous. The placenta was removed in pieces by peeling it from the cyst. The umbilical cord had become macerated and was not intact but part attached to child and part to the placenta.

liquor amnii: amniotic fluid

On examining the cyst, which had been kept well out of the wound to prevent any fluid getting into the abdominal cavity, it was found to be intimately adherent to the transverse colon, the omentum, the small intestine and pelvic colon, so Balls-Headley could not attempt to remove it. (Had he attempted to do so, she could have haemorrhaged fatally.) It was not sutured to the wound, and the abdominal incision was closed, leaving a glass tube into the cyst. The sutures used were silver wire internally and horsehair for the skin.[55]

It was a textbook operation for extra-uterine pregnancy, faithfully carrying out the procedures recommended by Alfred Lewis Galabin — like Balls-Headley, a Cambridge man — in his *Manual of Midwifery,* published in 1886. The mortality rate for abdominal pregnancies was fearful at the time, over 50 per cent for those left mainly to Nature; but a recent series of secondary abdominal sections had produced a mortality 10 per cent lower. Surgery was an acceptable risk, and no one wished on Mrs S. the years of passing *per rectum* the disintegrating detritus of her only baby, let alone the constant risk of grave pelvic or systemic infection. Part of the success of the operation was to allow those parts of the placenta and sac which were adherent to abdominal organs to undergo decomposition over the recovery period.[56] The nursing care was going to be critical.

Mrs S. was carried to the special ward. The operation had taken one and a half hours and the deep anaesthesia required to relax the abdomen for surgery was in itself a threat to life. She was therefore 'very low' after the operation, but after about three hours, 'rallied very well indeed but still was weak'. She now complained of great pain in the abdomen, which continued for several hours and at last, as she was getting restless, she had a hypodermic injection of $\frac{1}{4}$ grain of morphia, which had to be repeated several times during the next few days.

A good deal of dark red bloody fluid was drawn off from the cyst which gradually becoming scanty, seemed rather foetid, and then the cyst was washed out with Mercuric chloride 1-3000 twice and three times a day. The patient in the first week was in a very low condition, enemata being given of egg, milk peptised, as well as champagne and brandy freely by the mouth. (Champagne and brandy were standard post-operative care, as were the nourishing enemata. Saline infusion was known at the time, and would in fact be used, not very efficiently and with the wrong scientific understanding, in the great cholera epidemic that was to sweep Hamburg in 1892. Purging remained the basic treatment for cholera even in the late nineteenth century.[57])

peptised: pepsin added to make it more digestible

Mrs S. was in a desperate state and had to be watched constantly. Her temperature rose each night to 101° to 102°, but fell back to normal each morning. Her pulse was 108–130, respirations 28–32. A good deal of flatus collected but was got rid of easily with enemas. Her condition on the fourth and fifth day was critical, her bowels acting involuntarily. To control the diarrhoea, 'a mixture of chalk and opium' was administered. Some sutures were removed from the upper part of the wound on the sixth day — it seemed to have closed, but the edges of the cyst wall were showing signs of sloughing and turning black. They were cast off after a couple of weeks or ten days.

Second Week: June 28th–July 4th. The woman remains in the same low state, bowels acting (with mucous stools) very often; patient is low, restless, perspiring freely, tongue coated and side of abdomen sore. Temperature 101°–103° at night and 100–130 pulse. On thirteenth day some slight rigors probably due to small abscess forming in track of sutures which have been removed several days ago. The wound is being washed

Infirmary medical and nursing staff, *c.* 1890 Back: Dr G. H. Fetherston, Dr Walter Balls-Headley, —, Dr R. H. Fetherston, Sister Pat Waters, —, Dr Stephen Burke, Dr Thomas Rowan Front: —, Miss Findlay, matron and (?) Dr M. U. O'Sullivan *RWHA*

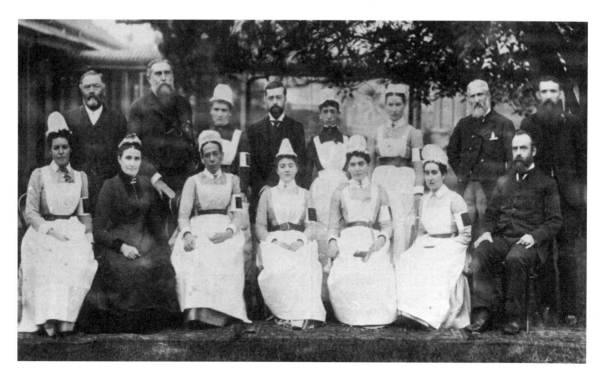

out frequently with Condy's solution, since the mucous diarrhoea it was feared was caused by Mercuric Chloride absorption; but its stopping had no effect on the diarrhoea. The sac remained adherent to abdominal wall. Treated with Quinine 16 grains a day, and diarrhoea much as before. She still received stimulants and nourishment, hot bottles etc.

Third week: She gradually began to pick up and get a little stronger, appetite improved and diarrhoea stopped. There was still a good deal of discharge from the sac, which is carefully washed out every few hours. The patient gets a Hypodermic of water at night to break her of the morphia habit. She perspires very freely at night. Still getting Quinine 16–20 grains a day and also a good deal of stimulants. Her temperature hovered between 100°–102° at night.

July 11th to August 2nd (four to six weeks after the operation): The improvement continues and she gradually gets much stronger, wound and sac contracting up very well and drawing the skin of abdomen inwards; able to take solid food. Sleeps well, temperature 100° at night. Pulse much better. Sides of sac adherent in places.

On August 3rd (just over six weeks after the operation): At 8 pm, after a very good day, she got a severe pain in calf of left leg, which rapidly became swollen and oedematous. On calf and front and at the side of the thigh there can be seen some veins which have become blocked and obliterated. All around these veins the cuticle is rising up in blisters; in a few hours the four places look very red and angry; pain still severe and also into abdomen. The red places look as if they were going to slough under the blisters.

The leg was raised, poulticed and treated as an acute attack of 'Thrombosis'. Morphia had to be given freely again. This attack threw her back greatly and she seemed to lose courage; she got very weak and began to vomit again. Temperature up to 102° to 103° at night.

August 5th (two days later): She was very low and almost in a dying state, urine passing involuntarily, and only kept alive by stimulants, hot bottles and great care.

She gradually got better and in a few days was much better and more cheerful. The veins that were sloughed by the thrombosis sloughed out and then left small ulcers which slowly healed.

August 10th: Nurse Archer who has been nursing this case night and day since the operation [seven weeks ago], having refused relief, developed a slight attack of Pleuro Pneumonia at the apex of both lungs from a chill caught at night. She completely broke down and had to be removed and kept in bed for some time. She left the case in a good condition and gaining strength rapidly, her care and attention were vital in the success of the case. From this time continued to improve and had no more bad symptoms. The wound (sac) gradually became closed and united forming one hard, firm cicatrise which still discharged a little pus on discharge from hospital . The temperature became normal and she put on flesh. The ulcers on the leg healed slowly.

September 21st: Mrs S. is still doing very well.

October 1st: Her temperature has been normal for some weeks. She is moving about a little. The wound is now only a sinus, but her leg swells a little when she walks and is painful if she is up too long.

On October 8th, four months after her operation, Mrs M. S. went home to Violet Town.

Mrs S. owed her life not only to her surgeon Dr Balls-Headley and to the Senior Resident, Dr 'Bertie' Fetherston, but also to Nurse Archer. Nurse Archer saved her life with 'great care': she became obsessed with the case, refusing all assistance. It was almost as though she willed Mrs S. to live. Yet it was unprofessional care, where the nurse transgressed the boundaries of the public and the private — the limits of proper professional detachment. Nurse Archer became too involved, she cared too much and destroyed her own health. It marks however, a turning point in the professionalisation of nursing, in the transition from private care, of personal commitment between private individuals, and the universalised care of the universal patient. The American historian of nursing, Susan M. Reverby, sees the defining dilemma of professional nursing as being 'ordered to care in a society that refuses to value caring'.[58] But even more fundamental is the awkwardness of being 'ordered to care' for strangers, strangers who might well be repellent in their behaviour, appearance or odour. 'Care' had to be regulated in order to be guaranteed. It could only be sustained and practised consistently if it was structured as a set of routines which had to be carried out on all patients, irrespective of who they were, and if nursing itself was constructed as a role. A hospital could not rely on raw human emotion and spontaneous relationships to guarantee appropriate care. If there had always been nurses in the past who cared too little, it seems there were also some who cared too much.

In Australian general hospitals, the final third of the nineteenth century saw the feminisation of nursing as a profession, the replacement of wardsmen by feminine agents of purification in all hospital care apart from the nursing of men with venereal disease and alcoholism.[59] The Women's Hospital was different because it was always staffed by female nurses and midwives. The only males permitted on the wards were doctors and

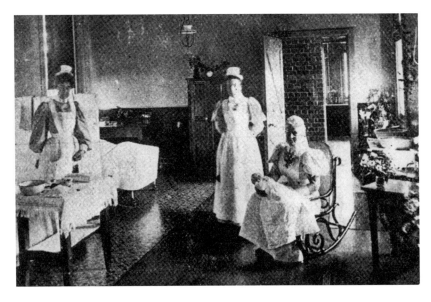

Ward in the Midwifery department, *Weekly Times, 1897, RWHA*

Infirmary visitors; otherwise it was a women's world. Further, midwives were usually married or once married women who had borne children: by definition they should not be virginal. They also enjoyed more professional autonomy than nurses, being traditionally practitioners in their own right and lay healers. Their task of midwifery was different from that of the monthly nurse who cared for a woman postnatally. It is unclear who delivered babies in the first decades of the hospital but, at least some of the time, midwives performed normal deliveries when the resident surgeon was occupied elsewhere. By the 1880s medical students and pupil midwives were conducting most deliveries, but all formal teaching of pupil midwives and medical students was under the control of the resident surgeons. The Women's Hospital was distinctive also in its pioneering nursing school, where women were trained ostensibly as monthly nurses, except that most received sufficient training in midwifery to practise privately later as midwives, claiming certification from the Women's Hospital.

By the time Nurse Archer joined the staff, the hospital was attracting respectable women as trainees, many of whom had already received two years training at another hospital. They paid either twelve guineas for six months training, or one guinea for twelve months training and received no remuneration. Mr W. H. Gibson, the superintendent, was proud that one of the eight staff nurses was the sister of a doctor of medicine and another was training to be a missionary. The further elevation of the training and status of nursing for women, he hoped, might absorb that yearning for a medical life that was tempting so many young women to enter the medical profession.[60] The doctors at the Women's had no doubt that women made the best nurses: Dr Rowan found that you could trust them, could rely on them to carry out instructions while male nurses were too often neglectful.[61] Dr Balls-Headley saw in woman's nature a vocation to care:

> I think women are fitted for nursing better than men; they sit up better and endure better, and I think they are apt to be kinder. Their hands are more delicate; they understand the feeding of people better than men, and they do not, as a rule, drink; in my experience, a great many men nurses do. Then they do not go out and smoke and loaf; they very often like their work. I think it is natural to every woman to be, to some extent, a nurse.[62]

Nurse Archer is the actor in the drama that we know least about. She appears only twice in the Board of Management Minutes, first in April 1888, when tension among the Infirmary nurses erupted in threats of resignation. The threats were withdrawn and Nurse Archer was made second nurse. Finally on 19 October 1888, with Head Nurse Atkins, she did tender her resignation. The dispute by then was over pay and Nurse Archer's replacement was given £45 per annum, an increase; none the less the level of friction among the Infirmary nurses suggests a workforce under strain. By mid-1890 Nurse Archer was back again on the staff and available to nurse Mrs S. Sometimes a grave post-operative case would require the employment of additional special nurses at three guineas a week, but Nurse Archer's devotion spared the hospital this extra expense.[63] The Infirmary nurses worked a twelve-hour day, the midwifery nurses a thirteen-and-a-half-hour day and the nurses chopped and changed, usually through plain exhaustion. In July 1890 the Board of Management officially asked the Matron, Miss E. Findlay, to reduce nurses' working hours, but after investigating work loads, she and the head nurse informed the Board that nurses' hours were not excessive. The Board then asked that the night nursing staff be increased to four, for a hospital of around fifty beds. Five months later Miss Findlay had changed her mind when she told the Royal Commission into Charitable Institutions that nine hours was quite enough for a nursing shift, but that the money was not there to take on more staff.[64]

Nursing was dirty as well as exhausting work. There were waterproof undersheets, but they were stiff and difficult to clean. Hot water would not be reticulated to the midwifery wards until 1892 and to the Infirmary's operating theatre until 1894. In the summer the Infirmary's water supply was apt to fail altogether. Candles were still used for lighting in many parts of the hospital, and in 1896 spilt ether ignited and a patient was burned.[65] The Infirmary surgeons insisted that everything required for special operations be new, and that any equipment used must not be used again. The straw palliasses remained in use until 1897 because they could be burnt after each case.[66] Consequently by 1890 the cost per patient in the Women's Hospital, with its heavy load of special surgery, exceeded that of the Melbourne Hospital by nearly £40.[67] The hospital was just about to build a steam laundry, but to date all laundering was done by external washerwomen, often the unmarried mothers-to-be in the Carlton Refuge. The cost of linen for aseptic surgery and midwifery was high, and when the new American Steam Laundry did arrive, with its engineer and voracious appetite for fuel, it only added to the financial pressures. In the first week of August 1891 the laundry washed 3470 items from the midwifery wards and another thousand articles from the Infirmary.[68] By the mid-1890s the Board of Health was insisting on new sterilising equipment and facilities, which were difficult as well as expensive to install in the 1858 building. Even the gardener had to be paid more because of what was required of him 'under the altered sanitary arrangements'.[69]

There were wards maids, so that nurses did not clean floors although they did dust, but their proper nursing tasks were far from easy. The irrigation of wounds and vaginas was tricky and needed to be done carefully on restless, feverish patients. Douches were meant to be 'long and hot'. In 1894 a patient died after being syringed with boiling mercuric solution by an ill-trained nurse.[70] Dealing with bowel actions, either trying to dry out diarrhoea or give massive enemas to the costive, were scarcely pleasant tasks. Glass, and later indiarubber drainage tubes, had to be watched, cleaned and kept in place despite delirium, pain and bed sores. The faith placed in absolute bed rest for as long as possible meant that many procedures which today would be performed by getting the patient up, had then to be done while they were lying down and that patients remained weak for long periods. The muscle strain, the mental anguish and the nauseating odours of the sick, infected and incontinent, made nursing a labour of love or desperation.

long hot douche: six to eight pints at least were given slowly at a temperature of 120°F

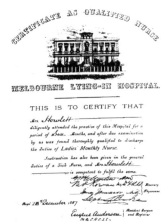

Nurse's certificate, 1887
RWHA

It was the nursing staff who bore the heaviest burden in the transformation of the Women's into a modern hospital. It was they whose work routines and personal disciplines were most affected, and the strain showed. A modern hospital could not function by permitting heroics like Nurse Archer's. Such self-sacrifice was too dangerous and unfair on both patient and attendant. The new costs hardened the rules: nurses now had to pay to replace thermometers they broke. Midwifery nurses were still expected to await the discharge of each woman whose lying-in they had attended and sometimes weeks went by without a day off. 'The terms for midwifery nursing are necessarily long', reported an internal sub-committee in June 1891, 'each patient requiring watchful care and attention for a certain period, during which time frequent changes of nurses would be imprudent or even dangerous'.[71] In the Infirmary the volume of work simply exceeded the available hours, and so the nurses stayed on duty. The Board of Management visitors were not as assiduous as Mrs Perry had been, and often they found nothing amiss; but every now and then they found the wards or nurses' bedrooms disordered, or the nurses themselves 'dispirited'. The nurses lost much personal freedom. Midwifery staff faced instant dismissal if they came 'near any infectious or contagious cases', even if that might be a dying close relative. Once it was understood that the floor was the most septic part of the hospital environment, nurses were sacked on the spot if they placed bedding or cloths on the floor. Nurses were now required to bath daily, under the supervision of the Resident Surgeon and the Head Nurses, and their grooming and dress were elevated into a religion. And as the nurses' physical imprisonment within the hospital buildings became even worse, they went for days without spending five minutes in the open air. To take a break from their work, nursing staff, it seems, had to resign.

The doctors were sometimes critical, but often supportive. Felix Meyer was to make nurse education and the advancement of the profession a lifelong cause, and 'Bertie' Fetherston, as Senior Resident Surgeon and the son of a former matron, understood. He resigned in 1891 to enter private practice, and in his final report he commended the nursing staff and the Board's resolution to increase their number. And surely he had Nurse Archer in mind when he wrote,

Nothing could have been more satisfactory than the working of the Nursing staff during the year. The number was increased, and now bears the same ratio to the number of patients as in the leading hospitals of the United Kingdom — viz., 1 to 3. It is now possible to allow each nurse a short time for recreation almost every day. The change has had a most beneficial effect, as is shown by the zeal and energy with which they have discharged their duties.[72]

But any hopes of continued progress in the early 1890s were to be soon dashed. In the 1880s financial speculation had made Melbourne Marvellous, driving new suburbs into the surrounding farmland, erecting tidy terraces for the working class, semi-detached homes for the upwardly mobile, villas for the expanding middle class and fantastical mansions for the rich. On a mountain of debt Melbourne became one of the great cities of the nineteenth-century world. By 1891 the speculative bubble was bursting, with building societies, property speculators and finally banks themselves failing. It was a depression worse in intensity and scope for Melbourne than would be the global economic collapse of the 1930s, for it afflicted the middle class almost as much as it did the poor. Sober good people of the church-going classes had invested all their savings and provision for old age in schemes promoted by prominent citizens who built coffee palaces to save the working classes from drink, and who presided over suburban Protestant congregations as elders, stewards, Sunday School superintendents and lay preachers. Now their blandishments had proved false and their probity was compromised. Lowland Scots had assumed the moral and business leadership of the Marvellous Melbourne in the 1880s; their fall in the 1890s, while hushed up for the next half-century, was never quite made up. Many middle-class men found themselves having to start all over again, and the young gentlemen who came of age in the 1890s were to become something of a lost generation, with hopes of professional or business careers, and even of marriage, abandoned. Melbourne became a sober, puritanical city, cautious and morally serious; that it had once been a brash, wild-spending, frontier town was remembered only in the florid architecture left to decay into rooming houses and institutions.

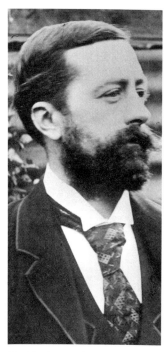

Dr R. H. Fetherston
RWHA

Among the very real achievements of colonial capitalism in Victoria was the voluntarist welfare infrastructure of which the Women's Hospital was part. The charity hospitals, benevolent asylums, orphanages, convalescent homes, lunatic asylums and places of reformation for the alcoholic, the diseased and the fallen, while inadequate and harsh, none the less had been built and continued to serve. But this voluntarist welfare infrastructure, while winning some government support, was still overly dependent on the commitment and generosity of private citizens. The Women's Hospital relied on its long list of subscribers who paid their monthly contribution to the Hospital's collector. It was also building a useful income from trusts and benefactions, and on the level of interest earned. The hospital was therefore particularly vulnerable to any deterioration of middle-class and upper-class private wealth and to any disturbance in the financial market.

The danger signs appeared early. The hospital's overdraft was £5000 by the end of 1891 and the Bank of New South Wales wrote to ask for it to be reduced. The Board decided to postpone plans for a new Infirmary building. There were hopes that a bequest from the late (and notorious) Dr Beaney would tide the hospital over, but by December it was clear that the Beaney investments had collapsed and his surviving brother and sister were destitute and contesting the will. The Beaney solicitor offered the Hospital £100, the Hospital accepted it, but the dispute was to continue for years. The *Age* backed a public Shilling Fund appeal and the hospital did well.[73]

But as the hospital struggled for its financial life, the demands for beds and midwifery fees for home births had never been greater. The respectable poor, who once would have eschewed its midwifery wards, were now desperate for admission. And as the depression deepened, the mean birth weight fell again. This time the decline was of about 0.4 lb

Dr James Beaney (1828–1891): surgeon, politician and philanthropist, honorary surgeon at the Melbourne Hospital

(~0.2 kg) from the late 1880s until the early 1900s. This was about two thirds of the decline in the mean birth weight seen in the Dutch famine.[74] It reached its lowest point in 1896, a fall which corresponds with the collapse of relief funds documented by Shurlee Swain.[75] As the depression dragged on and middle-class savings dwindled, the Ladies' Benevolent societies and the the Charity Organisation Society ran out of money. In 1897 there was a significant recovery, but the population of women seeking a place in the hospital remained underfed and vulnerable until 1904, when the records stop for sixteen years, suggesting a longer-term crisis for the very poor.

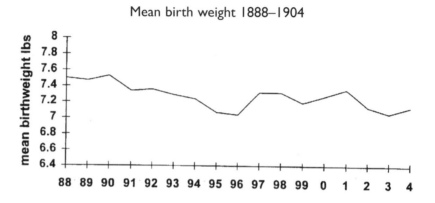

Mean birth weight 1888–1904

The character and public image of the hospital began to change: it was no longer the refuge of the single mother, the destitute or the degenerate. From 1894 onwards, married women would predominate in midwifery. It served all poor women of the colony and Victorian women needed the Women's Hospital even more in this time of economic crisis. By July 1892 the midwifery wards were packed, and yet now with antiseptic midwifery, despite grave fears of outbreaks, there was no contagious and very little endogenous puerperal infection. Tradesmen of all sorts came to the door asking for work, and income continued to fall. In July the Board cut the resident surgeons' pay to half and in August resolved that appointments would be for only twelve months. On 7 March 1893 the finance sub-committee recommended that the hospital follow the lead of the Melbourne Hospital by making the residents' positions honorary, and cutting the salaries of senior employees by 10 per cent and those of junior employees by 5 per cent. Economies were made in every part of the institution.[76]

But it was not enough. By March the hospital was practically insolvent, 'subscriptions are falling off to an appalling degree', so on 29 March, a meeting chaired by the acting governor at the Melbourne Town Hall heard the Bishop of Melbourne, Dr Goe, whose wife was president of the board, join with Dr Rowan and Dr Balls-Headley to urge public support and the finding of five gentlemen who would donate £100 each to deal with the hospital's immediate problem. The women, led by the Lady Mayoress of Melbourne, convened their own Town Hall meeting on 6 April. They invited 'influential ladies' from all over the colony, including all the mayoresses. The floor was taken by a relatively new player in the colonial charity scene, Janet, the wife of Sir William Clarke, Victoria's first baronet. Intelligent and forceful, she had been governess to his motherless children when she caught his eye. At an end of an era where the élite had played at being lords and ladies in Melbourne with liveried servants and great carriages sporting newly discovered or invented coats of arms, the Clarkes continued to live aristocratically and entertain lavishly. Janet, Lady Clarke proposed a week of denial all over Victoria, when everyone 'according to their means, should deny themselves something for one week'. It was to prove a stunning success, raising £6064 17s 1d, removing the urgent debts and paying for some expansion to the Infirmary wards.[77] The salaries of staff other than Resident Surgeons were restored in May 1896, but the Board resisted the many appeals for the return to paid residents until September the following year when, by a majority of one, it was resolved to pay residents just £50; (the house porter was paid £40 as a live-in servant).[78] This was in fact a decade of festering conflict between the Board and the medical staff, both resident and consulting. And caught in the tensions between the Board and the doctors were the hospital's first women doctors.

The entry of women to medicine was from the beginning a threat to those male practitioners who specialised in midwifery and the diseases of women. Surely women should treat modest women in intimate medicine, and women doctors might prove much more successful at the bedside. Indeed some of the support for women to enter medicine was so that they could supplant the male physician in the 'women's business' of parturition.[79] Hence when women doctors made their first appearance at the Women's Hospital this might signal the end of an era, and the beginning of a very different world. Yet the first female medical students do not appear to have caused any particular trouble, and neither did the first appointments to the resident staff. Dr Margaret Whyte was the first, elected over Dr Grace Stone and a Dr Henderson to be assistant resident surgeon

Committee of Management, 1897, Mrs Emma Goe as president, *Weekly Times, RWHA*

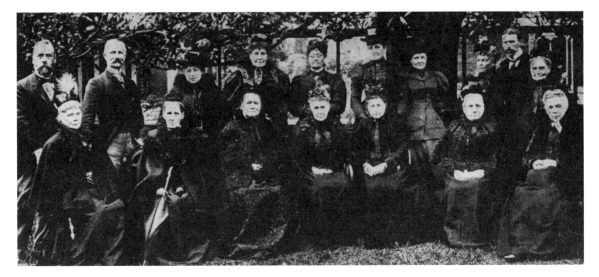

in Midwifery in January 1892. In her first week she had a baptism by fire when the Board investigated and reprimanded the medical staff and an honorary over the death of a woman who had haemorrhaged before admission. The Midwifery Honorary could not be contacted by telephone and Dr Meyer had to come from the Infirmary to deliver her instrumentally, assisted by the senior resident Dr Martell. Otherwise her first year was untroubled, and her locum when she took her annual leave was Dr Helen Sexton, who would one day be the first female consultant. Margaret Whyte resolved any of the hospital's misgivings about women doctors by marrying Dr Martell and retiring from practice.

It was not until 1895, when the Resident Surgeons were unpaid, that women were again appointed: this time Dr Amy Castilla as assistant in Midwifery. Then in September Dr Lilian Alexander was appointed Senior Resident Surgeon and the Women's Hospital had two. By December, when Dr Gertrude Halley wished to apply for an assistantship, the Board resolved that they had had enough of women doctors and denied her. It may be that the Board's reluctance to recommence paying the Resident Surgeons in 1896 and 1897 was driven by their discomfort with the women doctors. And it is not clear whether it was purely personal antagonism or anxiety at the changing boundaries of gender or fear of losing authority to the voice of professional women, but the Board did all it could to make Dr Lilian Alexander's unpaid senior residency a misery. They ordered her to wear 'washing frocks' when on duty in the hospital, and when in winter she asked to wear a woollen blouse with a print skirt, they said no. (The fussing over male doctors and medical students wearing white coats was still seven years away.) She was thirty-seven years old at this time and scarcely irresponsible. They policed 'rule 4' — an antiquated regulation which required the Board to be informed of each occasion that instruments were used in the midwifery wards and for instruments only to be used under the supervision of the honorary staff. The honoraries supported Dr Alexander without reserve. She was reprimanded for her admission of a dying woman with septicaemia, even though all precautions had been taken and the case was a success. Dr Alexander was promoted as was Dr Amy Castilla, but when they departed it was the beginning of a half-century's frustration for women seeking hospital residencies in obstetrics and gynaecology. Helen Sexton was elected an honorary to the outpatients in 1899, but that was an election by subscribers and she was popular in the profession, her earthy humour disarming much male prejudice. Violet Plummer served as a registrar without apparent incident, and Janet Greig was the first consultant anaesthetist. But the hospital, both medical staff and the Board, hardened over the next decade in its attitude to women doctors, and in fact was proud of its practice 'that other things being equal, to recommend the male candidate'. Thus Australia's first hospital for women closed the most significant career path in women's reproductive health in the nation. And it was such opposition which prompted the Stone sisters, supported by Lilian Alexander, to found the Queen Victoria Hospital, as a 'hospital by women for women'. If women doctors were to run hospitals for women, they would have to found their own — the Women's Hospital did not want them. The Board of the Women's Hospital was touchy towards the Queen

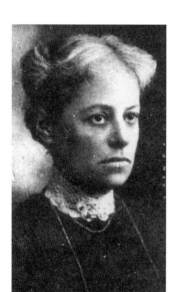

Dr Lilian Alexander
RWHA

Victoria Hospital as it appealed for funds from the public in 1897. They were rivals at once, and if the Women's was a hospital for women, it was to be the 'Queen Vic.' which would be the feminist standard bearer for women's health and medical practice.[80]

The conflict with the women doctors was also part of a wider struggle within the hospital for control of the institution. In part it was an attempt by the laity on the Board of Management to maintain its authority in the face of the advances which were making medicine more specialised and effective. Rather than relinquish authority to the scientifically qualified, the laity sought to reassert its control by policing the very antiseptic rules which now shaped the practices and culture of the hospital. Antisepsis both saved lives and imposed discipline, and that discipline easily degenerated into petty tyranny. The unequivocal truths of sepsis and antisepsis gave sanitary bullies irrefutable power. Honoraries could bully residents, residents could bully medical students, head nurses could bully ordinary nurses, ordinary nurses could bully pupil nurses, and everyone could bully patients. The culture of antisepsis, at its worst and under duress, licensed cruelty.

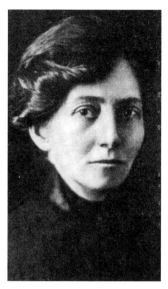

Dr Janet Greig *RWHA*

The Board at the top, if it were not to become more than a financial rubber stamp and fund-raiser, needed to control the doctors. And so the Board cast itself as the antiseptic police, demanding regular medical reports, querying every septic case removed to the cottage, fussing over women doctors' clothing while the men continued to visit patients in street clothes which were unwashable. Honoraries were called to account for alleged medical negligence, and the Board infuriated them when the hospital refused to pass on the medical and nursing students' fees to their lecturers and tutors. The Board still voted on the appointment of resident surgeons. Complaints by medical staff were rejected, and sometimes doctors' authority on medical matters was overridden. The Board refused the admission of patients with puerperal sepsis in 1890. In 1893 the Board went over the heads of the honorary staff in the Infirmary by asking the Melbourne and Alfred Hospitals to take abdominal surgery from the Women's. Accommodation in the Infirmary was now desperate and even the most urgent surgery was being delayed. The Board began insisting that the Consultancy Book be properly kept and signed by each consultant for each case. In 1896 the Board asked to see the consultation book and post-mortem results of Dr Mollison, the honorary pathologist: there seemed to be no concern over the privacy rights of the patients and their families. That year too the Board directed the consultants to have monthly meetings to discuss medical matters. In September 1897 Mrs Gurner moved that the honorary staff consider the motion that advanced cancer patients not be admitted because of the danger of infection; this time the doctors won, convincing the Board that cancer was not contagious. By December 1900 the consultants were in quiet revolt, refusing to sign the Consultancy Book, and the next January they asked the Board to consider reform to the rules which were now 'very old' — 'The progress of surgery since the rules were drafted now rendered them unnecessary'. In those earlier days the mortality from abdominal section was 30 per cent, now it was just 1 per cent, and the present system delayed operations. But the sub-committee appointed did not agree and the rules stayed.

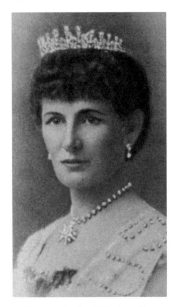

Janet, Lady Clarke, from the portrait at Janet Clarke Hall, University of Melbourne *RWHA*

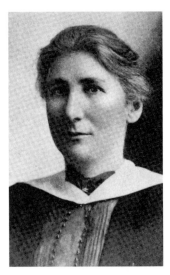

Dr Helen Sexton *RWHA*

The honoraries went into open revolt and refused to sign the book altogether.[81]

In May 1901 Mrs Emma Goe resigned as president of the Board because of ill health. Janet, Lady Clarke was invited to succeed her, and the offer was graciously accepted on condition that she be allowed to arrive late each meeting. Another festering conflict with the honoraries now also reached a head. The medical community had for long been severely critical of the modes of election by the subscribers of honorary staff at the Melbourne and Women's Hospitals. Illegal voting — faggoting — by the dead and the juvenile reduced to a farce what should have been medical appointments of the highest distinction and professional responsibility. Those candidates who recoiled from the indignity of canvassing and corruption found themselves consigned to oblivion. In 1894 Balls-Headley fell victim to his diffidence and dignity, even though he was by now the lecturer in obstetrics and gynaecology at the university: the Board had to rule that the lecturer automatically became an honorary so that he had access to beds for teaching as well as practice. In 1899 Dunbar Hooper failed to garner enough votes to remain on the Infirmary staff — a grave loss to the sick poor. The only consolation was that the subscribers did thus choose the first woman honorary in Dr Helen Sexton — if the Board did not want women doctors, the outside community did. A committee was formed in 1901 to investigate the by-laws and therefore the election of honoraries: it proposed various reforms but the honoraries' enemies on the Board argued successfully that it had exceeded its terms of reference and had sought to serve the hidden agenda of the medical staff.[82]

Then in January tensions finally exploded into an ugly and destructive public scandal. In late December a woman had died of septicaemia. The honorary staff had met and decided to isolate all the septic cases and fumigate the ward with formalin. Dr Cuscaden on behalf of the Medical Staff reported to the Board that the danger was under control. He was asked if the Medical Staff would take full responsibility if the hospital stayed open: yes they would. He was then asked if he could guarantee that no outbreak of sepsis would occur, and, quite properly, he said he could not. A sub-committee was then appointed to inquire into the matter.[83]

The next that Dr Cuscaden heard was that the Board claimed it was carrying out the wishes of the honorary staff and had closed the hospital; he sent a message back that the honorary staff did not want the hospital closed; the hospital's secretary, Mr Gibson, replied that the committee had decided to close the hospital. However the resident surgeons, Drs J. B. Lewis and J. Sandison Yule, refused to close the hospital, and Mr Gibson aided them by hiding the key to the building. All three were dismissed and the row hit the press. If the doctors were wrong in defying the Board, the Board were wrong for meddling in medical matters: two Board members were accused of months of intolerable interference in the medical department: patrolling wards weekly, bursting into labour wards during confinements, entering the residents' and students' rooms without knocking, and turning away an urgent case to get a reference without the Resident Surgeon seeing the woman at all. Janet, Lady Clarke found herself fighting for her public credibility for putting words into

Dr Cuscaden's mouth which he denied having uttered, and the Minutes report nothing of the alleged exchanges. Lady Clarke resolved her public embarrassment by going overseas for six months, leaving her deputy to brave out the Board's public humiliations. On the Board there were some practised antagonists, among them Colonel Goldstein, father of the feminist Vida Goldstein. He was combative, tactless and eager for conflict, and often when conciliatory gestures were made, he reminded his fellow Board members of the underlying rifts. Father O'Connell, however, the first Catholic representative on the Board, strove for peace but to little avail. Relations with the honoraries completely broke down, the wider profession placed a ban on the now vacant midwifery resident position, and the Board was forced to make do with Dr Shields, the son of a Board member and with Dr Margaret Whyte, now Martell, who came out of matrimonial retirement to save the hospital in its hour of need.

The annual general meeting and its elections would obviously resolve the struggle one way or another. The Board began to 'stack' the subscribers' list, enrolling *en bloc* fifteen members of the Toorak Presbyterian Church, until their solicitor advised them they were breaking the by-laws of the hospital. But as the meeting approached, the Board knew its days were over. At the annual general meeting, the doctors made their allegations public and called for a government inquiry. The premier declined, but the old board and its honorary officers knew that they no longer had the support of the majority of the subscribers and life governors of the institution. On the new Board the older members still controlled a majority of votes, but the new blood was led by Mrs D'Ebro, the daughter of the hospital's founder, Dr Richard Tracy, and straight-away she set about transferring power over medical appointments and medical matters to the medical staff.[84]

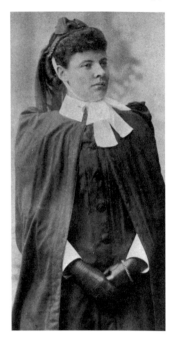

Nurse Jones *RWHA*

The reformers immediately confronted another public controversy. Since mid-1899 feminist groups and local councils had been calling for the removal of discriminatory bed cards which bore 'Mrs' for the 'honest women' and plain first and family name for the unmarried. Various local councils cancelled their subscriptions to the hospital and the hospital found itself widely criticised. The senior nursing staff insisted that the single women did not mind their lack of title; and the married patients were the most determined opponents of all to any removal of discrimination. The feminist campaign was led by Mrs Alison Pymm of Yarraville of the Women's Social and Political Crusade which was also calling for a septicaemia ward to be built at the Women's Hospital. The new Board wanted the matter quickly resolved. Mrs D'Ebro headed a small committee of investigation: the honorary staff considered the bed cards 'quite unnecessary and objectionable' and 'in many cases have found that single women have been subjected to cruel taunts, which are not only unkind, but also from a medical point of view attended with bad results on the progress of the patients'. Many subscribers wrote expressing their opposition to the cards: only the matron and nursing staff held firm. The committee then decided to abolish the cards and for patients' personal details to be kept in the nurses' pantry: a patient's marital status was her own business and it was up to her to inform 'the occupant of the next bed' of her circumstances. It was an interesting controversy, revealing a

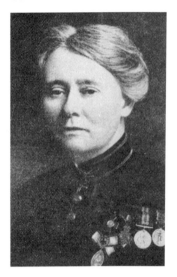

**Sister Hester Maclean,
first nurse matron
1900–1903** *RWHA*

significant level of tolerance in the community of unmarried motherhood — at a distance, however. Those women who shared their world with fallen women — married patients and ward staff, found in their sexual delinquency an 'other' to stigmatise and define themselves by. After two years of confusion over whose medicine was whose, bed cards were brought back, but from now there was to be no prefix as to marital status. Years later, all patients were treated as though married and the single women given cheap wedding rings to protect them from taunts.[85]

It was the beginning of a new era, however. The honorary medical staff gained control over the appointment of residents while the Board sought to retain control over the acceptance of pupil nurses and the appointment of trained nurses. The by-laws and the procedures of election of honoraries of the hospital were reformed. In December 1899 the Board finally approved the appointment of a trained nurse rather than a glorified housekeeper as Lady Superintendent and Hester Maclean served from 1900 until 1904 as the Women's Hospital first nurse matron. But perhaps most important of all was the regulation of the training and registration of nurses. In 1901 the Victorian Trained Nurses' Association was formed, and in 1902 it joined with similar organisations to form the Australian Trained Nurses' Association. In 1902 rules for the registration of general hospitals as training schools were approved and circulated, and thirty-six hospitals were thus registered and the first examinations conducted in December 1902. The Women's Hospital was registered as a 'special training school' providing certificates in gynaecological nursing and midwifery. The Victorian Trained Nurses' Association had refused to consider the introduction of a midwifery course without prior certification in general nursing because it knew that it would compromise the professional standing and competence of its members.

The curriculum for registered midwifery nurses in 1903 included:

1 — Hospital certificates stating that the trainee had seen not less than forty cases and had personally conducted not less than ten cases of labour. A minimum of four weeks had to be spent in the labour ward.

2 — Practical bedside instruction for six months by the resident surgeon to the midwifery department and by two sisters — one in the labour ward and the other in the after-treatment ward.

3 — Weekly courses of lectures for six months by the resident surgeon and matron, and a course of six lectures by the resident surgeon and matron, and a course of six lectures by the honorary surgeons to the midwifery department.

4 — A sound general knowledge of: —

(a) The elementary anatomy and physiology of the female pelvis and generative organs.

(b) The symptoms, mechanism, course of management of natural labour.

(c) Signs that a labour is normal.

(d) Haemorrhage — varieties and treatment.

(e) Antiseptics in midwifery and the way to use them.

(f) Management of the puerperal state, including the use of thermometer, catheter.

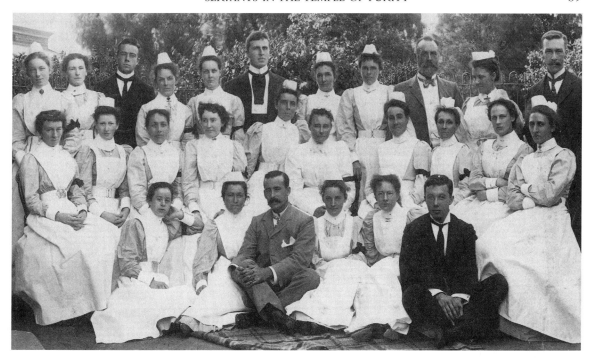

Staff group, *c.* 1900, Dr J. Hodgson Nattrass in middle front row
RWHA

(g) Management and feeding of the newly-born infant.

(h) Duties of the nurse with regard to the seeking of medical aid.

The gynaecological syllabus comprised:

1 — Practical bedside instruction for six months by the resident surgeon and sisters in the infirmary department.

2 — Weekly course of lectures for six months by the resident surgeon and matron in the infirmary department (of which three-fourths must be attended), and a course of six lectures by the honorary surgeons to the infirmary department (of which one full course must be attended.)

3 — A sound general knowledge of: —

(a) The special anatomy and physiology of the female pelvis and generative organs.

(b) Causes of and conditions that tend to disease of the pelvic organs, and the channels through which infection reaches the peritoneum.

(c) The chief germicidal agents used in gynaecology, the prevention of sepsis through hands, skin, instruments, sponges, dressings, sutures and patient's immediate environment.

(d) Preparation of the patient for operation; serious symptoms that may follow operation and their close observation; the nurse's duty in emergencies and her action pending the arrival of the surgeon.

(e) The technique of minor gynaecological procedures, hypodermic injections, passage of catheters, vaginal douching, rectal irrigation, sponging.

(f) The nurse's obligations in respect to her patient, her surgeon, her employer and her profession.[86]

The hospital by 1903 was delivering over 1200 women a year and had forty-nine midwifery beds and thirty-eight in the Infirmary. Further building and expansion was under way, but the institution had been transformed in the previous twenty years and it was in the nurses that the transformation was most evident. In 1903 a gushing journalist from the *New Idea* paid a visit to the Infirmary and revealed its aseptic and medical wonders to the magazine's genteel feminine readership. She was conducted around the hospital by Sister Munro-Campbell, who was just as she should be: 'fresh and spotless in the uniform of plain holland and linen, set off with shapely collar and cuffs, and the fascinating nurse's cap on the hair, in this instance having the addition of graceful streamers at the back, in deference to the rank of Sister'.[87] The hospital had now triumphed over the germ, Sister Munro Campbell explained as she took her into the operating theatre:

> . . . the theatre is a kind of sanctuary . . . a Temple of Purity. The atmosphere must be holy, strictly so, to our sense of duty, in being kept free from the taints and powers of evil in the disease-carrying microorganisms that threaten life under the surgeon's knife; or as nearly so as we can make it with every conscientious care and vigilance, and with all that science can teach us of ways and means.

This was total war, work 'without end':

> Oh, yes! if a germ mistakes himself so far as to intrude in here, he gets a warm reception. We try to scrub him, to scarify him, to boil or bake him, and to asphyxiate him. But for all that he is a very obtrusive fellow, and fond of bringing his myriad of friends and relations with him out of the dark corners of the earth. So you will judge, perhaps, what we have to do to fight him, and the efforts of all our hands put together can never be relaxed.[88]

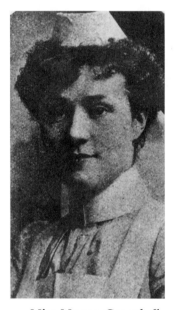

Miss Munro-Campbell, theatre sister, *New Idea*, 1903, *RWHA*

This war against the germ had become a gendered combat. The intruder in the feminised, sanitised and moralised world of the hospital was male. Similarly, the agents of the sickness of women were masculine lust and selfishness. The feminised world of nursing was united by its common masculine enemies: the male world of the doctors and their overweening authority; and the male world of sexual desire which brought disease and unwanted pregnancy to their patients. But as nursing evolved into a modern profession, control, discipline and routine consumed the psychic world of the career nurse: therefore, ironically, as nursing became more feminised, many of its career practitioners became less 'womanly'. As unmarried women, they did not share the pain of labour. Patients were to be treated all alike, therefore empathy and sympathy were rationed. Occasionally the tragic plight of a particular patient broke through their emotional reserve, but most patients became bodies which had to be processed. The object of all activity was cleanliness, efficiency and order. Even if the object of nursing remained patient care, the modern hospital required that it be controlled care.

III

Women and Doctors
1883–1913

The Sickness of Women Dr Burke's and Dr Fetherston's Case Books, 1883–1889

6

In 1883 the hospital changed its record taking in the Infirmary. Until then the more systematic honoraries had maintained their own case notes, but in 1883 the medical staff decided to have formalised case books printed which would record more than the patient's immediate medical care. She would now provide a history which would include place of birth and age at which, if foreign born, she came to Australia — important facts in a society of immigrants. Her full menstrual history would be analysed, as would the nature of her menstrual flows both early after the menarche and at the time of admission. The number of pregnancies would be broken down into deliveries and miscarriages, and the facts of her most recent confinement collected: the length of labour, the use of instruments and anaesthesia, the blood loss, her immediate recovery from labour and her long-term recovery from the lying-in. Next, her symptoms would be taken down: first as a narrative of when they first appeared and secondly of their character on admission. There were specific anatomical observations for the *per vaginam* examination, and finally a record of her heart, lungs and teeth.

The examining doctor made his own observations of her outward condition, but the narrative was shaped by a crucial leading question: 'Was quite well until . . .' which invited the patient to tell her story, and the doctors of a more literary bent often caught her voice and her exact words. Concealed inside the case history was a dialogue — brief, fragmented, but telling, and if medical discourse inscribed its meanings on the patient, the patient's narrative had some effect on the doctor's. For a moment the patient speaks on the historical record: there is a vignette of her life and the troubles which beset her. It is a moment of astonishing intimacy. The doctors say very little about her: not often do they categorise her as a human being, even more rarely do they criticise on the page, and they work hard at being neutral, at not passing judgement on lives and values very different from their own. Occasionally the notes for an obvious prostitute are unusually brief, as though her care mattered

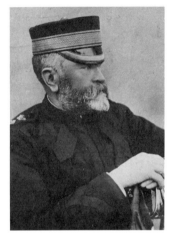

Dr G. H. Fetherston
RWHA

Dr Eugene Anderson
in 1889 *RWHA*

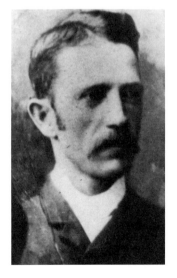

less and she was not liked, but other obvious prostitutes or women 'with a past' were given exemplary care and their notes are detailed. Often there is sufficient in the patient's story and in the doctor's clinical observations to hazard a modern diagnosis. Retrospective diagnosis, used prudently, has a place in the history of human health. If our interest is in the physical condition of people of the past, it may at the least open new questions. And the two case books to be discussed have been rediagnosed by Dr James Evans.

The case books were named for each honorary, but it was in fact the resident surgeon who admitted the patient and wrote the notes. The honorary was consulted for difficult cases and it was the honoraries who performed the surgery. The case notes of patients who underwent surgery and were nursed in the two 'special wards', were entered into another case book, but at various stages during the 1880s 'intensive care' records were added to the honoraries' case books. We have therefore a remarkable record of patients' lives and sufferings, of doctors' diagnostic thinking and responses to individual patients, and of the minutiae of nursing. The hospital comes to life.

What follows is an analysis of two hundred consecutive Infirmary cases who were admitted between 1883 and 1889 from the books of Dr Stephen Burke and Dr Gerald Fetherston, supplemented by cases from other doctors. Both doctors were popular members of the honorary staff, and both enjoyed esteem in their respective private practices. They practised in working-class suburbs, North Melbourne and Prahran respectively, but also had lucrative private practices, performing surgery on private patients either in the patients' homes or in their own private surgeries. Both referred private patients who needed hospital care to the Women's Hospital, so that local women feature in their case lists. (Major operations were still being performed in homes and surgeries: like Mrs Elizabeth Beck, who in 1877 had to walk home two miles on a bitter winter's day after having a cancerous mass stripped from her uterus by Dr Blair in his Collins Street rooms. She died of peritonitis.[1]) But the doctors' voices in these two case books are in fact those of the resident surgeons, Felix Meyer for Dr Burke and Eugene Anderson for Dr Fetherston.[2]

None the less it is the patients who take centre stage. They had to obtain a ticket of admission, just as for the midwifery wards, but many also came with referrals from their own doctors. Others had attended the outpatients' department. The most awkward applicants were those from the country and other colonies who simply arrived without warning: the hospital felt obliged to admit them at once, for to send them home again to wait was often inhumane, but they did thus jump the queue. There were only twenty-three ordinary beds and two special ward beds for post-operative cases, and since recovery from surgery could take months, the waiting lists were always long. In the 1880s the Women's Hospital was where the women went, so that many who were suffering non-gynaecological conditions were there as well. While these case books cannot provide us with incidences of illness that would satisfy an epidemiologist, they can tell us about the hospital's work and much anecdotally about women's health among the poor.

The first thing that is striking is the patients' youth. In both series 63 per cent were under the age of thirty; merely 17 per cent were aged forty or over. The Infirmary wards were therefore full of young women in their reproductive prime; but not all had been mothers: 36 per cent of Dr Burke's had never been pregnant, as was the case for 22 per cent of Dr Fetherston's. Few were still virgins, however. Even a fourteen-year-old admitted for period pain had no hymen.[3] The lateness of their menarches is also significant. While there is considerable genetic variation between families in the onset of menstruation, in a whole population it is an indicator of malnutrition. Whereas today the average age of menarche in Australia is twelve, merely 10 per cent of these women had menstruated by the time they turned thirteen, and 59 per cent menstruated after their fifteenth birthday. These women had had a very low body mass index in adolescence: they did not have enough body fat to stimulate the production of oestrogen. Even more significant is the fact that those born overseas but reaching menarche in Australia did not mature earlier than those who were still in Ireland or England at puberty. In other words, in the 'Workingman's Paradise' working-class women and girls were distinctly malnourished.[4] Soon after the menarche they began their sexual life, very many of them without a wedding ring to make it legitimate. The stories suggest impulsive experimentation and snatched opportunities for intercourse rather than 'affairs'. Of Dr Burke's one hundred, 70 per cent were married at an average age of 20.3 years, 36 per cent of the sample marrying under the age of twenty. And at least a third of the marriages appear to have been 'shot-gun' unions.

Women's reproductive health is necessarily divided into life-stages, and for those under twenty-five the conditions which brought them into the hospital were either unrelated to sexual behaviour or conversely the consequences of destitute motherhood and/or sexual delinquency. First there were girls and young women who simply had too little to eat, too much work to perform and few hopes for the future. They complained of difficulties with their periods, of headaches and weakness, of emotional disturbances or fits, but lying behind their stories was often the dread of tuberculosis. Miss C. C., a domestic servant aged eighteen, had been poorly ever since puberty. She complained of period pain and frontal headaches, insomnia and poor appetite, listlessness, continual fainting fits from the period pain, swelling of the abdomen and constipation. Dr Meyer wanted to know if she had spat blood — no, but she had been losing weight and sweating and coughing at night. He found her 'fairly healthy looking, with clear skin, but of nervous temperament', but her fears were not unfounded. Dr Burke performed a metrotomy, this time under an anaesthetic because she was so difficult to examine vaginally, and she later came down with pneumonia from the chloroform which may have 'tickled up' her tuberculosis.[5]

Tuberculosis was still a disease of the young, especially of women in their reproductive prime. More women died of tuberculosis than ever died of childbirth in nineteenth-century Australia and around the world, but their susceptibility to it derived from the strains their reproductive role placed on their immune systems; and they passed their everyday lives more than did men, in close, ill-ventilated places where infection was more likely. Lastly, working-class women ate less well than their men, both in quantity and quality. Tuberculosis therefore is a central feature of women's reproductive health in the nineteenth century. Most men and women would have had a brush with phthisis and it is significant how many autopsies for other causes of death uncovered major tubercular lesions; but as an actual killer, its victims were disproportionately young and female. Ten per cent of the patients of both doctors had obvious tuberculosis, either of the lungs or in the pelvic organs, and more cases were probable. The youngest victim of all was twelve, still a child, with a tubercular pelvic mass: 'rather weakly looking — trouble in breathing — mobility of chest much impaired'. Others were more far gone and had come in to die. L. L. was seventeen and dying of miliary tuberculosis. Her mother was blind, and the patient too sick herself to give a full history. She had been attended by a local doctor for seven months before admission. Meyer saw before him a 'wasted, sallow, cachectic' figure, with 'face very emaciated'. She gave off the strong mawkish odour of the advanced consumptive, but he saw the one lovely thing left of her: 'dark eyes, long lashes'. She could take no nourishment, but 'moans all day — will do nothing but drink'. After two weeks her 'friends took her away' and she died at home.[6]

Poor diet and close living exposed the poor to illness, but so too did the physical burdens of their daily work. There were no regulations about the weights women and children could not carry in workplaces, hence there was nothing to protect fourteen-year-old R. S. from having to lift a ten-gallon boiler. She strained herself and had to lie down all day afterwards. She got pains in her heart and lungs, and pain with passing urine and again a metrotomy was performed. The English gynaecologist Galabin blamed poor pelvic development on the carrying of heavy weights in childhood, as he equally condemned excessive running for narrowing the pelvis.[7] Lifting of all sorts brought on strains and bleeding. Other women eventually just wore out. Mrs B. had been on the diggings ever since coming to Australia in 1851. She had married soon after arrival and borne seven children, with one miscarriage in the next twelve years. Now aged fifty-two, she had been well until two years ago when she strained herself 'while lifting buckets of quartz'. She felt 'very weak' and had pain and a nasty discharge.[8] And Mrs H., Somerset-born, aged sixty-five, had had eleven children and one miscarriage, and until a year ago had assisted her husband in his blacksmith's shop. Then, 'when patient was using an eighteen-pound hammer on the anvil to straighten out a piece of red hot iron', something went, she felt a 'sharp, momentary pain and twitching about the womb. Patient felt no particular effect from this at the time. Two or three weeks afterwards a discharge of blood began from the womb and continued off and on for about two months'.[9] There were often life emergencies for which the poor had no one but themselves to turn to. Mrs C. D., a housewife of South Melbourne, was fine until a tree fell on her home a month after her first confinement at the age of twenty. She 'exhausted herself clearing away the debris etc and then complained of irregularly recurring intense pain in the right flank. This pain became aggravated in intensity and frequency during the last pregnancy'. She now complained of 'an ever-persistent severe pain in R. flank which is sometimes of an agonising nature'.[10]

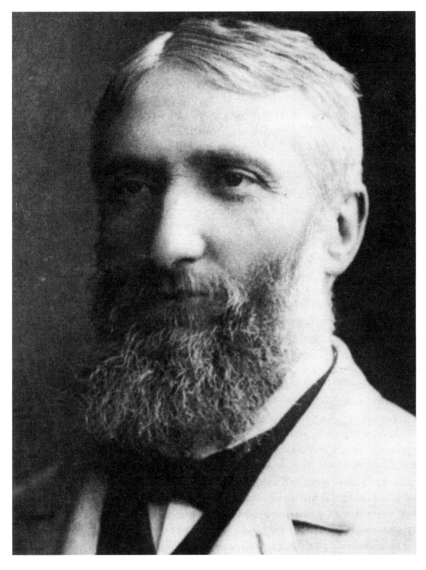

Dr Stephen Burke
RWHA

Among those under thirty, the most common condition not associated with pregnancy and childbirth was dysmenorrhoea. It is a scourge to those afflicted with it, and it is aggravated by tuberculosis, malnutrition and the cold. At its worst it can force a woman to take to her bed. By the 1880s there was more understanding of it — Jamieson was teaching at the university that it was thought to be caused by contractions of the uterus, but the remedies were perforce mechanical, that is surgical. Miss B. L., a nineteen-year-old tailoress certainly suffered, but she also had made a career out of her menstrual afflictions. Her florid case history tripped off the tongue with astonishing precision as to dates (she remembered that one menstrual cycle had gone six weeks when she was fifteen), and she had done the rounds of many doctors. She had been 'pretty well up to fifteen and a half; then she grew weak and pale, lost her colour, got blue lips, couldn't walk, frightful headaches, always taking medicine'. With each period now came frontal headaches and constant pain. Otherwise she slept and ate well, yet micturated often and suffered constipation. She was not a virgin, Dr Meyer noted, and perhaps her most distressing symptoms, which began two years after the menarche, were connected with an unwanted sexual experience. Certainly to the doctor's eye she looked 'healthy, dark, good colour and well nourished'. She was menstruating when she came into hospital, and on the second day threw a hysterical fit. Ten days later Dr Burke performed a metrotomy, and she was fitted with a small pessary and discharged after nearly a month's care.[11]

It is striking that many of these Infirmary patients were not working, even when single. A number of the single girls with menstrual problems appear to have stayed in the parental home, helping out with the house-keeping when they felt well enough. Certainly, the demographic historian Ann Larson found working-class girls staying at home and not working in greater numbers in 1880s Melbourne.[12] Miss M. M. of Richmond was a working-class chronic invalid. She complained of gnawing pains in the back passage — which were most likely endometriosis, but she too had had a busy round of trying doctors, eight all told in Melbourne, Sydney and Dubbo in just four years. One doctor gave her a pessary, but she had to take to her bed for seven weeks while it was in. Despite all this she had 'a healthy appearance — fair, clear skin; doesn't look thin but says she was much stouter. Pulse quiet, hands clammy and heart gets excited'. A *per vaginam* examination revealed nothing and after a week she departed.[13]

At the Intercolonial Medical Congress of Australasia in 1889 Dr Eugene Anderson presented an analysis of the menstrual history of 1200 patients in the Women's Hospital. In their early menstrual history just over a quarter reported suffering 'great pain' while only 42 per cent had painless periods. When he looked at the older patients, only a quarter reported no pain, with 43 per cent suffering severe distress. There had been an increase of 17 per cent, an increase that had everything to do with the damage and chronic infection inflicted by childbearing.[14] And since these working-class girls started their childbearing so early in life, the unfortunate could be condemned to chronic invalidism before they reached their twenties. Miss E. C. of Wangaratta had been delivered of her illegitimate baby in secret by her family. The baby was stillborn and she had never felt well since and had severe pains in the back. Defecation and urination were painful, and two months earlier 'she had tried to work but couldn't keep on'. She had received no medical advice until the last week. On examination it was found that her perineum was split to within half an inch of the anal sphincter and her cervix was badly lacerated. She had a chronic low-grade infection. There was little to be done but keep her in bed, feed her iron and tonic, insert a glycerine plug into the vagina at night and irrigate the vagina with hot water. After two weeks she went home, to a miserable future. She was just short of her nineteenth birthday.[15]

Miss J. McN. had borne a child out of wedlock at the age of seventeen, developed an 'inflammation' and was treated in the Infirmary. On dis-charge 'the patient went out and went about her work, gradually got weaker, had pains in back and difficulty in walking. Now she was in great pain in the side and the stomach, had difficulty in walking and was unable

endometriosis: the presence of tissue similar to the lining of the uterus at other sites in the pelvis. This tissue undergoes the periodic changes similar to those of the endometrium and causes pelvic pain and severe dysmenorrhoea (OMD). The pain is colloquially described as a 'red hot poker up the back passage'.

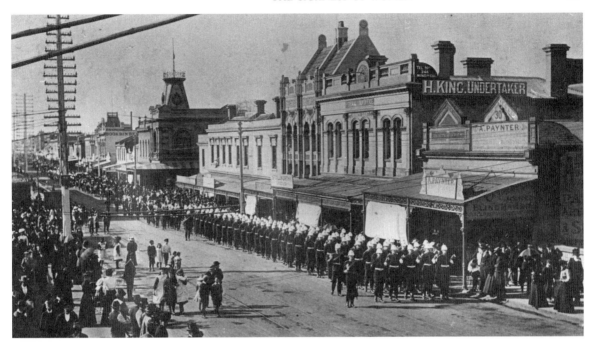

to lie down without pain'. She was losing flesh and had become 'much emaciated lately', her skin was florid and sweating. She probably had chronic pelvic cellulitis and there was absolutely nothing that could be done to cure her other than rest and good food. She was just twenty years old and she could well be sick for the rest of her life. Mrs E. S. of Coburg was also just twenty. She had married at seventeen, borne two children and was carrying her third. She had been well until her last confinement, when the baby was big and she lost a lot of blood. She was delivered at home by a midwife, but consulted a doctor later. Now her uterus had completely prolapsed and she was condemned to wearing a pessary already. She too would have little hope of relief in later life.[16]

The funeral of Dr G. H. Fetherston in Chapel Street, Windsor, September 1901 *RWHA*

Those who contracted venereal disease would also suffer for the rest of their lives. Both gonorrhoea and syphilis have latent phases and can become clinically apparent again later in life. Gonorrhoea can be almost asymptomatic in women, and its incidence can only be guessed at by the later extent of pelvic inflammatory disease. One seventeen-year-old was diagnosed with it, but it was syphilis which was easier to detect in the hospital. Miss E. S. of Clifton Hill aged eighteen had a suspicious labial ulcer and on a later admission to the Infirmary, condylomata, but she insisted that she had never had sexual intercourse and that she 'was not given to irritating labia in any way'. She was treated with mercury, three doses daily, for a month and the abscess with hydrogen perchloride. Mrs A. T. of Collingwood, like very many, acquired venereal disease as a wedding present from her husband. She had been quite well until she got married three and a half years before. Then she developed continuous toothache, weakening back pains, sores on the vulva, a sore throat and her hair fell out. She had never conceived. Now 'she always feels sick' and she was in agony with her menses. Dr Burke performed a metrotomy, for want of anything else to do. Mrs M. F. was the oldest syphilitic. She had married at nineteen and had nine confinements and eight miscarriages in fifteen years of marriage. Significantly, she had not had a pregnancy go to full term for five years. She was pregnant again and had been sick since her previous pregnancy. This time she also miscarried with a six-month foetus who had been 'some time dead'. And she had an umbilical hernia, hence she was advised to avoid 'hard food and <u>drink</u>'.[17]

The Infirmary was not always a parade of pelvic cripples for whom nothing could be done; there were women who were successfully treated. Burke's most common operation was the Emmet repair of the lacerated and infected cervix, lesions that were more commonly sites of infection which grew in the small tears most women suffer in confinements. Thomas Addis Emmet was the partner of J. Marion Sims and became the leading surgeon in their New York Women's Hospital. He had first published on the repair of the cervix in 1874 in America, and the technique was quickly brought to Melbourne by Dr Balls-Headley.[18] Felix Meyer reported on Balls-Headley's first case, a Women's Hospital patient in 1881, and a year later Balls-Headley himself published a paper on the vexed question of 'ulceration of the os' and Emmet's remedy. He painted a sad picture of the typical victim of the condition:

> The os having from some cause insufficiently expanded, the child in its passage splits it to some extent at one or both ends, or at one or both sides, or in each of these directions simultaneously. Some swelling occurring, the healing of the two edges is incomplete, and the cervical canal thus becomes exposed. Hence results cervical catarrh, with eversion of the cervical tissue. The angles of laceration being pressed perhaps by the weight of the uterus against the posterior wall of the vagina, some metritis occurs and sub-involution. Should the diseased action advance, pelvic cellulitis may supervene, or an inflammation may involve one or both broad ligaments, or also one or both of the ovaries. Finally the more acute conditions subside leaving a laceration of the cervix and a cervical catarrh, commonly designated cervical catarrh, complicated with leucorrhoea, perhaps some degree of fixation, and various sympathetic pains, as of the left or right side, the back, below the left breast, the left shoulder, or between the scapulae. Menorrhagia usually occurs in the earlier times, followed frequently by more or less of suppression. The patient is rendered an hysterical invalid and wanders among doctors.
>
> Yet it need not go as far as this. The laceration may be so extensive as to destroy health and comfort, but not enough to prevent pregnancy. Thus sub-involution may be a permanent condition, with cervical catarrh and leucorrhoea, and a chronic metritis, yet the woman may have children at short intervals, usually getting worse after each confinement, for each confinement splits her a little more.[19]

Emmet's operation could prevent all this, he argued. If the lacerated cervix is properly repaired, then inflammation and further tearing need not occur. Its effectiveness must have been limited, because what these patients suffered from was usually a more deep-seated pelvic inflammatory disease which may well have entered the bloodstream and the tissues via a fissure in the cervix after a confinement or an abortion, but which was doing its worst mischief far from the point of entry.

It was such infections which filled most beds in the Infirmary and would do so for another seventy years, but the surgeons had their successes, particularly when the patient was herself robust and well fed. Mrs E. R. of Drouin, 'a strong, healthy-looking woman', had borne five children in ten years, and had been well until the last one. No doctor had attended and she lost a lot of blood. Three days later the lochia ceased. She felt great weakness, but there had been no pain and now she was much the same. The examination revealed a cervix lacerated down the vaginal junction, and the parts were thickened, hard and oedematous. Her constitution won out, however, and a fortnight after the operation the sutures were removed and the union was perfect.[20]

Burke was a better plastic surgeon than abdominal operator, and in his private practice had developed a reputation for surgery for breast cancer. He was very good on repair of the perineum, and had a good result with Mrs J. C., another strong healthy-looking country woman. She was twenty-nine, and since the age of sixteen had borne nine children and suffered three miscarriages. The last confinement, fifteen months before, had been a nightmare. Her womb was now too tired and she laboured for two days, forceps were needed and she haemorrhaged afterwards. She had spent two months in bed, and now the pain was constant. On examination it was seen that the perineum was 'quite gone to within the margin of the anus — parts bluish and congested'. On 23 July Dr Burke operated, using silver and horsehair sutures, 'the parts came together well and there was a little haemorrhage from a spouting vessel which was ligatured'. Two days later the 'parts were looking well — not much constitutional disturbance', but she complained of rheumatism in her heels and she was given flannels. Two weeks after the operation the wound was perfectly healed and the sutures removed. A week later it was 'up today — very shaky', and eight days later she went home.[21]

Burke's case book covers the time when the hospital was in its worst septic crisis; one of his patients contracted a fatal streptococcal infection from a simple metrotomy, and others became infected simply from explorations with the uterine sound. In 1883 he performed a delicate operation on a sixteen-year-old with a congenital deformity of the vagina which had prevented menstrual blood from coming away, and when he excised the tumour via the rectum, 'a great quantity of foul pent up menses came away'. (The patient had to be placed in a ward of her own because other patients could not bear the smell.) The poor girl became infected with a staphylococcus which left her with a discharging abscess.[22]

Fetherston's case book, covers a period four to five years later, which was a better one for hospital sepsis. Fetherston, who attempted more abdominal surgery than Burke had in the earlier period, had only six post-operative deaths, five of which were inevitable. The one surprise was instructive. Mrs J. C. from Hotham was clearly a favourite among the hospital staff. The nursing notes are exemplary and her vivacity shines through the text. She was twenty-six and had just been delivered of her sixth child. She had also had three miscarriages in her brief reproductive life. In fact, she had been so often pregnant that it had been 'some years' since she had last menstruated. With this last pregnancy she had noticed that she was 'very big — twins her friends suggested'. She felt most uncomfortable, 'could hardly move at all, had constant pain in the abdomen and was feverish. The baby was very small at birth, with a small placenta, and lived only two days. After the birth, Mrs C. was 'astonished' that her abdomen was still very large, a girth of 38 inches. She had an ovarian cyst and was very ill. By the time she reached hospital her condition was only 'fair' and her heart action weak. For eight days her temperature rose so surgery could not be avoided. Five honoraries and the two residents assisted Dr Fetherston in the operation — the staff was desperately concerned for her. The tumour was exposed and punctured, 'giving suit to an extremely glutinous dark brown and greenish thick fluid containing numerous flakes and shreds. The weight of the tumour and contents was around $4\frac{3}{4}$ pounds, but at least $2\frac{1}{4}$ pounds more escaped by the abdominal wound'. In special care she did well, until day six when she told the nurse at 2.30 a.m. that it was hard to swallow. The doctor saw her at 7.30 a.m. and recorded that 'she swallows with great difficulty. On being asked to protrude her tongue, it is seen that she can hardly separate the teeth at all'. They gave her chloral hydrate, but to no avail. By 2 p.m. she went into spasm in the jaw and body. She was in agony, arching her back. They gave her a nutrient enema — brandy, egg and milk by rectum. By eight the next morning there were no more spasms, but her pulse was over 200, her respirations 70 per minute and her temperature 107°. Fifteen minutes later she died. It was tetanus, possibly brought in on someone's shoes — perhaps by one of the eight doctors who attended her operation.

chloral hydrate: a sedative and hypnotic drug

Another of Dr Fetherston's post-operative deaths revealed the immense difficulties surgeons faced in keeping wounds free of infection. Mrs C. of East Prahran was another of his local patients. She had borne six children and suffered one abortion, and now aged thirty-six was pregnant again and dying of cervical cancer. Ever since the child had quickened, the pain had become 'burning, lacerating in the vagina'. She could not pass urine unless she went on her hands and knees, yet she had all her children to care for. She was 'emaciated greatly — weak', and when she was examined vaginally, a cancerous mass was visible to the naked eye. The baby could not be delivered through it. The only course was to perform a caesarean, even though it would certainly kill the mother; but it was perhaps better for her to die insensible after an operation rather than slowly during an agonising obstructed labour during which the baby would surely die. On 12 June they operated and the child extracted (there is no record of whether it was alive or dead). An indiarubber drainage tube was passed from the uterus through the vagina, and ten days later the union of the abdominal wound was almost complete, there was little discharge from the tube and it was thankfully odourless. She was therefore ready to be moved to the general ward. Two days after she suddenly collapsed and was almost pulseless, and nine hours later she died. The post-mortem revealed that the uterine wound had not healed at all, and was gangrenous, so that she had died of peritonitis.[23]

This attempted caesarean section had failed because of the difficulty in suturing the uterine wound and keeping it free of infection. The 1880s saw the first successful caesarean sections performed in Australia, but the death rate was daunting. The first in Melbourne had been by Dr John Cooke at the Alfred Hospital in 1886.[24] The first at the Women's Hospital was by Dr Balls-Headley. For all his scepticism about Listerism, he was the outstanding surgeon of the honorary staff until Michael O'Sullivan was elected in 1888. Balls-Headley's first case was on C. C, a rachitic dwarf just 3 feet 10 inches tall and 'malformed'. She was seventeen but looked forty, and was so angry and frightened at her first admission to the Infirmary in July that she refused to speak. She was measured from head to foot, prodded and probed and required to be photographed naked. Her conjugata vera was $1\frac{1}{2}$ inches and it was obvious that a destructive operation would kill her as well as the baby. The decision was to operate closer to term and to perform Porro's Operation where the uterus was

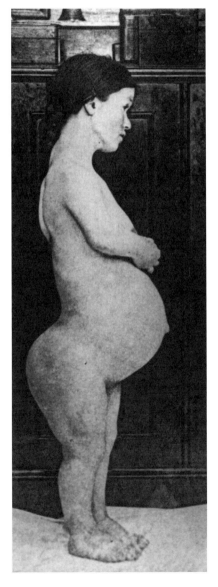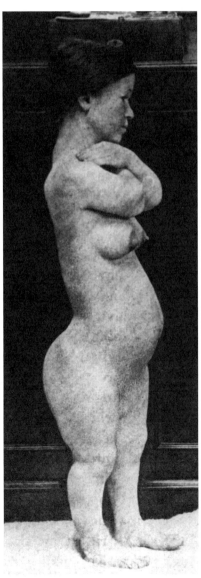

C. C., aged seventeen, before and after her successful operation *Walter Balls-Headley,* **Pamphlets** *(Melbourne, 1893), Brownless Medical Library Historical Collection, University of Melbourne*

itself removed and the stump clamped and brought out of the abdominal cavity to heal outside the body. On 14 October when the foetus was supposed to be between eight and nine months, the operation took place. Three honoraries assisted, as well as the resident surgeon Dunbar Hooper, with eight others watching. The incision was four inches, vertical between the umbilicus and the pubes. The bulging membranes were opened and the head expelled by the 'considerable uterine contractile force, and some external pressure around it, through the opening which was just large enough to let it squeeze through'. The child, a girl, 'cried lustily, and was enveloped in a flannel'.

> The hand then grasped the neck of the uterus, and Lawson Tait's uterine clamp was adjusted below the level of the opening of the ovaries and fallopian tubes. At this time the placenta was seen to be presenting at the uterine opening, and to be free from the neighbourhood of the neck, where by auscultation, it had appeared to be attached. A sound was introduced into the bladder, and as it appeared not to be included in the clamp, the latter was tightened up. The uterus was then cut away with scissors an inch below the level of the transverse incision, the abdominal cavity cleansed, and closed by six silver sutures above the stump, and one below it, and intervening horsehairs; the stump touched with solid perchloride of iron, and a strip of lint applied under the ends of the clamp wire, carbolic absorbent cotton over all, followed by Mead's plaster and a flannel bandage. There was practically no haemorrhage, except a little free bleeding when nicking the uterus, and what escaped from the uterine division after its constriction.[25]

It was a triumph. Mother and baby were well, the baby was wet-nursed and put on a pound in her first six weeks, and she was baptised in the hospital. Her mother named her Porrina Balls-Headley C—.

Such successes were few in the Infirmary, however. Most conditions could only be relieved, and even those who had been given surgical remedies seemed to be back in the hospital a few years later, the same or even worse since they had had their 'Emmet' or metrotomy. These were times when the poor lived with exhaustion and chronic pain, and the only relief to be found was in alcohol and opiates. Many more women were dependent on alcohol than the hospital realised, because alcohol was given so freely in the wards that delirium tremens rarely set in. (Mrs O'C. of North Carlton was kept alive on two bottles of stout a day while recovering from the removal of a vast ovarian tumour in 1884.[26]) Opiate addicts were remarkably few: Mrs P. was admitted in such a drugged state that she 'was quite unable to give an intelligent history'. Laudanum was denied her and for eight days she was 'constipated, vomiting and hysterical'. 'She often got out of bed and seemed to have no control over her actions, but was not in the least paralysed'. Suspecting her of shamming, Dunbar Hooper ordered her to bed to await a consultation with Dr Balls-Headley after she threw a five-minute fit. Suddenly she put on her clothes, telegraphed her husband, and left.[27]

The wards were not always places of quietness and order; the patients saw to that. Many were volatile, some very rough, some died very noisily,

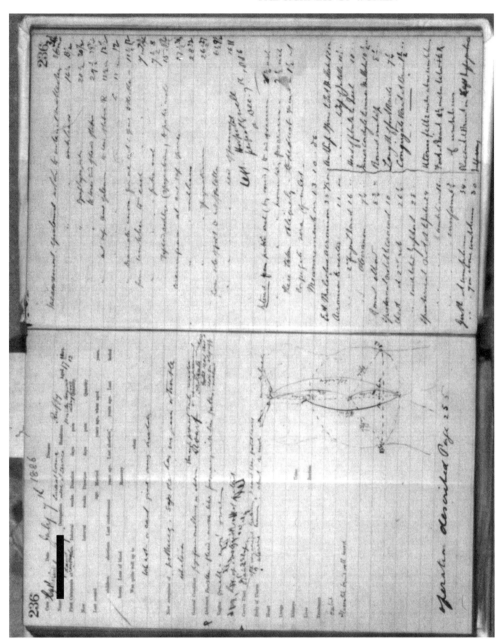

Balls–Headley's Case Book, C.C., adm. 7 July 1886 *RWHA*

many wept and screamed, and some even sang. Mrs F. D. of Richmond was twenty-six; four years before she had had a baby out of wedlock but, as often happened, she had married since. For twelve months a tumour had formed over her right ovary; it was not painful, but it was getting so big, she could hardly breathe. Her girth measured $43^1/_2$ inches. She was 'pale and anaemic, with a tired anxious look'. Her lungs were 'rather dull at both bases'. Dr Rowan operated with Dr Burke giving the anaesthetic, and Drs Jamieson and Fetherston assisting, as well as the Resident Surgeon. She took the anaesthetic very badly so that ether had to be substituted for it at times. She lost a lot of blood during the operation and became very pale and needed three hypodermic injections of ether to rally her. A five-inch incision revealed an ovarian cyst weighing six pounds and a gush of fluid which brought the combined weight to 20 pounds. The operation took an hour and afterwards she was 'very low — cold sweat, pallor'. She was given iced champagne. Suddenly in the small hours she improved: 'looks and feels wonderfully well — desires a little coffee, which is given and agrees well'. Later she took a little brandy and soda, and the next day some oatmeal and water. She was now even better: 'no headache, pain or sickness', in fact she was lying in bed 'singing!' But she was still helplessly weak, and each evening her temperature rose with her spirits. Not until a fortnight after her admission did the notes record that 'her old lung trouble' might be the cause of her feverishness, night sweats, and hectic happiness. She had tuberculosis, both pulmonary and pelvic and was doomed to die, but her operative wound improved enough for her to be discharged after a month.[28]

Yet if the admissions to the Infirmary for menstrual difficulties, infections and injuries from childbirth, cancer and infectious disease are to be expected, what is also significant is the number of 'social admissions', of women who were in fact not physically sick enough to warrant hospital treatment, but who were in sore need of a rest, good food and iron. The case books are a window into working-class unhappiness and suffering.

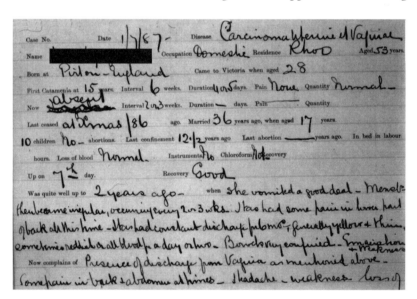

**Mrs H., adm.
27 July 1887** *RWHA*

Victims of domestic violence were admitted: one rested for two and a half weeks, recovering from a labial abscess where she had been kicked by her husband. The doctor never bothered to enter her name, however, and assessed her general condition as 'well, but querulous expression'. Nine per cent of Dr Burke's patients and 14 per cent of Dr Fetherston's did not suffer from a physical condition that warranted admission to a hospital. What they did suffer from was depression, fatigue, malnutrition and anxiety. Only a handful had the word 'hysterical' in their case notes, and those comments were made when the patient had actually become hysterical. The hospital was a stressful place, and not a few found the other patients a trial to their already frayed nerves. But, as Balls-Headley's account of the long-term effects of 'ulceration of the cervix' reveals, emotional distress tended to be explained by physical illness rather than the other way around. Some of these 'social admissions' were kept in for weeks, being restored with potassium bromide, food and iron, and purified internally by enemas. And potassium bromide, a mild sedative, was almost routinely prescribed for all patients at the first medical examination. Of course the rest, food and iron did work wonders with those who were simply worn out. But some of the very young patients were seeking refuge from unwanted life commitments: one new housewife, a keen tea-drinker even though she lived in Melbourne's roughest quarter in Little Lonsdale Street, clearly disliked coitus from the beginning. To Dr Meyer she looked 'healthy and pink' and he did find a urethral caruncle, which when removed may have reduced some of her discomfort. Another young bride, married a month but pregnant rather longer, had come down with 'twitchings of the hands' five months before when she 'got a fright and jumped out of bed. Ten days ' bed rest, an aperient and pot. Bromide improved her twitchings significantly'. And some of those at work clearly hated the strains of domestic service or factory drudgery.[29]

urethtral caruncle: a small red fleshy swelling in the urethra

Many women clearly had had more to cope with than they could manage. Mrs C., a boot machinist from Collingwood, had had eight pregnancies between the ages of twenty-two and thirty-four, but in her last confinement she had suffered a bad haemorrhage. Her menses had stopped four years before, and a year ago she began to feel sick, retain fluid, vomit blood and become jaundiced. Her abdomen had so swollen with ascites, that she could hardly breathe. Her eyes were yellowish, as were her tongue and skin. They tapped her and drew off nearly twelve pints of greenish, yellow clear fluid, but she was dying of cirrhosis of the liver caused by alcoholism, and three weeks later she was dead at the age of thirty-nine. She was unusual to be married and employed — if these married women had children and paid employment in the 1880s it signified that they were desperate. The respectable often proudly insisted that they were their 'own housekeeper'.

Mrs B. S., aged twenty-seven, with three children, was near to a nervous breakdown when she was admitted in February 1888. She had been well until 'twelve months ago when through not being able to get proper nourishment she got gradually weak, with severe pains in back, lower part of abdomen, extending into the vagina'. The doctor described her as 'soft and anaemic'. After six days in bed she was 'not so easily frightened', and she stayed in for a fortnight's rest, food and iron. The nurses could be very attentive: old Miss Maria Saddler was the second oldest patient at sixty-three and so deaf she had to use a slate. Her deafness made her 'rather irritable and peculiar', but so also did her cancer of the uterus, yet she was still nursed with kindness. Not so lucky were those who were judged rough and unrespectable, but even the brazen barmaids of Little Lonsdale Street were described as 'emaciated' or 'anaemic', already worn out before they were half way into their twenties. The Women's Hospital case histories reveal the private suffering of poor women: those afflicted with poor reproductive health led lives of inner misery, of endless pain and suffering; those who remained well suffered almost as much from their unfettered fertility. Mrs A., a Scottish-born nurse of Carlton, married at eighteen, bore seventeen children and had two or three miscarriages: she came in for a growth in the urethra; Mrs D., an Irish-born housewife of Kilmore, bore fifteen children and suffered two miscarriages: she came in for a rectal polyp. Mrs McT., Scottish born of Williamstown, eleven children and three miscarriages, was let off less lightly for she was dying of cervical cancer: 'rather emaciated, no teeth' noted the doctor. Mrs T., a dressmaker of West Melbourne, had ten pregnancies between the ages of fifteen and thirty — she had cervicitis. And Mrs P., aged only thirty-eight of St Arnaud, had twelve children and six miscarriages, and for sixteen years she had been sick with the remnants of a puerperal infection: her condition had 'fallen away a good deal lately'. Her teeth were good in her lower left jaw, however. And poor Mrs M., a sempstress of St Kilda, born in Ireland and coming to Australia at the age of eighteen, had married late for the time at twenty-seven. In thirteen years she had six children and one miscarriage. She had always been well until that first confinement when she had forceps without chloroform and her perineum had torn right through to the anal sphincter. She had faecal incontinence for twelve years and yet borne five more children. She had 'got much thinner of late'. But the surgery failed, because the wound did not heal, and the wound did not heal because she got diarrhoea after the operation and it was contaminated. Mrs H. had come down from Cowra in New South Wales to have her complete uterine prolapse repaired. She had had four babies and all of them died. At least her operation worked and after a six-week convalescence, she was restored.

**Mrs D., adm.
12 July 1887** *RWHA*

Medicine is a clinical discipline even before it is a theoretical one. Doctors' daily experience of women patients was that they were too often sick, and while their resistance to much infectious disease was superior to that of males, they laboured under disturbances or accidents to their reproductive organs. Cancer seemed to be a disease of women rather than of men in nineteenth-century Australia (men's mortality from accident

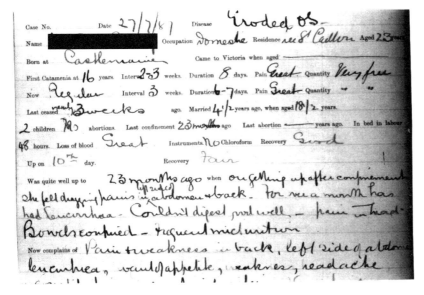

**Mrs C. C., adm.
27 July 1887** *RWHA*

and heart disease was very much higher).[30] But in women's reproductive health perhaps it is more important to comprehend the extent and nature of their morbidity in the past. In the 1880s women suffered greater mortality than did men during the childbearing years, but did better before and after. Their maternal mortality extended beyond the immediate events of childbed and the lying-in: young women who died of tuberculosis or pneumonia or typhoid or influenza were more likely to succumb because of the physical strains placed on them by their reproductive role. Many suffered from damage to the heart and to the kidneys from childhood infections — especially rheumatic fever — which compromised their reproductive health later. As Melbourne expanded and its drainage did not, many more women entered childbirth weakened by typhoid or dysentery, and died when they would otherwise survived. So much of women's reproductive health depended on the strength of their constitutions, and thus the poor — ill-nourished, over-worked, cold in winter and too hot in summer, frustrated and bored, and endlessly tired — fared worst of all. It constituted an associated or indirect maternal mortality and morbidity.

The doctors, when they philosophised, spoke from a daily immersion in sickness, dirt, pain and death. If they constructed females as sick, perhaps it is because that was what they saw. The great problem of late nineteenth-century gynaecology was why human reproduction caused so much pain and suffering. Surely the human race had somehow become unnatural if the natural functions of reproduction brought such sickness. Balls-Headley, in his *magnum opus*, a prolix exploration of *The Evolution of the Diseases of Women,* wondered if the sickness of women was in fact nature's method of population control. If women could have up to twenty pregnancies in their reproductive lives, well perhaps illness and damage were nature's way of preventing that. Balls-Headley and Jamieson have achieved historiographical notoriety beyond Australian shores for their respective warnings of the dangers of excessive brain work for young women (especially of would-be female medical students), but they were saying rather more than that.[31] The honoraries of the hospital discussed these issues at length, both in the Medical Society and privately. They were united in their condemnation of tight lacing and of the lack of physical exercise among young ladies, as they were of the excessive standing and heavy work of working-class girls. Balls-Headley:

> The second class of women compete for a living in two ways, mental and physical. If her work be mental, she is in special competition with men in large numbers, with the prejudice of custom against her; and therefore to attain her end, she must excel, which infers excessive work with its disadvantage to the female. If physical she is liable to be affected by a combination of overwork, whether constant standing or bending or mental strain, late hours, deficient sleep, of which she requires so much, defective meals or unsuitable food or drink; and in Australia, particularly by the drinking of excessive quantities of very hot strong tea as a nerve stimulant; whence result undue brain-waste, debility, loss of appetite, constipation and anaemia. With them, too, the wearing of stays and deficiency of marriage at suitable ages detract from healthy womanhood.[32]

Balls-Headley also, with sentiments not unfamiliar among later medical practitioners, blamed the rise of socialism and trade unionism for vitiating manliness, and thereby husbandly duty. The agents of the sickness of

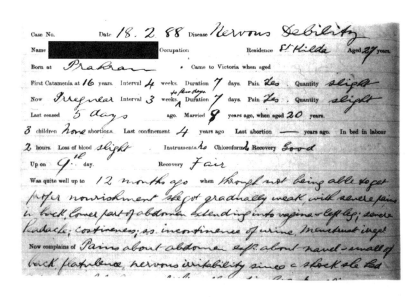

**Mrs B. S., adm.
18 February 1888** *RWHA*

women, again, were masculine moral deficiencies. But clearly women's lives and modern civilisation must also be at fault if women were so sick.

    Women coped best with reproduction if they were well fed, rested, clean, loved, physically athletic and did not wear stays, the doctors said. If the race was to be preserved, then women needed to be healthy and the best specimens among them should breed the most. Jamieson, as a medical philosopher, was more moderate and reasoned. He told his university class in 1887 that women, especially in a modern, civilised society, lived longer than men but were more often sick, and that it was their reproductive function that brought them down:

> There is danger resulting from the possession of specialised organs, such as the uterus and mamma, working sometimes at high pressure, and again, as regards function, almost in a latent condition. Perhaps it is partly this intermittent activity which causes the special liability of these organs to be affected with malignant disease in its various forms.

Normal married life, therefore, imposed 'a burden of disease and death' that made public life impossible. Further, if the best and most intelligent women entered public and professional life, they could not also bear children which would then deprive society of its most valuable maternal stock.[33] The only real solution lay in birth control, a measure no doctor mindful of his public reputation and private practice would dare to promote. Women themselves, however, had begun to take matters into their own hands.

Patient Histories

This small sample of case histories brings the women to life.

Mrs Margaret McT, Bootmaker, Clifton Hill
aged 48

> *First catamenia:* 14
> *Now:* irregular
> *Married:* 31 years ago aged 17
> 7 children, last born 12 years ago
> 2 abortions, last $1\frac{1}{2}$ years ago, 2–3 hours labour, well after 14 days
> *Well* until 30 years ago when first child was born, after which treated for ulcer of womb. Second child born nine years after when passage had to be cut to allow it to pass. Thirteen months after third child was born, after which she was confined to bed for 3 months for infection of womb and complete loss of power in L. leg which was much swollen. Other confinements normal except has had flooding after all. Been in hospital 4 times, twice operated on.
> *Now* dragging pains, sleeplessness, frontal headache
> *General Condition:* Well-nourished—been getting stout during last 3 years
> *Cervix:* ulcerated
> *Fundus:* tender in anterior fornix
> *Dr Balls-Headley's Case Book, no. 1, adm. 29 July 1885*

Mrs. K. D., teacher, State School (rural)
aged 45

1st Catamenia: 16
Now: haemorrhage
Married: 27 years ago aged 17
11 children, last 3 years ago, 2 hours, moderate loss, up on 5th day
2 abortions, 8 or 9 years ago
Well until 18 months ago when she began to break down with symptoms as below: she was nursing at the time and lost her husband by sudden death, flooded then followed discharge from vagina, now discharge between periods and too frequent menses.
Weakness and pain across back and in leg occasionally
General condition: good but thinner than she was.
Emmet, disch. 26 May 1886
Dr Rowan's Case Book, no. 1, adm. 11 March 1886

Mrs M. H., housewife, Albert Park
aged 35

Married: 15 years ago aged 20
6 children, last $1^2/_3$ years ago, very good
3 abortions, last 3 years ago
Well until birth of 4th child — she fell away in health, felt very nervous and became disinclined for work. There was a profuse discharge from the vagina and she was treated for ulceration. Three miscarriages but carried last child to term.
General condition: sanguinous, bilious temperament, well nourished
Abdomen: lax, linex Albicantes [stretch marks]
Went away (while being prepared for operation) her baby being very ill.
Dr Balls-Headley's Case Book, no. 1, adm. 7 July 1885

L. R., waitress, Carlton
aged 21

1st Catamenia: 16
Now: regular, not so much pain, scanty
single
no pregnancies
Well until 2 years ago when patient complained of pains in lower part of abdomen and back — had a strain just before this and was in great abdominal pain and passed blood by the bowel. Was in hospital in March and went out in May — at this time had pain, tenderness and swelling in L. side of abdomen.
Now some enlargement of L. side of abdomen — pain, tenderness and throbbing there — frequent and painful micturition — can't lie except on back. No leucorrhoea — sweats at night.
General condition: rather thin and drawn
Treatment: 12/9 needed morphia to sleep...had pyrexia from 12/9 to 23/9 [raised temperature]

Operation: 24/9 Patient having been prepared for operation by liquid diet — warm bath — sponging abdomen with corrosive. Hst Dom. Alb., enema and vaginal injection, she was removed to special ward. Urine drawn off just before operation.

<u>Patient</u> anaesthetised with chlo. by Dr Burke, and then kept under by ACE mixture.

Operation at 4pm by Dr Rowan, assisted by Dr Balls-Headley and RMO. Incision made in Linea Alba — bleeding points force pressed. Peritoneum picked up and divided on a director, operator's carbolised hand introduced into Abdominal cavity where the tumour was plainly felt. While trying to free it from adhesions some most foetid pus escaped. The abdominal and peritoneal incisions were then enlarged to admit the hand, and after much trouble the tumour was brought to the surface and found to be a dilated fallopian tube containing foul pus and much new tissue. The Omentum was so adherent as to be part and parcel of it. This was separated carefully by the fingers and wrapped up in hot flannels — the growth was then transfixed and ligatured with carbolised silk as near the uterus as possible — the ragged portions of the Omentum were then carefully ligatured and many portions by carbolised silk. The pedicle was cut short and returned to the abdominal cavity. On the Right side an irregular semi-broken down mass was discovered in site of R. ovary and tube — this was also transfixed, ligatured and the pedicle dropped back in the abdomen.

The abdominal cavity was then sponged out as far as possible — it was then well washed out with warm carbolised water and then sponged clean. The abdominal wound was closed by deep silver wire and superficial horsehair sutures — a Reith's glass tube being inserted into Douglas' pouch between the two lowest sutures. Idoform dusted on — CW — strapping and flannel binder — sponge over mouth of tube and this wrapped up in oiled silk.

Patient was sick twice during operation and the wound had to be supported with hot sponges.

Put to bed with hot bottles and half grain morphia Supps given.

Operation took about 1 hour and 10 minutes.

Slept a little up to 7.30 pm when the tube was examined and 4 drchms of clear thin red fluid drawn off.

10 pm 3 v. fluid drawn from tube. Rectal tube used and Foments applied.

25/9 12 am 99.6–26–125/98.2–20–120/98.6–32–130/99.6–138

26/9   99–18–120/100.4–18–89/98.4–18–118/98.6–16–118

27/9   99.6–132/99.2–17–127/100.6–15–130/103–160

25/9 Vomited some watery fluid - 3 drachms of fluid drawn off from tube at 3 and 7 pm — tube washed out during the day (every 6 hours) with warm carbolised water till it became clear — in evening discharge was brownish red and offensive — Vomiting of dark gummous fluid commenced — Enema given regularly of Brandy with milk or beef tea — every 4 hours

26/9 Much dirty discharge from tube and dark vomit — Some distension of abdomen

27/9 Much dirty discharge all day — Vomiting almost incessant.

<u>Died at 10 pm</u>

Dr Rowan's Case Book, no. 2, adm. 11 September 1888

Mrs Thunderbolt, domestic, Walhalla
aged 24, born Carlton

1st Catamenia: 13, now fairly regular, some pain, lasts 2–3 days
Married 8 years ago aged 16
2 children, last 5 years ago, instruments used for first child 7 years ago
Some abortions, last 8 months ago, normal loss, up on 11th day, recovery fair
Well until last confinement when flooding came on and had difficult and painful micturition. Bearing down sensation in vagina, pain in lumbar region, also hypogastric and both iliac regions—Free discharge at times
Now losing some blood p.v. nearly every week—Pain under L. breast, Leucorrhoea at times, frequent and painful micturition, Menses regular until last month when she was unwell for 14 days right off and marital intercourse brings on loss of blood.
General condition: good
Cervix uteri: lacerated bilaterally, partially united on Left side, ulcerated round edges of laceration
Treatment: rest in bed—aperient
Hot irrigation.
9/10: Left hospital at her own wish (Couldn't bear being separated from her husband).
Dr Balls-Headley's Case Book, no. 2, adm. 6 October 1887

Mrs C. F. home duties, Sunbury
aged 60, born Ireland

1st Catmenia: 11
Menses ceased 26 years ago
10 children, last 26 years ago, never instruments, recovery always good
1 abortion (of twins)
Well until 12 months ago—fell on her right hip, was very weak, has been almost helpless for last 6 months
Now general weakness, pains in back and right leg
General conditon: old and feeble
Uterus: prolapsed
Treatment: to wear ring pessary
Dr Fetherston's Case Book, no. 2, adm. 21 February 1890

Mrs E. D., 'Invalid', Richmond
aged 44

Married 27 years ago aged 17
12 children, last 2 years ago — instruments all confinements
9 abortions
Well: never well since last confinement — has not been able to do any work, general weakness
Now: general weakness, pains in back (sacrum), inguinal region and down thighs, headache
General condition: weak, delicate
Os: lacerated and congested
Cervix: blue
Fundus: uterus heavy
Treatment: rest, tonics, Glycerine plugs, hot douching with occasional scarifying of os.
Dr Fetherston's Case Book, no. 2, adm. 9 September 1889

S.M., barmaid, Melbourne
aged 23, born Bacchus Marsh

1st Catamenia: 16, now regular, some pain, free loss
single
1 child, 12 months ago, in bed in labour 4 days, no instruments, chloroform for manual removal of placenta; up on 28th day, recovery fair
no abortions
Well until time of accouchement, when after a long labour and an adhered placenta, she had some pelvic inflammation. Ever since then she has had pain in L. side of abdomen and at hypogastrium. No leucorrhoea. Bad for 3 weeks now. Caught cold when menses were on.
Now pain over the abdomen especially on Left side — also some in back. Tenderness in L. ovarian and hypogastric region. Painful and difficult micturition. Loss of appetite.
General condition: rather emaciated
Diagnosis: pelvic cellulitis
Treatment: rest in bed, Poultices, Glycerine plugs and hot irrigation.
Discharged 27 January after 25 days medical treatment
Dr Balls-Headley's Case Book, no. 2, adm. 2 January 1888

The Natural and the Unnatural 1887–1914

7

The Women's Hospital, with its university connection, was now the dominant specialist women's hospital in Australasia. And when Melbourne hosted the first Intercolonial Medical Congress in 1887, Dr Balls-Headley starred, with sixty medical men cramming into the Women's operating theatre to watch him perform. The medical community delighted in this opportunity 'to shake off a little of the narrow provincialism which we are all apt to suffer from . . .'[34] The chairman of the Gynaecology section, Dr Joseph Foreman, from the Prince Alfred Hospital, Sydney, gave a historical review of the discipline, and reflected on the inadequacies of antisepsis and the superiority of 'extreme cleanliness'; on the evils of tight lacing, higher education and overcrowded homes and workplaces, and on the virtues of physical exercise for young women. Then he came to the vexed question of 'oophorectomy'. The initial horror at its introduction had abated, he argued; it was appropriate in cases of diseased ovaries, but it was indefensible as a cure for 'nervous affections'. He remained puzzled, however, over what to do with prolapsed ovaries: 'the intense misery they cause is sometimes unbearable', but should they be removed or repositioned? If healthy, then the latter was the better course, he believed; if diseased, removal by a vaginal rather than abdominal operation was safer.[35]

oophorectomy: surgical removal of an ovary

His successor in the next congress two years later, the able New Zealand doctor Ferdinand Batchelor from Dunedin, took this problem of the diseased and displaced uterus and its appendages as the subject of his presidential address. Batchelor was certainly no victim of 'narrow provincialism' and he treated his peers to a world-class analysis of pelvic infection. He suggested a reconception. He argued that the gynaecologist kept himself in the darkness if he relied upon the speculum, the sound and the finger. A bi-manual pelvic exploration, however, could reveal the inter-relatedness of diseased pelvic organs. Those who relied on the speculum saw only the lacerated and infected cervix, and did not see that, while it may have been an entry point of disease after a confinement, 'cervical

bi-manual pelvic examination: using one hand in the vagina and the other externally to palpate the abdomen ulceration' was not the patient's worst problem: the real mischief lay deeper in the pelvis, in the appendages of the ovaries, but above all, in the fallopian tubes.

> Possibly some of you may think I have a hobby, and am riding it to death, but when I see, as doubtless many of you see, cases of oophoritis, and pelvic peritonitis, and salpingitis, which have been treated for months, and sometimes years by pessaries, applications to the cervix, intra-uterine stems, and what not besides, and the true cause of the patient's sufferings not even suspected; and when we remember that until six or seven years ago, the most eminent leaders in gynaecology throughout the world had apparently altogether overlooked a disease viz. salpingitis and its complications, which we now recognise almost daily by this method of examination alone, I feel I need make no apology for dwelling thus at length on the absolute necessity there exists for every one who attempts any gynaecological work whatever, to perfect himself in this most important method of investigation.[36]

The other source of illumination was the laparotomy — the abdominal exploration operation. Batchelor had sharp criticisms of the American Thomas Emmet whose procedure for the resection of a lacerated cervix had been the favourite operation of Doctors Burke, Rowan, Fetherston

Infirmary medical staff, 1897
Back: Dr R. H. Fetherston, Dr Ward Farmer, Dr George Horne, Dr F. W. Morton, Dr J. D. K. Scott (resident surgeon) Front: Dr Rothwell Adam, Dr M. U. O'Sullivan, Dr W. Balls-Headley, Dr Felix Meyer, Dr Dunbar Hooper *RWHA*

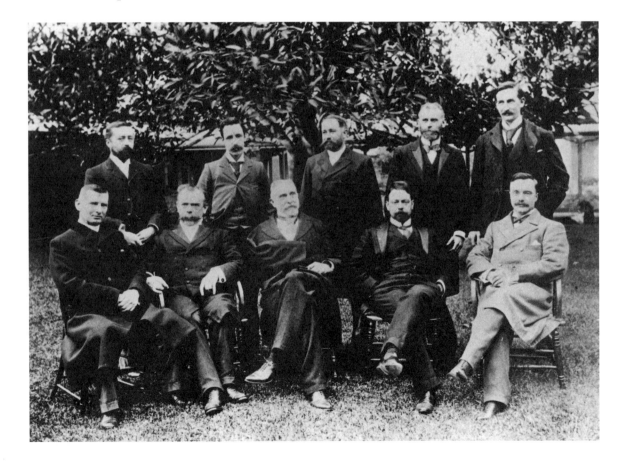

and Balls-Headley at the Women's Hospital for the past decade. Emmet had formed his theories before the laparotomy became safer. From abdominal explorations the great Lawson Tait realised the significance of tubal disease and the inflammation which spread through the perito-neum, producing the dense, tender masses of adhesions which pushed the uterus out of position. It had seemed logical before that, when examination by the uterine sound revealed a uterus oddly flexed and the patient in much pain, that the malposition was the cause of the pain. Hence that 'Victorian speciality' — the retroverted uterus. Batchelor also deplored the fashion for hysterical ovarian disease and those doctors who profited by it; the removal of ovaries for hysterical conditions, he insisted, was as indefensible as the excision of a hysterical knee-joint. However, the removal of pus-filled tubes and genuinely diseased ovaries brought the most wonderful relief to women incapacitated by pelvic pain, for it was now clear that 'the most common causes of severe pain and chronic suffering with the diseases peculiar to women are morbid conditions of the ovaries, Fallopian tubes, and surrounding pelvic peritoneum'.

This new comprehension of pelvic infection and its adhesions threat-ened a number of fondly-held and lucrative theories about diseases of the uterus and its appendages, and was likely to meet with understandable resistance. And it did, the very next day, when Felix Meyer, not long elected an honorary at the Women's, presented a paper arguing that far too many of the diseases peculiar to women were the result of 'unscien-tific' and hasty obstetrics. Meyer was an environmentalist also, but of a more subtle and scientific kind. Obstetrics could not be left to the ministrations of 'what is often sneeringly termed old women's work' because 'the conditions of life . . . bring about so many deviations from the natural process, as to render it very often pathological' and that it was the task of obstetrics, more than any other in medical science, 'to bridge with the smallest span the distance between the natural and the unnatural'.[37] Those who rendered the natural unnatural, tried to deliver before the cervix had fully dilated, and especially those who introduced forceps too soon or unnecessarily, had much to answer for:

> If the use of forceps is abused in the first stage, it is much more so in the second. The how and when of their application cannot be taught theor-etically; but this is certain, that to their misuse and unskilful application are due, very often, lacerations of the perineum, rectocoele, cystocoele, vesico-vaginal and recto-vaginal fistula, pelvic cellulitis and peritonitis — the latter very commonly the first link in a chain of pathological process, leading up to ovarian and tubal disease. Formidable as this list appears, it is a true bill; and in taking the history of every woman who attended either as an in-patient or out-patient during my time of residence at the Women's Hospital, how often has the stereotyped reply come, 'I have never been well since my first confinement; I was hurt with instruments'. I yield to none in my appreciation of the value of forceps, but in the hands of many, they are a thing of evil.[38]

rectocele: bulging or pouching of the rectum into the posterior wall of the vagina from uterine prolapse; cystocele prolapse of the base of the bladder

He recommended the use of anaesthesia, the drawing off of all urine in preparation, and the careful removal of blades to allow the uterus a role

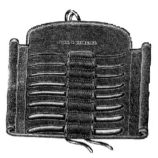

Hegar's dilators, set of eight in khaki drill roll
Allen & Hanbury's, p. 438

dilatation and curettage: an operation in which the cervix (neck) of the uterus is dilated, using an instrument called a dilator and the lining (endometrium) of the uterus is lightly scraped off with a curette.

in the final expulsion of the child. He had been greatly interested in Dr Batchelor's ideas, but did want to impress upon his audience that there were indeed lacerations of the cervix which were not secondary to graver internal disease and which deserved operative intervention.

As was his wont, Dr Balls-Headley opened the discussion in order to control it, and he chided Dr Meyer for raising the question of the lacerated cervix for it was outside the scope of the paper. He did believe that, in certain cases, disease of the ovaries and appendages was due to parturition, but lacerations of the cervix were 'a wise provision of Nature for the prevention of too many children' — that is, again, nature's contraceptive was the sickness of women. Dr Batchelor cut in to disagree with Dr Balls-Headley; their views were diametrically opposed, 'with all due deference'. Others disagreed with him also. Dr Foreman reported that a lacerated cervix was not a bar to impregnation, but there was another issue raised by Dr Meyer which no one else had canvassed. Women who had received an Emmet repair of the cervix, suffered difficulty with the cervix being unable to dilate fully; that is, they were in danger of a full rupture of the cervix if not the uterus itself. Meyer emerged from the fray with dignity.

These exchanges marked a turning point in the evolution of gynaecology and the scientific understanding of 'women's troubles', as well as the medical politics of the Women's Hospital. But what was happening in the wards? Dunbar Hooper was also now a member of the honorary staff, and he remained, like Meyer, a student of his own medical records. His case book from June 1894 until March 1898 contains 191 cases, for which Dr Robin Bell, a medical epidemiologist, in consultation with Dr James Smibert, could make 163 probable diagnoses. Fully one third of the 163 cases fell into the Pelvic Inflammatory Disease (PID) category, by far the largest single condition suffered by the patients. Twenty-five of these fifty-three cases were clearly the result of parturition, another nine were likely venereal infections, but of the remainder it is too difficult to say. Twenty of the cases received surgery, but only five were also given an Emmet repair; now the operation of choice was a Dilatation and Curettage (D & C), as it was for almost everything else that involved the uterus. Ovaries were only removed in cases of ovarian tumour, not yet for 'salpingitis'. For the rest of the admissions, prolapse was common, tuberculosis and hydatids now more likely to be admitted to a general hospital. Cancer was problematic. It was seen as a 'women's disease' rather than a men's, because many of the carcinogens which endanger men in particular, were still less significant in private habits and the workplace than today. It was also seen as a disease of the poor and the sexually active. Women, including quite young women, fell victim to cervical cancer and, when older, cancer of the body of the uterus and of the breast. But as men and women began to live longer, more contracted the disease.[39]

Even so, there was no question that bad or non-existent obstetrics had caused the sickness of many of these women, and the Women's Hospital, because of its teaching role, took very seriously its responsibilities to the practice of obstetrics both within and without its walls. Felix Meyer's position as an honorary, backed with his extended clinical experience at the hospital, gave him authority to speak as he did on the abuse of forceps, but this role as a monitor of the profession locked the hospital into careful, even conservative practice. The inevitable shortage of money for a charitable institution similarly drove the medical and nursing staff to work always on a shoe-string: so that what was done was the cheapest and simplest option. The wards, especially on the midwifery side, were always crowded and always short-staffed.[40] The financial stringencies of the 1890s prompted the Board to take risks like replacing a qualified (and therefore salaried) midwife as the night nurse with an unpaid pupil midwife, and yet the Visitors' Committee complained when few nurses were to be found on the wards during their inspections. At the same time the Victorian Government attempted in 1896 to force hospitals to observe the eight-hour day for nursing staff.[41] There were accidents and disasters and nearly always the cause was revealed to be the consequence of too much to do and too few to do it. In August 1899 an eighteen-year-old single girl from Camperdown was admitted under Dunbar Hooper's care for a diseased left ovary and tube. She had been in pain for three years and now she had stopped menstruating. She was always feeling exhausted. She was very ill and the doctors advanced the operation by twenty-four hours, but the nursing staff were not warned. The morning of the day before she asked to see a priest; the nurse was so busy she forgot to pass the request on to Sister until late in the day. The priest was never called and the next day she was relieved of a cystic ovary the size of a mandarin. Six days after the operation she suddenly died, without taking Communion. Her family and Father O'Connell were out-raged and complained to the Board, so that the nursing staff were rep-rimanded. (The tragedy had a distressing footnote: Dr Mollison's post-mortem revealed that she had died of heart disease and an embolism in the lung: 'All the organs showed congenital syphilis'.)[42] And for all the national, even international repute the Women's Hospital's honorary staff now enjoyed, it was a pinched, mean and shabby place, where 'good care' was efficiently delivered to patients' bodies, sometimes at the loss of their dignity and peace of mind. The few cases of complaint brought by former patients who had the courage or the outside help to brave the Board, reveal the hospital's 'Dickensian' culture. In November 1898 Miss Ellen Maher, with the support of the Infant Asylum, alleged that her savings had been stolen by a nurse:

> It was stated that the infant had been sent clothed only in a cotton gown, no flannel or binder, but a small quantity of cotton wool on the infant's chest.
>
> It was also stated that the mother was not in a fit state to be discharged from this hospital.

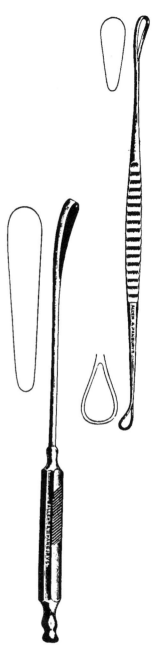

Sims's sharp and blunt uterine curettes
Allen & Hanbury's, p. 441

Nurse Wells defended herself. The baby had been wrapped in its mother's cape; there had been adequate cotton wool around the child, and when she had given the mother her purse, she had said that all the money was there. The matter was never quite resolved, and the Ladies' Committee asked for better security for patients' possessions.[43] That same month a woman died of a ruptured uterus because the hospital was slow to find an honorary and the honorary in question was censured for not attending

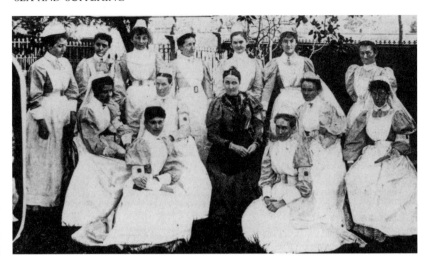

the hospital at once. The honorary responded by calling for a special operating theatre for the midwifery wards, because operative emergencies were still conducted in the busy labour ward.[44]

If poverty were to remain the hospital's defence for its rough efficiency, there was also a more insidious deterioration in the psychological and social management of the patients. As the hospital grew, the face-to-face relationships between all staff, patients and the managing committees inevitably became more distant and more 'routinised' than they had been in Tracy's time. Fewer people came to know each other well. Nursing staff turned over so fast and worked such long hours and enjoyed so little recreation, that a body of common feeling among them was difficult, and those who did stay developed fiefdoms that they defended fiercely. As the antisepsis and asepsis disciplines imposed more rules, there was more opportunity for 'disobedience' and censure. The hospital inevitably became more authoritarian, and overworked people became unavoidably crisp and short, brooking no nonsense, tolerating no delay, forgiving no sloppiness. Patients were slapped, forbidden to sit up in bed, bullied and abused. The good order of the ward became more important than the comfort of the patients. Poor female patients were too often depersonalised, and while some of that was simply the result of a staff under stress, the agent of part of it was the march of medical science itself.

In the twenty-five years from the end of the 1880s through to the outbreak of World War I the new science of bacteriology transformed the medical understanding of the agents and the processes of infection. And once those agents and processes were identified, blame could be apportioned and judgements made about the behaviour and prospects of the afflicted. There were two constellations of 'women's diseases' which came under moral scrutiny: disease and disability contracted from sexual intercourse or from a deliberate attempt to destroy an unwanted foetus. These were medical and moral problems which would dominate the work of the Infirmary for the next half century until the discovery and development of antibiotics. These changes to the medical culture did not emerge instantly once Pasteur's work was broadcast; rather, they came gradually, timed by the individual discoveries of infecting agents: the spirochaete of syphilis, the gonococcus of gonorrhoea, the bacillus of tuberculosis, the streptococcus and the staphylococcus. Second came the discovery that both syphilis and gonorrhoea had latent phases where the disease was apparently cured, but in fact was only awaiting the infliction of even worse damage. The concepts of infectiousness and congenital blight therefore raised difficult moral issues about the civil rights of the sick: should the syphilitic be allowed to have children, should the tubercular be permitted to cough all over their babies, should the infected be incarcerated for the protection of the uninfected? What moral power did medical knowledge confer on doctors; and what did this mean to the sick and suffering women who found a bed in the Women's Hospital?

In 1892 Dr C. H. Mollison replaced Dr George Syme as the consultant pathologist for the Women's Hospital. Mollison was already appointed to the Melbourne Hospital and he soon became the leading pathologist in Victoria. Between 1897 and 1912, 77 279 medical specimens were examined in his bacteriological laboratory at the University of Melbourne, with a phenomenal growth in the last three years, where there were more examinations done than in the preceding thirteen. That dramatic leap was in part, but not entirely, due to the introduction of the Wassermann test for syphilis. In 1895 the medical school started six week crash courses in bacteriology for graduate doctors, and in 1898 the honorary staff petitioned the Board for a new bacteriological laboratory and pathological museum — a wish that would take painfully long to fulfil.[45]

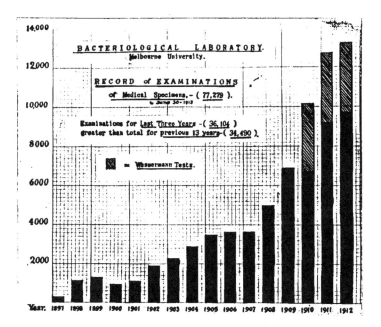

Bacteriological Laboratory, University of Melbourne Record of examinations of medical specimens, 1897–1912
Felix Meyer Collection, Syphilis box, University of Melbourne Archives

Yet as important as syphilis and syphilology were to become, gonorrhoea played a crucial role in the reframing of sick women during the 1890s. While a venereal and unpleasant disease, gonorrhoea had so far provoked none of the horror of syphilis. In 1890 Rothwell Adam opened a paper before the Medical Society of Victoria with,

I should perhaps ask pardon for taking up the time of the Association
with so trite a subject as gonorrhoea in the female, but since Noeggerath
enunciated his well-known views in 1872, gonorrhoea has gradually
become recognised as playing an important part, if not the most important
part, in the causation of acute disease of the uterine appendages.[46]

The difficulty was that gonorrhoea can be almost asymptomatic in
women, especially in those with poor hygiene. Once it was known to
have a latent phase and to continue to do its mischief in the fallopian
tubes, it took on a far more malevolent aspect, in Dr M. U. O'Sullivan's
words: 'Claiming a remote antiquity, it would seemed to have gained
fresh strength from generation to generation, until today it has become
a veritable scourge amongst our womankind'.[47]

O'Sullivan was now chairman of the Honorary Staff at the Women's
Hospital, and speaking in 1896, as president of the Victorian Branch of
the British Medical Association. He surveyed the new discoveries of
bacteriology, the current thinking on malignant tumours, and then
warmed to philosophical reflections on the role of bad heredity (the cause
of 'much of the disease which afflicts civilised communities'), and the
sickness of women (which had many causes, none of them being excessive
childbearing). He deplored 'the ever-increasing invalidism which would
seem to have become the heritage of civilised woman'. Women should
not indulge in bicycle riding, higher education or sewing with machines.
Bicycle riding through crowded city streets over-stimulated the mind,
just as did intellectual pursuits, 'and remembering the close kinship existing between the brain and the generative organs, the almost inevitable
result must be increased instability of nerve power and derangement of
uterine function'.[48]

But Dr O'Sullivan also argued that some of women's ailments had a
more specific aetiology: gonorrhoea was now known to be one, as was
criminal abortion, which 'performed generally by illiterate and unclean
charlatans of either sex, claims numberless victims, or consigns them to
permanent invalidism'. But worst of all was the 'prevention of conception',
for this 'lamentable Neo Malthusian practice has found its way into all
classes of society'. He condemned the contrivances and artifices resorted
to, the frustration of natural law, the degradation of the ethical standard
of the 'sexual relations obtaining in civilised life'. Why is it, he asked,
that so many women under forty are sick or sickly? It is because they
'offend against the laws of nature by deliberately impeding their sexual
organs in the due discharge of their allotted functions'. For O'Sullivan,
a Catholic, this was sin, and sickness was its just retribution. (O'Sullivan,
however, did induce abortions for medical reasons, such as in a thirty-
four-year-old para twelve, mother of eight, who had suffered 'a severely
lacerated perineum and cervix for fourteen years'.)[49]

O'Sullivan had many supporters among non-Catholics, and similar
notions of the natural and the unnatural pervaded medical discourse.
Even for secular patriots, the deliberate restriction of population in a new
country was a heresy, and yet the sick and suffering women crying for
relief were the victims of their uncontrolled fertility and their poverty.
Most of the gynaecologists treating them were entirely absorbed in the

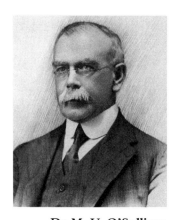

Dr M. U. O'Sullivan
RWHA

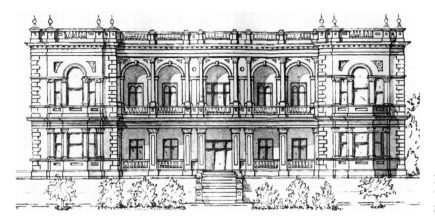

Dr O'Sullivan's house, 'Eildon', Grey Street, St Kilda *RWHA*

pathology of reproduction. The social dimension to the sickness of women depended on society's recognition of natural law: that women are there to reproduce the species and men are there to impregnate them, and later protect them as they brought forth and raised the next generation. This biological burden was so complex and so precious that women had to be relieved of all other public burdens so that their energies could be entirely devoted to maternity. Doctors were there to intervene when nature took the wrong course, but they were not there to wrest control from nature. Sex was part of nature, and as long as it conformed to the 'laws of physical life', it was a life-force and good. Thwarted sex produced illness also, therefore the celibate woman was unnatural. When such women appeared in the hospital, the doctors took careful note of their 'depression of spirits' and Dr O'Sullivan and Dr Morton both performed surgery for a retroverted or prolapsed uterus in single women who claimed to have never been pregnant and were suffering from depression.[50] Many of these celibate women gave a history of invalidism since adolescence; and a significant number were teachers and governesses, so reduced in their circumstances as to be 'distressed' and within the income restrictions of a charity hospital. But denial of full sexual function resulted in disease, the doctors insisted — cystic ovaries and uterine fibroids, the fruit of the 'disappointed womb'.

Then there were those who transgressed both nature's and God's laws. One unmarried schoolteacher aged thirty was admitted in 1907 with an infection after using a vaginal douche the Thursday before: 'she had an attack of acute pain across the lower abdomen' which made her 'double up'. Her love affair was scarcely happy, and the doctor found her 'anaemic, not too well nourished'. She had an infection, so Dr O'Sullivan performed a D & C, and swabbed out the uterus with pure carbolic and alcohol, all without an anaesthetic.[51] Miss N. R. aged just twenty-one from Northcote, was delivered of a macerated seven month foetus in the Midwifery wards at the age of nineteen: she had then been covered with syphilitic condylomata which 'soon cleared up under Hg [mercury] treatment'. Fifteen months later she was back: she had been well until her last period, which had been 'very little' so she 'took a powder to bring on her courses'. Stricken with acute pain in the lower abdomen, shivering fits and vomiting, she had post-abortal sepsis, but lived to be discharged three weeks later. Her nursing notes were scanty, a sign that the staff found her unacceptable.[52] Most of the syphilitics were young, perhaps pretty, certainly naive, and therefore easy prey to 'rakes' whose promiscuity exposed them to infection. Others may have been seduced or procured by syphilitic men in the hope that intercourse with a virgin might cure them. Another syphilitic patient was a nineteen-year-old tailoress, and she already had pelvic inflammatory disease: at least she was unlikely to ever risk danger from septic abortion for she was surely infertile already.[53] And Mrs A. P.'s marriage was off to a bad start: she had had a yellow discharge for a year, had married six months ago and now was covered with condylomata: she was given a right partial oophorectomy. She was twenty-one.[54] By 1909 the staff were instructed to wear gloves when treating Mrs F. K. aged twenty-nine, mother of five, and covered with a 'hard, nodular, tender' rash on the vulva which was to be shaved and bathed with 1 in 4000 perchloride of hydrogen.[55]

The gravest contravention of the natural was the deliberate and criminal induction of abortion. Urban Australians began their fertility transition a decade later than the English and the Scots, but the birth rate was falling significantly by the 1890s, receiving a further blow from the 1890s depression. The women who reached childbearing age during the 1890s were to prove to be the least married in modern Australian history, but the very poor were in fact the least likely to be practising contraception.[56] To use condoms or pessaries, women and their partners had to know how and where to buy them as well as be able to afford them. Very few doctors would help. The women of North Melbourne in the 1890s were blessed with the presence in the Errol Street shopping centre of Mrs Brettena Smyth, who sold devices and offered advice from her draper's shop, wrote books and pamphlets, and gave public lectures. A widow, six feet tall and a superb speaker, she longed to become a doctor but was rejected as a candidate by the university.[57] Andrade's Bookshop also sold pamphlets and various health and contraceptive products but the bohemian radical sub-culture of Melbourne was scarcely representative. Condoms were very expensive for the passionate, caps were useless for women with prolapses and had to be fitted properly or they didn't work. The poor and the ignorant who wanted to avoid pregnancy and who had patent tubes and healthy uteri, had to resort to the time-honoured practices of abstinence, withdrawal and abortion.

The national demographic data shows that family limitation began with women deciding that they had had enough children and thereafter preventing pregnancy. Most women by the 1890s began childbearing as soon as they commenced sexual relations, had a number of children close together, then stopped. The gynaecological survey of the Women's patients confirms that pattern. The question is, *how* did they stop becoming pregnant. The stiking fact is that once they stopped, they stopped completely — few had 'accidents', that is few later pregnancies separated by a significant gaps. Since mechanical contraceptives were not only expensive and hard to find, they were also unreliable, this suggests that barrier contraception was not significant in working-class marriages of the 1890s and 1900s. Withdrawal also was apt to fail. Abstinence, therefore, seems to have been unhappily common: women were tired, unwell and cross, they

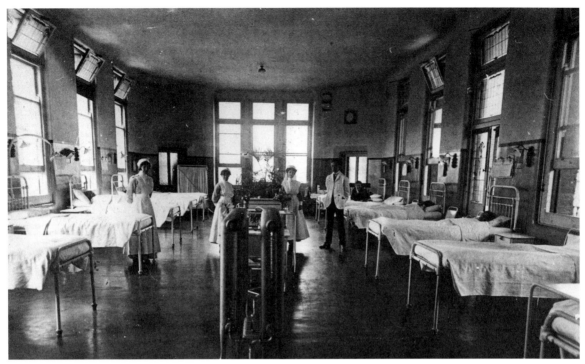

Infirmary ward, *c.* 1912
RWHA

had 'had enough' and their men were expected to find consolation in beer and betting. Their medical attendants often assumed that once a woman reached her late thirties and early forties, her sexual life was over. Older women were not sexual beings and certain medical decisions were to be made in that mistaken belief until after World War II. (Dr Gytha Betheras can recall older gynaecologists admitting that when they performed a Manchester repair at the Women's Hospital, they deliberately made the vagina too small to permit intercourse, just to ensure that their working-class patients would not have another pregnancy and need another repair.[58]) Even among the better-off, the maturing into being a matron — a mature mother and eventually a grandmother — was assumed to mark the end of a woman's own sexual desires and desirability. Most women put on fat and became heavy of limb and face: (they were difficult to nurse, particularly in the labour ward because of their bulk). That middle-age signalled the loss of libido was of course not true, and one wonders whether doctors viewed their own wives in that light, but when it came to other men's wives, especially those of men who were shiftless, drinkers, bashers and poor providers, it was a different matter. When the women took matters into their own hands and refused to have 'any more to do with it', they exerted considerable power, as a number of historians have demonstrated.[59]

The British historian Simon Szreter has also raised the issue of infrequency of intercourse as one way the British people effected their fertility transition from the 1880s onwards. He cites new medical research which has found that occasional intercourse so statistically reduces the chance of conception that the 'once-a-month' or 'once-a-fortnight' couple inevitably spaced their family or stopped having children altogether. This

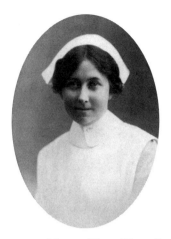

**Nurse Mary Hassall
(Mrs Eiseman) in 1909**
RWHA

was not total abstinence but rather a culture of abstinence of which sex was only one part along with the moderation of alcohol, gambling and spending on pleasure.[60] The culture of abstinence rose with the rising respectability of the urban working class, a newly ordered, rational and premeditated private life made posssible by the increase in regular over casual employment.[61]

The other way in which women took matters into their own hands was to induce an abortion. The induction of abortion is an ancient practice: powerful emetics and drugs like ergot known to cause contractions have long been used, and were advertised in newspapers and sold by chemists and shady midwives everywhere. In fact the one form of fertility control that *was* widely broadcast and within the reach of even the poorest was abortion. Very old women still until this day, when asked about birth control, sometimes assume that you mean abortion, not the full range of practices and methods to prevent or terminate conception. A few doctors were willing to perform terminations, and certainly among the honoraries at the Women's Hospital, Felix Meyer for one did so for private patients. Brave doctors could perform discreet and safe terminations under the label of a therapeutic D & C; but those who were less choosy and careful were also cheaper. A number of prominent Melbourne doctors found themselves accused: the ultimately philanthropic Dr James Beaney in 1866 and Dr Stephen Burke of the Women's honorary staff in 1887. Burke was exonerated after powerful support from his colleagues, but doctors called in to treat women bleeding or infected ran the risk of being implicated in the original crime.[62] The poor more often sought help from a midwife or a local woman who 'knew about such things'. They sold emetics, but they were also prepared to dilate the cervix, perforate the amniotic sac and injure the foetus so as to induce a miscarriage. One technique was to insert slippery elm bark into the cervix, which slowly swelled in the moist environment until the cervix was sufficiently open to stimulate contractions. The cunning digitally dilated the cervix slowly over a number of days so that they could not be accused

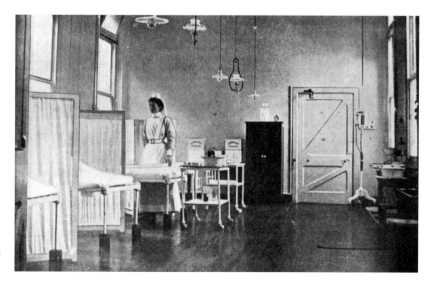

Labour ward, *c.*1900
RWHA

of anything more heinous, until the woman began to bleed, whereupon she presented herself at a doctor's surgery or a hospital to be curetted. They came in droves to the Women's Hospital with threatened or incomplete abortions; the hospital suspected the worst, but the women would rarely tell. As the admissions grew, often simply for day surgery without anaesthetic, and the lies continued except from those infected and haemorrhaging who were dying, so the hospital came to assume that almost every woman who came in with an infection following a complete or incomplete abortion, had sought to murder her foetus. By the 1920s all medical staff were instructed to assume that every post-abortal sepsis case was the result of a criminal abortion.

Abortion was dangerous. Women with retroverted or displaced uteri could easily suffer puncture wounds from knitting needles or curettes wielded by the untrained. The breaking of the waters and the introduction of any unsterilised foreign body or hand introduced pathogens which could kill. The houses and private hospitals run by self-trained midwives, especially those who offered 'special services', were frequently filthy, with patients sharing beds, befouled bed linen, close, damp rooms, and contaminated cloths and dressings. Sefton House, just up the road from the Women's Hospital in Madeline Street, was found in 1888 to have a bathroom which was 'very dirty, it is used as a dog kennel' and the cellar floor was inches deep in foul water. Mrs Hendy of 156 Nicholson Street, Fitzroy, advertised that she 'received ladies' at a cost of £3 for nine days, plus 9 shillings board. Patients were four to a bed and her own daughter died of a septic abortion there in January 1896.[63] In 1890 the Board of Health recommended the regulating of private hospitals, but the worst places often evaded detection. Women who went to be aborted in such premises endangered their lives, but they also did so when they attempted to abort themselves.

The one birth control device that was a good financial investment for a working-class family was a Higginson syringe. They were sold everywhere, they 'lasted for years' and they had many uses: for syringing out sore and infected vaginas, for douching after intercourse and, ominously, for administering enemas. They hung behind washroom, toilet or bedroom doors in tens of thousands of Australian homes. Their rubber tubing cracked so that dirt lodged permanently in the fissures. Few knew to boil them hard before use, and those who induced abortion by inserting the nozzle through their cervix and injecting soapy water or lysol into the uterus, risked infecting themselves with some of the bacteria most lethal to human beings. Yet they were viewed as a device for better hygiene rather than as dispensers of death. Not just chemists and birth control campaigners sold them, so even did the Women's Hospital's own dispensary after 1894 and at cost price.[64] The syringing cases of post-abortal sepsis grew slowly, and at first the offenders were more likely to be 'fast women' with 'knowledge'. N. P., a barmaid from Hotham, came in under an assumed name in 1884. She was twenty-four and had had a stillborn child eight years before. Since then she had had four abortions, the last four months previously. She had been well until two months ago when she caught a 'chill' after 'syringing herself with cold water'. Severe pains came on in the lower abdomen, but she 'had medical advice and got well

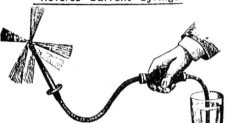
1898 advertisements for syringes and pessaries Supplement to Stewart Warren, The Wife's Guide and Friend (Will Andrade, Melbourne, 1898)

until three weeks before she had come in'. For the past fortnight she had taken to her bed and 'suffered much' so that she had been forced to take morphia. To the doctor she looked 'fairly healthy', but she had a 'dull, listless expression — drowsy — under the influence of some opiate'. A week later she was well enough to get up, but there were some 'suspicious red spots on her left leg'. Five days later she was free of pain and discharged.[65] But doctors themselves were teaching women to use a syringe and women could err in trying to do the right thing. In 1910 an extern midwifery case concluded in an emergency admission because the patient had been nursing a child with a septic leg and, anxious to protect herself from infection, had syringed herself with Condy's crystals just before the midwife arrived, only succeeding in inducing labour. Two days later her temperature was 104.6° and she had rigors. After careful nursing and treatment with quinine, she was out of danger in four days.[66]

Through the 1890s post-abortal sepsis began to emerge as one of the hospital's gravest challenges. The lay Board was apprehensive: it was not only sordid and stigmatising, it drew the hospital into police investigations. By February 1889 the number of post-abortal sepsis admissions had risen to such numbers that the Board decided to begin informing the police.[67] In 1901, fearful of growing scandal, the Board wanted the hospital to take no more, but the honorary medical staff insisted that such cases were fully entitled to admission as lying-in patients. Moreover, where else could they go? All hospitals sought to avoid infectious or septic cases as detrimental to the hygiene of their operations.[68] In 1909 the hospital was censured by the coroner for not ridding a post-abortal sepsis victim of vermin: she had been found in a dying condition by a neighbour and was in a 'filthy state when admitted'. All normal treatment had failed to clean her of lice; once she lost consciousness, the hospital could not shave her hair, because to do that they needed her consent.[69] The hospital was vulnerable now that coronial inquiries into abortion deaths were becoming more frequent. And yet the case record of that patient shows a different story. She looked 'septic' and very pale on admission, and her discharge was not offensive, so it was a more deadly aerobic infection. Long hot vaginal douches were ordered, saline per rectum and quinine four hourly. Scrapings from inside the uterus were cultured, a staphylococcus grown and a serum vaccine prepared by Dr Bull at the university. On the third evening after admission, she was given the vaccine by hypodermic injection, after which her temperature fell and remained about normal until the last two days of life. A week later she was drowsy, the next day comatose with loss of muscular control down her left side and passing everything in the bed, and three days later she died. The post-mortem revealed a large piece of placenta still adherent to the fundus and three brain abscesses.[70]

Medically the cases were a challenge, but they were dire emergencies and often offensive. In March 1909 Miss M. R., a twenty-two-year-old machinist, was admitted in a 'septic' condition. She had presented as an outpatient twenty days before with a threatened abortion, was curetted and sent home. A sudden rise in temperature now saw her in the Infirmary. Her immediate treatment was to be placed in Fowler's position and given long hot douches, frequent fluid nourishment and purgatives. The douches were then stopped and four days later she was treated with strychnine, brandy four-hourly, and with Aspirin and Veronal at night. The next day she was operated on. A laparotomy revealed numerous pelvic adhesions, a curious tumour-like mass in her left side, pus, 'also a lot of stinking breaking-down substance (like placenta)'. With drainage, a second operation after her wound broke down, and great care she survived, but it was almost two months before she was discharged.[71] The fulminating infections stank, and any who set foot in the septic wards never forgot the vile smell.

The laboratory was now offering both new knowledge and new therapies. The discovery of the immunological functions of serum offered for the first time actual intervention in the process of infection. The first reports from England of the injection of anti-streptococcic serum for puerperal septicaemia appeared in the Australian literature in June 1897. By October came the first instance of its successful use by G. T. Howard, an Outpatient Honorary at the Melbourne Hospital.[72] The administration of serum proved difficult, however, and the initial hopes were soon dashed by the constant failures. Not until 1907 could Dr Cairns Lloyd report some partial success in treating puerperal infection with serum at the Women's Hospital, and he attributed its possible efficacy to the production for the first time of the serum specific to the staphylococcus infecting the patient.[73] More effective was the actual identification of bacteria, and this knowledge persuaded doctors to be bolder when the laboratory revealed that salpingitis was often caused by gonorrhoea and even by tuberculosis. Since the doctors now realised that the women were probably already sterile, and that local treatment might have little effect, the removal of diseased fallopian tubes and ovaries seemed a rational choice. The poor could not afford repeated readmissions to hospital, therefore the treatment they were to be given needed to last a lifetime, and by 1900 the oophorectomy replaced D & C in most of the hospital's salpingitis cases. The endocrine significance of the ovaries was recognised by now, even if it was far from being understood. The doctors knew that a

Miss Louisa Mann, matron 1906–1911
RWHA

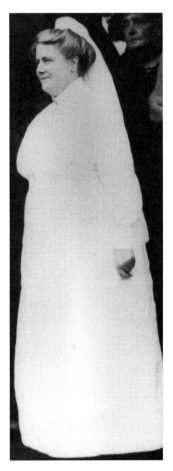

young woman deprived of her ovaries would not only be sterile, she would also suffer a premature menopause which would bring its own discomforts. Rothwell Adam noted that it was not uncommon for the removal of ovaries to lead to 'an increase in the mental aberration'.[74] He believed that full consent was necessary and in 1898 actually sewed up a twenty-eight-year-old married woman with such severe fibroids that only the removal of her ovaries would reduce her suffering, so that he could allow her to decide for herself. We do not know whether patients were always apprised of the possible removal of their ovaries and tubes before surgery — anecdotal evidence over the years suggests not. Another of Adam's patients was still anxious to have a child, so he preserved as much of her left ovary as he could.[75] The complete oophorectomies in the surgical statistics and case books seem shocking to modern historians, but what those sources do not necessarily enable us to appreciate was how many of these patients were in intolerable pain from their pus-filled, coiling, gnawing, 'hot' uterine appendages. A. M. was sixteen when Dr Morton removed both her ovaries and tubes for a double pyosalpinx, chronic appendicitis and a retro-fixed uterus in 1909. She had advanced PID and would otherwise have been an invalid for the rest of her life.[76] Mrs P. was nineteen and married only nine months when she had both ovaries and tubes removed by Dr O'Sullivan in 1904, but her PID was caused by tuberculosis.[77]

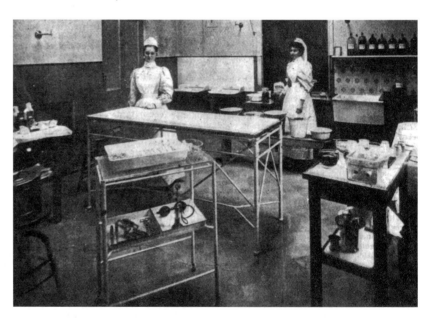

Operating theatre, 1897
Weekly Times RWHA

In 1907 O'Sullivan was again finishing a turn as the president of the Medical Society of Victoria. His presidential address returned to the themes of his speech a decade earlier, but with a new ferocity and certainty. Bicycle riding, university studies and sewing were dropped from the list of culprits in the sickness of women. Medical science now afforded better explanations: 'the greatest evils of modern civilisation are — specific infection of venereal disease, criminal abortion, and the prevention of conception'. Gonorrhoea was now clearly the greatest offender, and the guilty were not women but the selfish and profligate men who gave it to them: chronic infection, sterility, extra-uterine pregnancy, genital malformations and blindness in the newborn were now blamed on the gonococcus. And gonorrhoea was everywhere. 'Reliable authorities' now estimated that three quarters of the male population had suffered from it at one time or another and that at least 30 per cent carried 'the latent germ to the nuptial couch'. Syphilis was the curse of the poor, for it 'attacks 30 per cent to 40 per cent of the poorer classes' and in England 'it is given as 80 per cent'.[78]

O'Sullivan condemned criminal abortion and argued persuasively that the caesarean section had become safe enough to render unnecessary the operation of craniotomy. The third of the greatest evils was deliberate contraception. The truly alarming fact about the falling birth rate was that it was falling most among those who were 'the very class capable of begetting the more desirable citizens'. He even quoted with approval the analysis of the decline by Sidney Webb, the English Fabian socialist, although the two men may not have agreed as to its significance and remedy. O'Sullivan's remedy was continence. The 'carnal union' was 'redeemed' of its 'grossness' by the higher purpose of procreation. Young men had to be taught self-control, and those who had sinned must now submit themselves to medical control:

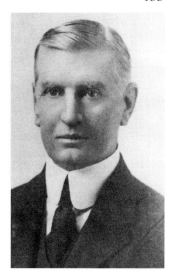

Dr Rothwell Adam
RWHA

> Let us have the courage to tell the man who comes to us more honestly with an apparently cured gonorrhoea, and a question whether he may not now marry, that it by no means follows that his apparent cure is real, that because he now has no discharge or discomfort he may not therefore infect his young wife and set alight the train of symptoms, the end to whose pain lies only in the grave. Let us insist on repeated and careful examinations ere pronouncing him perfectly clean.[79]

But it was syphilis more than anything else which united the medical reformers.

The campaign against syphilis was led by doctors of a different philosophical bent from O'Sullivan. They were men of modern science, who worshipped a secular deity of natural health, life-forces, social progress and scientific certitude. Understood as 'vitalists' or 'progressives', they were thoroughly modern and rational. James Barrett, a consultant at the Eye and Ear Hospital, and later Chancellor of the University of Melbourne, and Professor Harry Allen, the long-time holder of the chair of Anatomy and Pathology, began their campaign in tandem in 1904.[80] Barrett commenced with a presentation to the Medical Society of Victoria at the May meeting of a series of case notes on patients whose eye disease he believed could be traced to syphilis. In September Allen published a powerful paper analysing one hundred consecutive autopsies at the Melbourne Hospital, looking for the internal signs of syphilitic damage unrecognised by most medical practitioners. He drew a terrible conclusion: fully 34 per cent of these patients showed clear signs of syphilis, another 19 per cent doubtful signs. The most frequent, apart from facial scars, were lesions of the arteries and the heart. Few had the obvious external signs which doctors normally went by; the damage syphilis

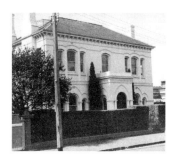

Dr Adam's house, East Melbourne *RWHA*

wrought was hidden deep inside the body, safe from medical detection: 'Its baneful influence is hidden behind the names of many common fatal diseases, such as granular kidneys, Bright's disease, nephritis, uraemia, anaemia, dropsy, cirrhosed liver, arteritis, aneurism, apoplexy, myocarditis, chronic endocarditis, locomotor ataxy, general paralysis etc.' (He was blaming syphilis for everything — illustrating the contemporary nostrum, that to know syphilis was to understand the entire human body.) He hastened to add that his collection of cadavers was not representative of the population of Melbourne: the Melbourne Hospital was the final refuge for a large proportion of the 'flotsam and jetsam of the metropolis' and he had deliberately avoided those who had died of pulmonary tuberculosis. Therefore, his sample was not even representative of the normal population of the hospital; nevertheless, the results were 'more grave' than he had expected. Allen admitted that many colleagues believed he suffered from a 'monomania' about syphilis; but now the scientific moment had come to persuade society that a pestilence did exist and was sapping the vitality of the nation and that its victims needed to be controlled. (New South Wales was busy with a Royal Commission into the falling birth rate, it too feeding on race suicide panic.) Allen's supreme purpose was to persuade society to accept Fournier's 'marriage law' forbidding marriage less than three to four years after completion of treatment. In other words science now gave doctors a new authority to suspend civil liberties. In the discussion that followed, Dr Mollison spoke of syphilis being the underlying cause of eclampsia in multiparous women at the Women's Hospital and Dr Adam reported that apparent uterine malignancies revealed themselves under the microscope after surgery to be syphilitic disease which should have been treated chemically.[81]

The Intercolonial Medical Congress of 1908 devoted an entire session to the red plague. Professor Allen was president and his position gave added authority to the papers on syphilis. He opened with the results of another one hundred consecutive but selected autopsies, this time finding 32 of them syphilitic and 30 'more or less doubtful'. His rough one third of the public hospital morgue population was echoed by the only other Victorian speaker, Dr P. B. Benne, an honorary at the Children's Hospital. He testified to his growing awareness of the extent of syphilis infection, to the point where now he estimated that a third of his patients were so afflicted, and from this he deduced that around 10 per cent of the children of Victoria were 'syphilised'. Melbourne, it seemed, was as diseased as Paris, London or Berlin.[82] The Sydney-based *Australian Medical Gazette*

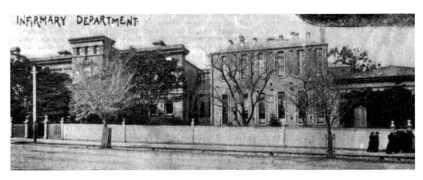

**Infirmary department,
1897** *RWHA*

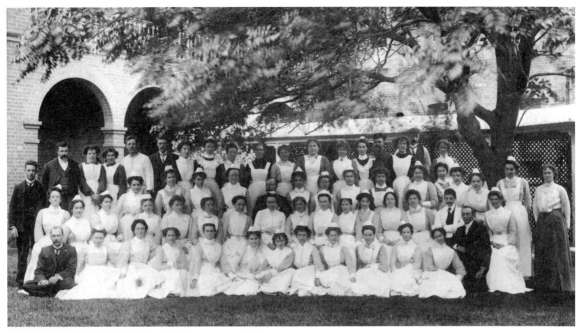

Medical and nursing staff, c. 1900 *RWHA*

had its doubts: 'We should hope, for the sake of the future of Victoria, and its capital, it is, to say the least of it, a gross exaggeration'.[83] The vitalists succeeded, however, in the passage of a resolution that syphilis 'is responsible for an enormous amount of damage to mankind, and that preventative and remedial measures directed against it are worthy of the utmost consideration'. Armed with this, a delegation visited the Victorian Premier the next day and eventually succeeded in persuading the state government to support an investigation into the accuracy of the new Wassermann test. Konrad Hiller, an Out-patient Physician at the Melbourne Hospital, had been working hard on the new procedure and devised a scheme for its testing in the field. The campaigners were really hoping, however, for a measure of the actual incidence of syphilis in Melbourne. The Victorian Government declared syphilis to be a notifiable contagious disease for 12 months from June 1910 to May 1911 for all patients within a ten-mile radius of the GPO. Doctors who had diagnosed or suspected syphilis were required to send blood samples to Dr Hiller who then applied the Wassermann test. But the results when they finally came were inconclusive. The tests confirmed that the procedure identified around 60 per cent of the cases, as others had reported. As to the incidence in Melbourne, while the Eye and Ear Hospital Outpatients' clinic showed an incidence around 13 per cent, the only figure they could calculate for the whole of Melbourne was merely 0.5 per cent. 'The gravity of the matter' remained 'beyond question' insisted Dr Barrett, and he went on to use his own Outpatient figures in public discourse and said no more about Dr Hiller's findings.[84] When finally the Women's Hospital produced its own survey early in 1913, there was less reaction, even though the results really were alarming: they had tested one hundred consecutive admissions, not chosen for their likelihood, marital status or anything else. They ranged in age from fifteen to forty-nine, and just under half— 46 — appear to have been primiparas. The results were bad: ten positives and six partials, hence given the inaccuracy of the Wassermann test, a possible tally of at least 16 per cent. To make matters worse, one patient who died of eclampsia had a negative test but at autopsy was found to have signs of congenital syphilis. In fact of the 84 negative reactions, the doctors had suspicions about eleven of the patients. They drew the obvious conclusion that a Wassermann test should be made of every pregnant woman.[85] But in a sense the damage had been done. The Hiller survey and its 'disappointing' results had been 'quoted all over the world', and the *Australian Medical Journal* tactfully editorialised in May 1914 that the main discovery was the 'large margin of error that must obtain in any inquiry of the kind and the wide difference of interpretation that might quite reasonably be placed on the result'.[86]

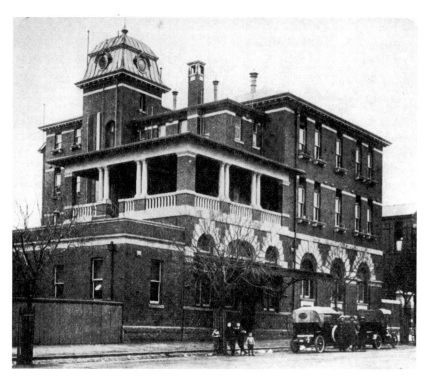

New Outpatients department and Nurses Home (1909) *RWHA*

Action was still to be taken, however. The Victorian Government agreed to fund the opening of a twenty-four-bed ward for syphilitics at the Alfred Hospital and a twenty-five-bed one at the Women's, and £2500 was put aside by the Treasurer for twelve months. When the Minister for Health visited in October 1912 there were just six cases at the Women's and twenty-one at the Alfred. Twelve months later the government began to back out, criticising the two hospitals for wasting money. At the Women's only twenty-one of the twenty-five beds first planned had been funded, and in them at present were eighteen patients. Now that the syphilis panic had subsided, the government thought that six beds was more than enough.[87]

Barrett scarcely missed a beat. He widened his campaign to include gonorrhoea and quoted freely the gynaecologists who claimed that

80 per cent of all surgery on the uterus and its appendages was the fault of the invading gonococcus and that 'the clap' caused half of all puerperal infections. He pictured hundreds of thousands of unknown diseased men and women stalking the great cities of the world: '60 to 90 per cent of males of urban populations contract gonorrhoea at some period of their lives', he claimed. The agents of disease were men, not bad women, in Barrett's mind; hypocritical men who brought pain and sterility to the mothers of the nation; sexually frustrated men who could not afford to marry; uneducated men who could benefit from proper instruction. The solution, therefore, was not to lock up the prostitutes. The old Contagious Diseases Acts had failed, he argued, 'because of the intense opposition to them roused in the minds of the people who do not fully understand the facts'. Further, 'The method . . . is exceedingly distasteful, and as it cannot be applied equally to men and women in practice, it seems futile'. The solutions needed to be more democratic: the encouragement of earlier marriage through the raising of male wages and reduction of female remuneration to reduce the temptations of independence; sex and hygiene education for the young, syringing for women and washing before and after intercourse for men; the banning of unqualified therapists, full treatment for all the afflicted, and detention of 'persons found to be suffering from contagious diseases, and punishment of those who wilfully or negligently communicate them'.[88] Nine months after he spoke these words at the Australasian Medical Congress in New Zealand, the world was at war and the war would bring changes which were unthinkable in peacetime. Also since 1910, doctors had been trying out a new drug — Salvarsan, Paul Ehrlich's 'magic bullet', the first germ killer specifically targeted at a particular enemy. The initial results were mixed, for it was very painful to administer and dosages were not properly understood. All that could be said was that it was 'encouraging'. None the less, it marked the beginning of a new age.[89]

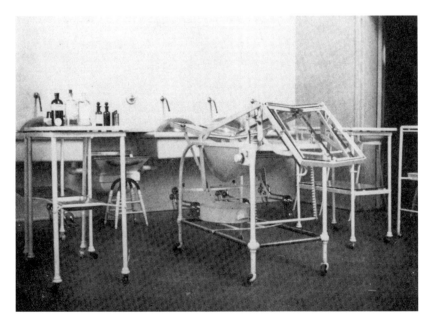

Infirmary operating theatre *RWHA*

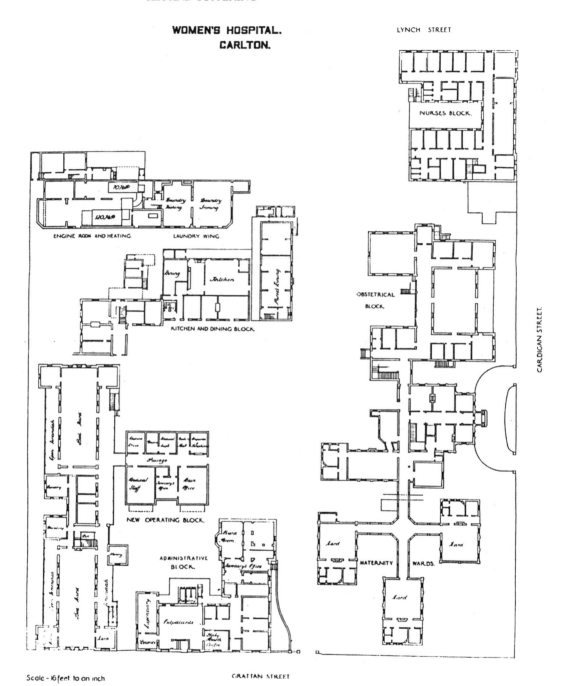

Map of hospital in 1908
RWHA

Dr Hooper's Case Book

Consecutive cases bring alive more than statistics the patients and the doctor and we begin in late June 1894.

29 June, Mrs S. T. housewife, Ascot Vale

Born in Jersey, aged 42, she migrated at three and married 13 years ago at the age of 29.

She had menstruated first at 16 and a half, and had no problems.

Now her periods were regular, but painful and profuse.

In thirteen years of marriage she had had five pregnancies and four confinements.

Two years ago she had 'a mishap' at 4 months and had been unwell ever since with constant pains in the lower abdomen and back. Then came heavy periods, a feeling of obstruction and difficulty in passing urine.

She had a fibroid tumour in the uterus and the miscarriage had in fact been deliberately induced in the hospital's midwifery department 'because' as she stated herself, 'a fulltime child might have caused great difficulty and danger to woman in delivery'.

She was getting sicker and sicker. The pain was worse, she could feel the mass building inside her, she had constant headaches, could not eat and was getting thinner. She had had 'floodings' and was anaemic from loss of blood.

Eight days later Dr Hooper operated. The fibroid was so huge, it almost filled the pelvis. The stump was treated outside the peritoneum to reduce infection, but the patient suffered 'a good amount of haemorrhage'.

She died four days after the operation from acute peritonitis and 'exhaustion', that is insufficient blood.

15 July, Mrs A. R., housewife, Fitzroy

Aged 29, she had married at 15 and a half and borne six children by the age of 23. And had suffered between seven and eight miscarriages. Therefore at 29 she was a G.14, P.6.

Her periods were regular and painless (she had reached menarche at 14)

She had been well until her last miscarriage four months before. Ever since, however, she had been in pain, and when pain came on she could not do her work and had to lie down. She was feeling better now she was in hospital, she said.

The doctor, however, assessed her condition as 'very fair', that is not good, and he could feel the mass of adhesions, the coiled and distended tubes, the swollen ovaries and the anteriorly displaced uterus of PID.

She did have a previously lacerated perineum and a currently lacerated cervix and was therefore a recipient of an Emmet repair; but the only other procedure was a D & C, and despite the 'good result' scrawled across the bottom of the page, her real problems remained untouched.

16 July 1894, Mrs M. W., housewife, Port Melbourne

Aged 40, Mrs W. had been born in Dublin, but brought to Australia as a two-year-old. She reached menarche at fourteen, married at fifteen and a half and in twenty years had seven children and six miscarriages (thirteen pregnancies). She had been well until three years ago when she had a slight facial paralysis, became weaker and lost appetite, suffered much from indigestion, pain in back and abdomen. She had attended as an outpatient and 'relieved'. To the Resident Surgeon then and to Robin Bell now, her ailments were not gynaecological in nature. Perhaps it was gastritis, or a peptic or duodenal ulcer. Certainly the 'general and local treatment' decided upon improved her condition.

29 May 1894, Mrs A. W., housewife, Malvern

Mrs A. W.'s case was written up out of order and without a proper case history. She was thirty and had had 'some children'.
She did have a perineum lacerated down to the anal sphincter and 'no control over faeces'. We do not know how long for, however.
Dr Hooper operated the day after her admission, catgut sutures being used for a perineorrhaphy.
However, 'operation not successful. Sutures apparently gave way. Could not control motions afterwards. T° normal for 18 days after operation. Then went from 99.6° to 103.6° for period of eleven days. T° 100.2° when discharged.
Two days after T° rose, became very queer in the her speech and actions, especially at night. This condition became worse, and she had almost from the first to be watched by a special nurse. Physical condition improved after a time, but mental became worse and worse, and finally she was quite irresponsible for her actions. All the patients in terror of her. Phthisical history on father's side, and mental instability very marked on the mother's. In consequence of the serious disturbance she was creating amongst the other patients, the lack of any accommodation for such cases, and the fact that there were not nurses available to special watch her, the Honorary Medical Officer advised that she should be taken home by her friends and looked after there, which apparently could be done as well as in the Hospital. She went away in charge of husband and father.'
Dr Robin Bell: Incontinence of faeces, peritoneal wound broken down, pain, discharge, infection, septicaemia. You do not need to invoke mental illness to explain her state of distress and episodes of apparently psychotic behaviour.

21 July 1894, Mrs E. K., housewife of Hotham (North Melbourne)

Mrs E. K., age thirty, was born in Lancashire and brought to Australia at eight. She had a very early menarche at eleven, married at nineteen, but had borne only one child ten years ago.
She had made a slow recovery from that first confinement, then six years ago, fell ill, went to doctor who told her she had 'ulceration and falling of the womb'. She now complained of pain, neuralgia, indigestion and general weakness. She 'had difficulty in getting about and doing her work'.

She had a femoral hernia, but she also had the swellings and tenderness of PID; however its onset and the fact that she had had only one pregnancy suggest gonorrhoea and consequent infertility. Here perhaps was a case to support Dr Balls-Headley's theory that 'ulceration of the womb' was Nature's way of restricting unwanted babies.

No operative treatment was considered worth while.

30 July 1894, Mrs C. McH., housewife, South Melbourne

Now aged 22, she had been born in Glasgow and emigrated at the age of twelve. She had reached puberty at fourteen, married at seventeen and borne three children in four years. She had not menstruated at all for four years until eleven days ago.

She had been quite well until her last confinement a year ago. The labour was difficult, concluded with instruments under chloroform.

'Very soon after getting up felt great pain across the back and as though something were pressing on back passage. Had great difficulty with bowels. Then had trouble with micturition, unable to pass it for hours together. Bad headaches, pains over lower abdomen and bad leucorrhoea. Often had to go to bed and quite unable to work.

The doctor assessed her only as 'fair'; she was in great pain, and the 'tube and ovary on left side swollen and very painful and tender on pressure'. Her cervix was lacerated 'in one or two places and two silver wire sutures were inserted for a slight laceration'.

Otherwise she received a D & C and again, her class PID, contracted after an instrumental delivery, went on as before.

30 July 1894, Mrs E. M., housewife, Middle Park

Mrs E. M. was twenty-six, born in Tasmania and brought to Victoria at the age of eight. She reached puberty at thirteen, married at twenty-one, and had a child within the year. Her labour had been only two hours, but she had been delivered with forceps under chloroform (perhaps precipitously). Five months later the symptoms of infected tubes were felt, and now the uterus was displaced anteriorly by the inflammation, and the pain, headaches and leucorrhoea often left her 'unable to perform household duties'. She was feeling better that she was in hospital, however, and no operative treatment was thought necessary. She also appeared to be infertile.

5 August 1894, Mrs H. D., housewife, Fitzroy

Mrs H. D., aged thirty-two, had been born in Calcutta and married at fourteen, a year after she reached puberty. Between the ages of fourteen and nineteen she had five children, and since then four miscarriages. She was 'rather inclined to corpulency'.

She had been well until 'twelve months ago when she first felt severe pain of an intermittent character over the lower abdomen. Pain across back and bearing down pains. Leucorrhoea rather bad. Was able at first to get about and do her work. Weak and suffered much from intestinal colic, accompanied by vomiting. Had a mishap four months ago? since that time has been very much worse than before. Since then subject to severe and frequent floodings, in fact had hardly been well for a day since. Pain is now mostly felt over the left lower abdomen and down the left leg. Other pains as before. Is much weaker than before and unable to do her household work. Poor appetite.'

On examination she was a mess. The perineum was lacerated almost through to the sphincter, the cervix 'apparently lacerated', and on the left side the tell-tale 'thickened, coiled and painful tube and ovary'.

Perhaps she had been inducing her 'mishaps'; certainly she now had PID and severe anaemia from the chronic blood loss. She was given a D & C and the uterus was washed out three days after the operation.

A decade later, the bleeding would have aroused the suspicion of secondary syphilis.

18 August 1894, Mrs A. G., dressmaker, South Melbourne

Mrs A. G. was now twenty-seven, and had been married for seven years but had apparently never become pregnant. She had reached puberty at fifteen and had no problem with her periods.

For the past fortnight she had been unable to pass urine, the doctor was having to catheterise her twice a day. A large soft tumour could be felt in the abdomen, and a harder one behind it to the right, high up.

A month later she was operated on, in which a left parovarian cyst with dense adhesions to surrounding structures was removed. The right ovary was healthy and left alone.

24 August 1894, Mrs W. P., housework, Eastern Hill

Mrs P. was an emergency admission with peritonitis from a multi-ocular ovarian tumour with a twisted pedicle, and was operated on the next day. She was thirty, born in Westbury, England, and had been in the colony only five years. She had married the year after emigrating, and had a single miscarriage within the year. She had been unwell ever since, with severe dysmenorrhoea, bearing-down pains, headaches, weakness, and three months ago, floodings. Prior to admission, she had been in bed four weeks with violent pain all over the abdomen, but especially on the left side. She had to lie on her right side and was vomiting all yesterday. Dr Hooper removed a large multilocular right ovarian cyst, with its pedicle twisted two and a half times. The cyst wall was dark and haemorrhagic, and twenty-two ounces of fluid was drawn off with trocar and cannula.

She recovered.

Dr Bell: Outstanding treatment and result.

3 September 1894, Mrs J. W., housework, Carlton

Mrs J.W. at fifty-nine was the oldest of the group. She was also one of the few Australian born, having come from Tasmania to Victoria at the age of thirteen. She had reached the menarche at thirteen and married at eighteen. She then had three children by the age of thirty-three and no miscarriages. She had reached menopause at fifty-one.

For eighteen months now she had had a reddish and very foetid discharge which lately had included clots. She was in no pain, but 'thinner and weaker'. Dr Hooper suspected cancer of the cervix, did a D & C and sent a specimen to Dr Mollison at the university. He could discern no malignancy and perhaps it was tuberculosis. There was nothing else to do, as it was. A decade later some doctors would have suspected syphilis as the cause.

7 September 1894, Mrs E. L., dressmaker, Albert Park

Mrs L. was thirty, born in Scotland and had come to Australia as an eight-year-old. She reached puberty at sixteen, married at twenty-one and had three children in the next five and a half years.

Two years ago she began to get thinner and weaker, with pains in her lower abdomen. 'Had a "fit" about three months ago. Soon recovered. Menses have been irregular during last two years, leucorrhoea, bearing down pains, pains in head and lower abdomen and back. Cold feeling in hands and feet.' The doctor assessed her condition only as 'moderate'. The clinical examination apparently revealed only a lacerated cervix, for which she was given an Emmet after a D & C. Perhaps her symptoms indicated PID; perhaps their cause was non-gynaecological.

8 October 1894, Mrs M. W., waitress, City of Melbourne

This was another childless young married woman. Now aged twenty-three, she had come to Victoria from Sydney three years before. Reaching puberty at sixteen, she married at seventeen and had never been pregnant.

She had already been in the hands of doctors, having been operated on at seventeen for dysmenorrhoea (a metrotomy?). She had felt better for a while and then got bad again. She had pain, leucorrhoea and frequency of micturition. Vaginal syringing had improved her condition.

Her symptoms and infertility suggest PID or perhaps endometriosis. She received no further operative treatment.

13 October 1894, Miss L. T., housework, Ascot Vale

Aged twenty-seven, Miss T. was not obviously ill although she felt so. She had had a painful, heavy period ten weeks ago, and she had had bad headaches. 'Has not been able to do any straining work for last two or three months'.

She had improved a lot in hospital, but still had pains in lower abdomen and back. Her condition was 'Pretty fair'.

Nothing abnormal could be felt or seen, but she was very tense during the abdominal examination, exhibiting 'abdominal guarding'.

There was no treatment for this unhappy soul other than good food and rest.

20 October 1894, Mrs A. B., housework, Footscray

Mrs A. B. was twenty-seven. She reached menarche at fifteen, married at twenty and had three confinements in seven years.

This last confinement had actually been a procured abortion of a seven-months foetus. A post-mortem and inquest were held.

About a week after getting up she began to have pains across the lower abdomen. It went away then returned and was very acute. She had retching and loss of appetite but no night sweats or shivering. She came to the hospital for treatment for the pain in her side. That night her temperature was 103°. She was sweating, pulse quick, tongue coated, sordes on teeth. Her condition was 'rather bad' but with 'general and local treatment' she survived.

IV

Class Relations
1914–1931

Improving the Race
1914–1929

8

A hospital devoted to lying-in and the diseases of women, situated ten thousand miles from the battle-lines, was none the less directly and profoundly affected by World War I. After the Gallipoli tragedy, the Australian respectable classes enlisted in droves, among them senior nurses, young medical graduates and established practitioners. Of the honorary medical staff who shaped the hospital for the next half century, only a handful of medically unfit men did not serve in one or both world wars. Even Helen Sexton, having retired to Europe in 1910 because of ill health, took a small hospital staffed entirely by women to the front and served in the French army with the rank of Majeur. She was by then over fifty. Many displayed immense personal bravery, dedication and medical genius under appalling clinical conditions. Several endured some of the worst experiences inflicted on military personnel during each war.

As doctors and nurses of women they had particular competencies which were needed in war medicine. While they knew little of orthopaedics and amputation, they were good at wound infection, sudden and catastrophic haemorrhage, emergency intervention and the plastic repair of lesions. Temperamentally, they were quick to make hard decisions and thrived on emergencies; one distinguished World War II veteran would confess that he loved casualty at the Women's because it was 'exciting', and it was just that sort of medical courage which was needed in war. They were also accustomed to treating patients in the prime of life but temporarily injured or sick, rather than diseased and decayed people at the end of their allotted span. But the war also extended their own skills. Doctors and senior nurses learnt to be administrators of medical units and many more acquired an experience relatively early in their careers that in civilian life might have come more slowly. Sir George Cuscaden managed the entire military medical service; others, like E. ('Teddie') Rowden White were commanding officers of field ambulance units. The medical administrator, the doctor turned bureaucrat, was a development accelerated by war and it diminished the control of

Sir George Cuscaden
RWHA

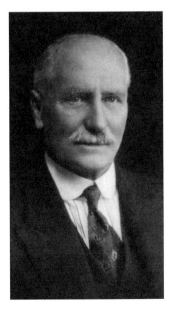

hospitals by the honorary staff and a more or less acquiescent lay Board. Clinically it extended the doctors' knowledge of trauma, plastic surgery, haemorrhage and infection — the observation of gas–gangrene infections would later have particular relevance to the Melbourne Women's Hospital. And when they returned from service, they were given preference in civilian appointments.

But the war also had more subtle cultural effects. The rigid discipline and strict hierarchies of the hospital were sympathetic to the military method. The hospital had an unquestioned etiquette which cemented the structure of authority: the honoraries were the generals, the residents the lesser officers, the medical students the officer cadets, the matron the NCO, the charge nurses the corporals and the pupil nurses were the privates. The orderlies who cleaned, carried, cooked and served were merely a labour corps. These structures were enacted daily in ward rounds, with each rank in the appointed place, so many steps behind the next rank above, and this performance of medical authority is still defended by some who remember it as a necessary discipline for the staff and a comfort to the patient. Uniforms had to be perfect, as did body language. There were places you could and could not go, and ways you could and could not talk. Doctors dined in one room, the charge nurses in another with matron sitting apart, and both had silver services; but doctors were served alcohol on special occasions and, later, at formal dinners, luxuries like oysters and lobster. All medical and nursing staff sat down to starched linen table cloths and napkins and were waited on by maids. Servants, porters and kitchen staff ate separately again. When a doctor entered a room, nurses had to stand to attention and speak when spoken to and nurses must never pass through a door before a doctor or a more senior nurse. Entering the dining room, a pupil nurse had to make way for her seniors, and if a large crowd of charge nurses entered she might be five or ten minutes waiting for them to pass and permit her to get her meal. The observances of deference to authority were those of the nineteenth-century country house, where servants became machines who went about the housework silently while the 'real people' pretended that they weren't there. But the hospital was also, like the armed forces, intended to operate as a well-oiled machine that reacted instantly and perfectly in a crisis. When a woman in labour ward needed to go to theatre, she was there in minutes. But the transition to such efficiency was painful.

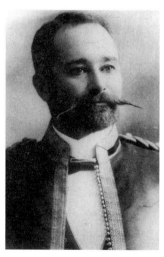

Dr George Horne
RWHA

The worlds of the nurses and the doctors were entirely separated and, now that Helen Sexton had retired, apart from the occasional female resident, divided between the female and the male. The war deepened the masculinist cast of the doctors' culture. Devoted to serving women they might be, but most were 'men's men', interested in sport, good dining and fine wines. A number were cultivated, with interests in the arts and George Horne was a pioneer anthropologist; Felix Meyer was a fluent writer, was widely read and had a very good eye for paintings. There were hearty and lavish dinners, in evening dress, with carefully chosen wines, witty and sometimes *risqué* speeches; and when Dr Margaret Mackie became a consultant in 1948, as the only woman on the honorary staff, she would go home just before 'port' so that the men's stories could still be told. Nearly all the senior doctors were locally born, bred and educated, and as the century went on, most had come from a small group of just five boys' private schools, especially and in order, Scotch College (Presbyterian), Melbourne Grammar School (Anglican) and Wesley College (Methodist). In the senior echelons of the medical profession, many had known each other since boyhood, so that university and medical practice were socially extensions of school. Victoria had little secondary state education, it cost around £1000 still in the 1930s to get a medical degree, and thus men who had risen from the 'lower ranks' were few indeed. Most honoraries had undergone some overseas postgraduate training, but they were now very much Australian doctors. And they were, after 1918 until into the 1950s at the Women's, overwhelmingly Protestant.

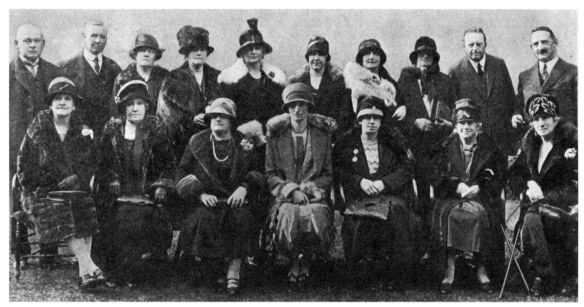

Committee of Management, 1926–1929
Top row: Mr Colin Colquhoun, Dr Allen Robertson, Mrs W. J. Earle, Mrs A. McCracken, Mrs C. Cowper, Mrs A. F. Kimpton, Mrs T. A. Tabart, —, Mr Gilbert G. Gobbins, Mr H. Pride (Hon. Treasurer)
Bottom row: Mrs George Langridge, Mrs J. J. Brenan, Mrs James Alston (Vice-President), Mrs Herbert Brookes (President), Mrs D. A. Skene (Secretary), Mrs W. Fitzpatrick, Mrs Brodie Ainslie *RWHA*

In January 1918 the Committee of Management, which had Catholic members, appointed Dr Gerald Doyle as Medical Superintendent. The honoraries were enraged. Here was a member of the flock of the traitorous Archbishop Mannix who had supported the Easter Rebellion in Ireland and opposed conscription for 'an ordinary trade war'. It had been the militant Protestants' great opportunity to isolate and stigmatise Catholics as unpatriotic. To older colonials who had known a more temperate and unsectarian Melbourne, the prejudice was disgraceful. When Mrs Moss stated that there were twenty doctors in the hospital and only one of them was Catholic, Mr Ievers almost walked out of the Committee meeting, declaring: 'He had been sixty-three years in Carlton and never asked a man, woman or child what religion or denomination they belonged to'. Mrs Fitzgerald was reported to have warned Mrs Brenan: 'If I were you I would not take too prominent a part in the matter, because everybody has been stirred up by Dr Mannix'. The crux of the matter was disloyalty and Dr Doyle had to answer why he was not in the war. But

when he insisted that he had enlisted only to be rejected as unfit, it still
did not save him and he lost the job.[1] Catholic nurses were barely toler-
ated, and certainly discouraged by the reluctance of the hospital to provide
sufficient non-meat food on Fridays and Holy Days.[2] Frank Hayden, as
a resident doctor in 1934, felt the Protestant cold shoulder and deplored
the stuffiness of the older honoraries.[3] But Catholics were expected to
'stick with their own', and in the 1930s senior doctors at St Vincent's
Hospital worked hard to build up a clinical school.[4] Melbourne was two
cities, one Catholic and one Protestant, and you could progress from birth
to death without casting your shadow over the threshold of a single
school, hospital, welfare home, cultural institution or university college,
let alone place of worship, of 'the other faith'. The next Catholic senior
appointment would not be until the 1950s. As for Jews, there were four
appointed honoraries out of seventy-eight between 1856 and 1966.[5] The
consequence was often that exaggerated consciousness of 'difference'
that comes from living in a very small, homogenous world.

The world of the nurses was almost as Protestant, but it was exclu-
sively female and perforce celibate. Although of more mixed social origins
than the doctors, very few came from the same world as the patients
they nursed in public hospitals. If the nursing staff knew their place, stood
to attention, deferred to doctors and spoke only when spoken to, they
none the less resented their inferiority. While some would still today
champion that hospital etiquette, and while doctors and nurses worked
together effectively, it has always been a fact of hospital life that nurses,
underneath, much of the time, resent doctors. From the doctors' point
of view, the control and reform of nursing was not just an exercise of
male professional power over a female servant class, it was also necessary
to the institutional creation of the modern hospital. The reshaping of
nursing practice after the introduction of antiseptic midwifery and aseptic
surgery was far from completed by the dawn of the new century.

Professor Harry Allen used his presidential address before the
Australasian Medical Congress in 1908 to call for the reform of private
midwifery with a Midwives' Act. Since the coming of antiseptic midwifery, puerperal sepsis deaths had fallen only in hospitals: in the community both doctors and nurses had not taken the lessons to heart. There
were doctors whose 'grip of aseptic methods' was imperfect, 'but the lack
of progress depends chiefly on nursing'. 'It is not too much to claim that
out of every ten deaths from puerperal sepsis, nine are probably preventable'.[6] From 1904, when the Royal Victorian Trained Nurses'
Association was founded, the control of nurse training and registration,
especially in midwifery, was its greatest object. The Women's Hospital
attempted to alleviate the nurse shortage by providing both basic and
postgraduate training, but lost its registration to do so in 1913. Within
the hospital tensions had been running high between medical and nursing
staff, the doctors alleging incompetence, the nurses rudeness and bullying.
In early April 1912 an anonymous letter to the Committee of Management complained of patient conditions: that they were washed only once
a week by staff and that they were expected to wash themselves at 3 a.m.,
in the middle of the night; that basic facilities were lacking and that
patients in general were poorly treated. By 12 April the matron had

resigned and the nursing staff with her. The staff withdrew, but then the Honorary Staff made an official complaint to the president, alleging indiscipline and poor patient hygiene.[7] A new matron was appointed, but the tensions continued, especially in the operating theatre where six theatre sisters resigned in a space of months because of rudeness from doctors. A real issue was a shortage of skilled nurses. The general nurse training provided by the Women's was felt by doctors to be insufficient to equip them professionally; and there was a shortage of applicants for midwifery training because the hospital was perceived to 'give too little time off'. (Matron retorted that each Midwifery sister had three hours a day off duty and one clear day each week.)[8] The outcome was the return to postgraduate training for most, and a full year's training for those without previous qualifications but who wished to become midwives only. In 1915 Victoria passed a Midwives' Act, which once amended, registered midwives, prescribed their training, regulated their practices and placed them under the surveillance of the public health system. They were to observe aseptic rules, to submit to restraint from practice if in contact with infectious disease, to measure pulse and temperature daily during the puerperium and consent to having their instruments and appliances inspected.[9] The act licensed independent practising midwives and they were to remain part, albeit a steadily diminishing one, of Victorian childbirth until after World War II.

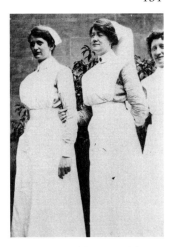

Nurses, *c.* **1915** *RWHA*

Within the hospital the conflict between doctors and nurses continued and the honorary staff were convinced that standards could only be raised by the appointment of a resident medical superintendent. Finally by June 1916 the Board passed a resolution to do so, but deferred the matter until after the war. It was therefore not until August 1919 that the Staff moved again for the appointment and the first incumbent was Dr W. A. Birrell at a salary of £300 in the first year, to be raised to £350 in the second. Birrell resigned after six months, but the Board by this time was committed to the concept of a medical administrator and a new appointment was made.[10] The medical superintendents, men (and one woman) still in the early stages of their careers, were to become in many ways even more important than the honorary staff in determining the character and functioning of the hospital over the next half century.

The nurses lived and worked apart from the world. Even in a public hospital the culture of vocational celibacy drew on the ideal of the religious order. Nurses were 'Sisters' and in private life required to be as spotless as they were on the ward. Those who made nursing a lifetime career spent decades living in hospitals, and at a public hospital witnessed the consequences not just of poverty and ignorance, but also of sadism, selfishness and sexual delinquency. It was not difficult to begin to hate men in general as well as some in particular. Nurses suffered the condescension and authoritarianism of male doctors (and some women doctors copied their braying clinical voices and supercilious ways), but they also saw the worst of what men could do to women. They saw young girls impregnated and infected with syphilis. They saw women who had been battered, even genitally mutilated; they saw pregnant unmarried women who had been seduced by lies and abandoned, then driven to destroy their babies at the risk of their own lives. They were appalled when sick women discharged themselves from hospital too soon because they were afraid their husbands might drink all the money and the children would starve. All the time they saw exhausted women who had had too many children, who should never be having any more but were; whose husbands spent some or even most of their income on drink and gambling; whose lives were a misery, it seemed, because of male lust, selfishness and irresponsibility. There were too many dirty little working-class men with dirty little habits. 'Husbands', one nurse told a journalist in 1921, 'don't talk about husbands here! We see too much of them. Of course there are some decent ones, but . . .'[11]

To those who worried about the dirty little habits of working-class men the war was a godsend. The scandal of the war was the high infection rate among the troops with venereal diseases, and, as Judith Smart has shown, the appearance in the streets of venereally diseased soldiers provoked legislative action where the diseased women of the back lanes before the war had not.[12] The gynaecologists warned that the return of thousands of 'grossly infected soldiers' would do untold damage to their women and the nation. The already frightful toll of salpingitis would rise further, robbing women of their health and the nation of their potential babies, for nearly all infections which reached the tubes, warned Dr William Chenhall of Sydney, were 'induced by filthy sexual intercourse or deliberate interference with the natural processes of reproduction'.[13] In 1916 the Victorian Government passed a Venereal Diseases Act, and it was an act more sensitive to the civil rights and privacy of the afflicted than the old-style Contagious Diseases acts in the United Kingdom. The diseases were notifiable and victims had to consent to full treatment, but their identity would remain with the doctor unless they refused proper treatment. Women could request a woman doctor to examine them, but there were fines and even forced detention for those who refused or avoided treatment. Persons knowingly infecting others or conducting a brothel with diseased prostitutes, could be fined or gaoled for up to twelve months.[14] There were thus sufficient concessions to feminist concerns to win support from many women's organisations and the Labor women.

As many have noted both here and overseas, World War I delivered knowledge of birth control down the class system and sexual licence up it. Also, for many Australians, it was the first major dislocation in time and space experienced in their family history since the act of immigration. The venereal disease among the troops forced military authorities to issue condoms, thereby teaching an entire male generation about barrier contraception. The problem was that many still contracted disease, were not cured and did infect their wives, fiancées and casual sexual partners. It was now clear that Salvarsan only halted but did not cure syphilis, and gonorrhoea remained intractable. Some parents even discouraged their daughters from going out with returned men because of 'soldiers' diseases'.[15] And the terrible things that the doctors warned of did happen. On Armistice Day 1926 Ian Wood, a resident medical student at the Women's, and Sister Bryce from the District Nursing Society, were called to a home birth in North Melbourne. The woman was forty-two. Before her husband went to the war she had borne three healthy children, breast-fed them and reared them successfully. Since his return, she had suffered eleven miscarriages and produced six stillborn macerated foetuses, and the student and the midwife then delivered her of her seventh. Her husband was 'in good health', but she was a 'pale, anaemic, worried woman — wasted'. She had no idea that she now had syphilis.[16] In 1921 the serological investigation of public patients continued, and, with more careful use of the Wassermann test in collaboration with the new Walter and Eliza Hall Institute of Medical Research, the Women's labour ward patients again revealed a 10 per cent incidence of syphilis. It was a shocking figure. Further, they now believed that syphilis was implicated in a third of stillbirths occurring around the seventh month and perinatal deaths. Most of the cases were latent; how many of the mothers were themselves congenital syphilitics rather than having acquired the infection, they did not know nor speculate upon, but they believed infection to occur largely before marriage. Later, Robert Fowler who conducted this survey, would operate on the figures of public hospital patients displaying a frequency of luetic pregnancies of 'not less than 7.5 per cent' — one in thirteen.[17] The Venereal Diseases Act did not recognise the Wassermann test as a legal proof of infection, therefore latent cases could not be compelled to accept treatment. The conclusion was that all pregnant women should be tested, adding to the case for antenatal care.[18]

The war accelerated social change and to hospital staff it was clear that people's sexual behaviour was different. The large-scale entrance of women into male occupations — although less conspicuous in Australia than in the United Kingdom — the growth of female trade unionism and political activism, especially in opposition to conscription, all betokened a freer, more independent womanhood. What historians have perhaps appreciated less is that women by the 1920s had begun to look different. By the end of the war the decline in the birth rate had affected an entire reproductive generation, and with fewer pregnancies in their childbearing years, women could look younger by the time they reached their forties. The new fashions made poor women look better: shorter hems and simpler styles used less material, and the innovation of the paper dress pattern and the cheap sewing machine enabled the working-girl and the older housewife to own more than one or two outfits. By their late thirties they could be less worn, better dressed and cleaner, so that the contrast with those still drained by childbearing and poverty became sharper.[19] While it is obvious from the literature of the department store and the women's magazines that a new woman had been discovered as a lucrative market, it is less obvious that women did look and were different from their mothers and grandmothers. There was also a new sexuality, and the person, more than any other, who brought that into the lives of ordinary people, was Marie Stopes. Her medical reviewer in the *Medical Journal of Australia* had no doubt that the epidemic of venereal disease during the war had focused the public mind on the 'sexual problem' in a new way; as had the writings of Freud. Marie Stopes' book *Married Love* had appeared at just the right time at the end of the war: she preached that sexual happiness was the right of every man and woman, and sought to teach married couples about the natural rhythms of the female libido and the art of making love. For the reviewer the 'sexual problem' was women's apparent frigidity, therefore for married couples to find joyful sex was a profound liberation from a conflict between men and women 'which has caused more heart-burnings and difficulties than any other problem in life . . . Every man and every woman may learn something of the nature of their love from this delightful and romantic essay on the married state'.[20] And they did, reading Marie Stopes in their millions for the next forty years. But if they wanted to practise the new marriage, the technology of birth control was still expensive and unreliable. As individuals struggled with their private lives, they made mistakes, acted on impulse or more often in ignorance. If there was a growing acceptance of human sexuality and female libido, there had to be a more conscious pursuit of sexual fulfilment. If there was more knowledge of barrier contraception in the community, there had to be more sexual experimentation and therefore more accidents. And if young women wanted to slow down their childbearing, whereas their mothers had borne their brood quickly and placed an embargo on marital sex ever after, the daughters wanted to keep having sex and spacing their babies. Hence there had to be more unwanted, because ill-timed, pregnancies, and therefore more induced abortion.

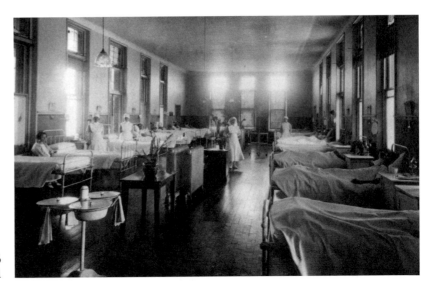

Infirmary ward, 1926
RWHA

The hospital had to pick up the pieces. In 1912 the Women's had opened its new Infirmary wing after finding financial support from the Druids' friendly society. The long-felt need for a proper septic ward was now met: there were two floors of sixteen gynaecological beds each and the third floor of sixteen beds was entirely for septic cases. There were surgical examination rooms on each floor, electric light and lifts and hot water radiators for heating. Within the year there was a 35 per cent increase in admissions.[21] In the financial year 1913–14, 103 women were admitted to the septic ward, fifty suffering from septic abortion (of whom three died) and fifty-three suffering from puerperal sepsis (nine died). Felix Meyer was now the senior honorary gynaecologist, and his first medical report was the most detailed and analytical report in the hospital's history. The septic ward had 'proved invaluable', and was always full; but it had been decided that the special venereal diseases ward was unnecessary. Salpingitis was only fifth on the table of conditions suffered by

Infirmary patients; plastic repair of the cervix and perineum the most common procedures. Removal of tubes or ovaries comprised 12 per cent of the operations, curettage a third. Septic cases accounted for just 6.8 per cent of admissions.[22] Yet by 1917–18, after three years of war, sepsis cases had multiplied six-fold and constituted 41 per cent of total Infirmary admissions. Of the 626 septic cases, seventeen had died of post-abortal sepsis, and seven of puerperal sepsis. Surgery on tubes had multiplied four-fold, while the removal of diseased ovaries had decreased a little.[23] It would have been a reasonable deduction for hospital staff to believe that the war had brought an epidemic of 'filthy sexual intercourse or deliberate interference with the natural processes of reproduction'. The behavioural changes in the wider society could well have been less dramatic, but the clinical evidence before the eyes of doctors and nurses inevitably shaped their responses.

The intellectual leadership of the medical profession emanating from the University of Melbourne had clear ideas of what needed to be done. Professor Richard Berry, who had taken the chair of anatomy so that Professor Allen could concentrate on pathology, influenced not just his students, but also the wider medical profession. In 1918 he was president of the Victorian Branch of the British Medical Association, and in his speeches and papers he married his research interests with his fears of 'the many evils and dangers threatening the social fabric', above all the social cancer of the 'unrecognised mentally deficient persons' — that is 'morons'. Berry's passion was the measurement of heads as an index of intelligence, which he supplemented with Binet-Simon intelligence tests. He was honorary alienist (psychiatrist) at the Children's Hospital where he had access to what were believed to be a large proportion of sub-normals, congenital syphilitics and 'poor types'. With S. D. Porteus, the Superintendent of Special Schools, he had examined nearly 10 000 Victorian schoolchildren, and was convinced 'of the prevalence of moronity and mental dullness amongst the school population' and,

> our most recent researches have forced upon us the conclusion that a large proportion of the lower class population never attain the mental levels above the age of twelve years, while at least 15 per cent of the population would be in one or other of Goddard's five classes of subnormal mentality.[24]

The 'most dangerous' was the high-grade moron: mentally deficient but deceptive, because he can be 'no way different from the intelligent man, and not only in outward appearance, but in conversation and bearing, these people often pass for normal'.[25] The expert could diagnose them, however, and if you went in search of them, you would find them in brothels, in venereal disease clinics, in hospital septic wards, in public mid-wifery beds, in refuges for fallen women, in prisons, in pubs, in gambling dens and two-up schools, on the wharves and in labouring gangs, in prisons and in the back lanes of Fitzroy, North Melbourne, South Richmond and the Collingwood flat. These people could not be morally trained; they could be putty in the hands of 'Bolsheviks' and militant unionists. And society was oblivious of the danger:

It permits individuals of extreme mental backwardness, many of them not more mentally developed than the boy of eight, ten or twelve years of age, to vote on problems of great and vital national importance, to impede the effective work of the schools, to become sexual plague spots in the community, to propagate their kind in legitimate and illegitimate ways, and generally to act as a virulent social poison.[26]

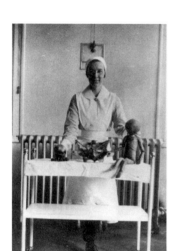

Miss Jean Headberry
RWHA

Behind all this was fear, fear of a politicised, empowered and over-numerous working class. As the English eugenicist, Karl Pearson, had argued and the authors of the 1911 British Census had contrived to prove, the educated classes were restricting their fertility and the masses were outbreeding them.[27] But infant mortality was still too high. The losses of young men in the war were still lower than those of young babies: 'Of the British forces engaged in the war in 1915 there died, on average, nine men every hour; but in the same year there died every hour twelve infants under twelve months old'.[28] If the losses fanned anxieties over race suicide, they also impressed the concerned with the concept of 'wastage': of the nation losing potential citizens and soldiers to disease and poor mothering. Therefore the response was less one of advocating mass sterilisation and institutionalisation than of intervention to prevent the wastage of infant and maternal lives and to correct bad mothering. The growing shortage of babies required the salvaging of working-class babies — saving their lives, protecting their health, educating their mothers, training their minds and bodies and thereby raising the *quality* of the poor. If heredity was crucial, it was still possible to offset the worst results with manipulation of the environment. And if the environment could not be improved, then the nation had the right, even the duty, to remove that child — Aboriginal or 'slum white' — from its degenerate environment and train it for better things or adopt it out to an acceptable home. The 'slum' discourse, which stigmatised and disenfranchised the poor and the outcast so that their children could be stolen by the state, was part of the wider discourse about national degeneration.

The nation needed more babies and better babies, and to achieve this it needed healthier and better mothers. From early in the war through to the 1920s and 1930s, the constellation of reforms and movements to improve the quality of mothers and babies — the maternity allowance, antenatal care, infant welfare centres, free kindergartens, all with their experts brimming with hygiene, good nutrition and science — did imply a new valorisation of motherhood.[29] Kereen Reiger has conceptualised the intrusion of the trained expert into the family as 'the disenchantment of the home',[30] and it was; but it was also a new value placed on motherhood which embraced the poor because the nation needed better babies. (If you can't abolish the working class, you may as well improve them.) In Tracy's hospital, it was women who mattered; the babies were scarcely mentioned and even neo-natal deaths went unrecorded; from the 1920s onwards, babies began to matter.

In the mental world of the Women's Hospital there came a new respect for the battler of the back lanes, as opposed to the smart young thing, who played around and 'brought her troubles on herself'. The 'slum mum' was the innocent victim of male lust, selfishness and fecklessness. Since

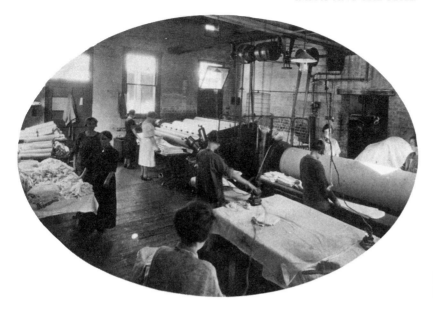

Laundry workers, 1927
RWHA

the 1890s the proportion of married women delivered at the hospital had been rising, and if the Infirmary wards disclosed the sexual delinquency of the single and the young, in the midwifery wards the staff had welcomed an increase in 'the better type of working class who find it necessary to go there', or so the hospital told the press in 1921 for its £50 000 appeal to build a new Infirmary wing. The hospital represented itself to the public as sanitary and suburban, just like a hospital that any reader of the *Age* and the *Argus* would happily enter. It had

> . . . spacious and airy, well-lighted, and fresh-looking midwifery wards, tastefully decorated with the flowers of the day, with dainty white beds and little white cots in which sleeping quietly, or exercising their tiny voices, lie the little mites whose coming has brought to the mother either the crowning glory of her womanhood or merely the anxiety of having another mouth to feed, another body to clothe, when there is little food or clothing to spare; amongst whom there are some who have come into a world that offers them neither home nor name.[31]

The *Age* was moved by the babies: many babies were beautiful, fat and contented, but some

> . . . tiny wrinkled faces most uncannily bear the impress of worry, they look as if they belong to people reaching a hundred years, and one wonders what life has in store for them. Then a glance at the bed of the mother tells all one needs to know. The mother, too, is careworn, haggard, suffering. One woman looked over sixty but is thirty-eight: 'Poor thing', said the compassionate nurse, 'she has had a terrible lot of worry and has such a big family'.[32]

The cause of all this suffering were men, in particular working-class husbands: 'The high wages, with the constant strikes, have left the women much worse off than in the olden days, when there was some continuity of income. Then there is the menace of drink'.[33] It is scarcely surprising that a decade later dole payments during the Depression were usually paid to wives because husbands could not be trusted.[34] The appeal, therefore, was to women, to help their 'suffering sisters' — to cross the barriers of class and support the Women's Hospital as one of 'those charities that soothe and heal and bless'.[35]

The doctors framed their attack on infant and maternal mortality at both prevention and the reform of medical practice. It was all very well to preach the dangers of race suicide, but interventions and reforms could be implemented now. And whatever their opinions of women in general and the poor in particular, doctors of course liked many of their patients, did want to relieve their suffering and mourned their deaths. And it was Rothwell Adam who led the call to institute an antenatal care programme at the hospital — following the examples of Adelaide and Sydney (Adelaide claimed its 1910 antenatal clinic was the first in the world, Sydney's the third). In May 1914, before the war had started, he had argued,

> An Antenatal clinic is for the definite purpose of observing and treating pregnant women who are suffering from pathological conditions which may prevent their pregnancy proceeding to a successful issue, and for the care of the unborn child so that it may be born healthy with a good prospect of surviving and becoming a useful citizen.[36]

He cited successful ventures in Scotland and America, and since the Board was now planning a new midwifery wing, it should incorporate a proper antenatal clinic. He provided an outline: the establishment of a distinct department under an experienced physician, six or seven beds for antenatal treatment, a close relationship with the department of clinical pathology, and supervision from the honorary obstetric staff when not on duty in the wards.

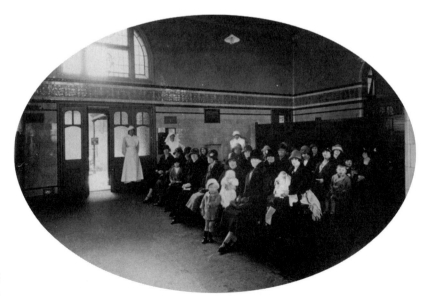

Outpatients waiting room, 1927 *RWHA*

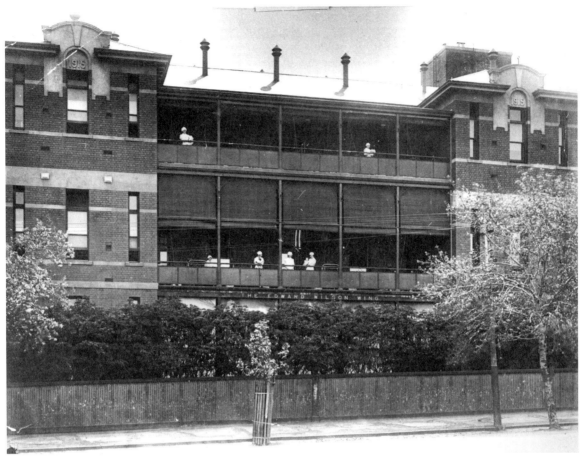

Edward Wilson Wing, Cardigan Street, built 1917, third floor added 1924, demolished 1969
RWHA

In early 1917 it was opened, as was a new midwifery wing, and the numbers of attendances more than justified its inauguration. The ante-natal clinic continued to grow, recording over five hundred attendances a year by 1919. By mid-1923, it was near three thousand. And there was the Baby Health Centre Clinic: that same year there had been 6350 attendances compared with 4910 the previous year. The first Baby Health Centres, as 'Schools for Mothers', had begun in the inner suburb of Richmond in 1917.[37] Then in December 1918 the Victorian Baby Health Centre Association applied to the Board of the Women's Hospital to establish a clinic, and in 1924 opened a Model Training School for the Baby Health Centre Association in the same building, so that midwifery training could be followed and complemented by Infant Welfare training. In 1926 a postnatal clinic was started. All these were new preventative interventions which doctors hoped would both reduce the mortality from labour complications and eclampsia. But what was also important was the enthusiasm young mothers felt for 'better mothering' and better care. As the soldiers returned from the war, married and started families, the hospital again was overtaxed and its expansion continued. The £50 000 fund of 1921 resulted in a new nurses' home and another storey added to the Edward Wilson wing with thirty beds. In 1924–25 the hospital confined 2534 women and the Infirmary admitted 2079. It was now a very big and complex institution, extending the role of professionals in women's reproductive health well beyond the delivery and lying-in.

The theory and practice of antenatal care developed rapidly during the first half of the 1920s, and the younger men among the honoraries at the hospital — Arthur Wilson, Robert Fowler and R. N. Wawn — published and lectured both to the wider profession and to postgraduate classes conducted at the Women's. From Brisbane came the work of Dr R. Marshall Allen, who in 1925 was appointed the Director of Obstetrical Services at the Melbourne Women's Hospital and commissioned to undertake a full survey of obstetrical practice and services in Victoria. Antenatal and neo-natal care had to become part of the maternity hospital, he had argued in 1922 — the time had long gone when 'lying-in' was the sole responsibility of a women's hospital.[38] On 8 July of that year Arthur Wilson, R. W. Chambers and Robert Fowler presented papers to the Section of Preventative Medicine of the British Medical Association (BMA) — a section initiated by senior staff from the Women's as well as other hospitals. They each enumerated different aspects of the intent and conduct of antenatal care. Maternal mortality was stationary, and when analysed, revealed that too many deaths were preventable, as were so many of the disabilities that plagued childbearing women and filled the gynaecological wards. If infection was still the greatest killer of parturient women, it was usually the consequence of interference. Aseptic technique now required that vaginal examinations be only for emergencies, but emergencies still arose and their mismanagement led to the possibility of infection. Therefore if emergencies could be anticipated, emergency intervention might be obviated or at least reduced. The antenatal regime, therefore, was to discover early if there was any likelihood of obstructed labour, to advise on diet and constipation, to record any history of heart or kidney disease or previous obstetric difficulties, to diagnose venereal disease and institute treatment. Fearful of infection, pelvic examination was to be kept to a minimum and much attention paid to constitutional health.

It was still common for women, even when confined by a doctor, to

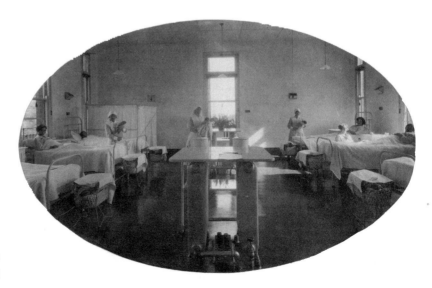

Midwifery ward, 1927
RWHA

be seen for the first time when already in labour. Doctors constantly walked into obstetric emergencies in complete ignorance of the woman's medical history. Bearing their chloroform and their forceps, they were summoned by desperate relatives and friends to a woman often exhausted and in agony: 'Doctor, do something — put her out of her misery — take the baby away'. And they did, with forceps often applied too early. Antenatal surveillance, however, should reduce the temptations to impulsive interference. Antenatal knowledge could also change the management of the woman with tuberculosis, heart or kidney disease, and that pre-knowledge opened the possibility of early therapeutic abortion when there was very real fear that she would not survive a delivery.[39] It was not unexpected, then, to read in a paper by Fowler three years later, that should a woman be too sick to risk pregnancy, it was now the doctor's duty to advise her on methods of birth control.[40] The acceptable medical discourse had changed very fast.

But driving the antenatal care movement, even more than preventable infection, was eclampsia. Australian doctors believed that its incidence was higher in Australia than in the United Kingdom, and that it was especially so in Melbourne. Again, the fact that the medical staff of the Women's Hospital led the Victorian profession on women's health shaped its perception as to its incidence and gravity. It was the emergency most likely to come to the hospital and they saw more of it than any other group of Australian doctors other than their equivalents in Sydney and Brisbane. They blamed the changeable climate, 'inefficient clothing', and the rich Australian diet (too much meat), but essentially remained mystified.[41] In the hospital's statistics, however, it was now the most common cause of maternal death. They took a wide definition of the predisposing toxaemias of pregnancy, including hyperemesis or uncontrolled vomiting, chronic nephritis and pyelonephritis. Of the true eclamptic cases, as Arthur Wilson admitted, the mortality was 'appalling': 'During the last fourteen years at the Women's Hospital, the maternal mortality was 24 per cent and the foetal 50 per cent'. He hastened to add that none of these women died after a caesarean operation: 'Indeed, both maternal and foetal mor-

pyelonephritis: bacterial infection of the kidney substance, which when chronic may result in kidney failure (*OMD*)

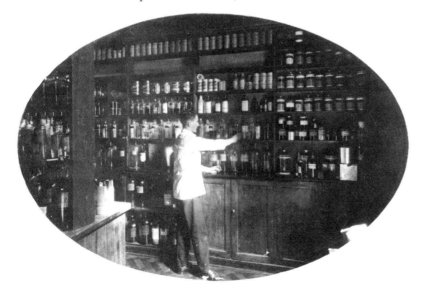

Dispensary, Lady Weedon Wing, 1927 *RWHA*

acidosis: condition in which the acidity of bodily fluids and tissues is abnormally high (*OMD*)

acetonuria: (ketonuria), presence in urine of acetone. This may occur in diabetes mellitus, starvation, or after persistent vomiting and results from the partial oxidation of fats. (*OMD*)

talities after operation have been slightly less than in those patients treated by conservative measures'. The most successful cases of all were those given antenatal care: and in fact not one toxaemic woman given antenatal care at the Women's had suffered a convulsion.[42] Antenatal care married the clinic with the laboratory: in addition to the Wassermann test were the analysis of blood for jaundice, acidosis and acetonuria; of urine for albumin, salts, 'nitrogenous waste products' and sugar for diabetes: a regime encapsulated in Robert Fowler's brilliant 1925 paper on the 'Clinical Conduct of Pregnancy'.[43] If it meant the increasing medicalisation of the natural process of reproduction, it also represented growing confidence in the capacity of modern medical science to anticipate and prevent the pathologies of parturition. Interventions increasingly worked, but they needed to be judicious. Older interventions could do as much harm as good: the solution, therefore, was careful scientific observation. The new generation warned their fellow practitioners and lectured their students that 90 per cent of pregnancies were normal and required only 'watchful expectancy' and 'careful management'. As Arthur Wilson explained, 'The word "careful" has been used advisedly, as in the art of obstetrics, carefulness counts much more than skilfulness'.[44]

The treatment of eclampsia was in dispute. There were two schools of thought by the end of the war: the Rotunda in Dublin believed that 'toxin was elaborated from the food taken in by the mother, owing to some fault in her metabolism', and advocated 'conservative treatment'. The other school of thought, known as the English or Continental, blamed the foetus as the source of the toxic response of the mother. An early theory was that

the symptoms are due to placental albumin finding its way back to the maternal blood stream in quantities greater than can be dealt with by the antibodies which are elaborated to deal with it. It is on the presence of these antibodies in the maternal blood that Abderhalden's serum test for the diagnosis of pregnancy is based.[45]

Treatment was therefore either to purge the mother, sedate her with morphine, remove all stimulation, place her on a water diet, and wait for the toxins to be eliminated; or it was the removal of the offending foetus as quickly as possible. The honorary staff at the Women's were still much influenced by the Rotunda and leaned towards conservative treatment. Sedation with morphine or chloral hydrate, a light diet, darkness and absolute rest could reduce symptoms, but once the patient started to have fits, the sooner the uterus was empty the better.[46]

But the debate involved another volatile area of obstetric intervention, the caesarean section. Should an eclamptic woman be delivered by caesarean despite all the risks? In March 1921 Arthur Sherwin, an honorary outdoor surgeon of the hospital, gave a paper to the Melbourne Gynaecological and Obstetrical Society arguing for fewer caesareans — the 'mania' of 'belly ripping' — and the induction of labour as a safer option. He attacked the practices of the indoor staff at the hospital, questioned their lack of reporting of 'albuminuria' and of any conservative treatment (in 1914 the hospital had reported the incidence of albuminuria:

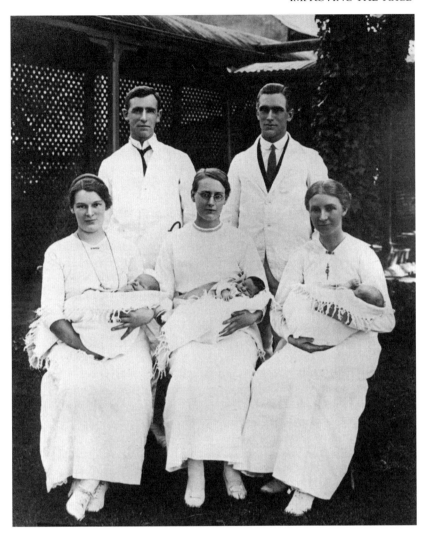

'The Three Caesars'
Back: Dr Arthur Wilson,
Dr Anderson
Front: Miss Wisewould
holding Baby McCorkell
(placenta praevia), Miss
Bennett holding Baby
Cusach (contracted
pelvis), Miss Balaam
holding Baby Challiner
(contracted pelvis)
RWHA

300 out of 1391 deliveries) and deplored the deaths of six of the thirty-one eclamptic cases. He compared the Women's Hospital with the Queen Charlotte Hospital in London, where he had been a resident from 1910 until 1912 before he joined the Montenegrin contingent in Northern Albania. The Queen Charlotte's astonishing record amidst the poorest women in London deeply impressed him, and he was devastated to find a caesarean rate at the Women's more than double that in London, and a maternal mortality nearly ten times greater than the Queen Charlotte's.[47] His audience that night did not take offence, and revealed themselves to be equally cautious towards the caesarean solution, and looked to better antenatal care as the real answer to toxaemia.[48] But 1919 and 1920 were bad years for the hospital and scarcely a fair comparison. The Spanish Influenza epidemic reached Melbourne in the winter of 1919, and in the last week of July the hospital was overwhelmed, with three wards full of influenza cases. With many staff themselves stricken, thirty beds were set aside in midwifery for influenza victims in or nearing labour.[49] Altogether twenty-nine midwifery patients died from influenza, blowing

out the maternal death rate to figures not seen since the 1880s. Incomplete, threatened or inevitable abortions also rose, with 1092 in 1919–20, comprising 36 per cent of midwifery 'deliveries'. Perhaps it was an epidemic of induced abortion in the emotional chaos of the immediate post-war years, and a sudden leap in post-abortal sepsis deaths in the Infirmary would support this; but many must have been spontaneous, the result of the influenza itself.

Once the influenza retreated, the pattern was set for the 1920s where eclampsia and death from kidney disease of various sorts, began to outpace deaths from sepsis. In addition to pre-eclampsia and eclampsia, many women suffered chronic nephritis as the result of past, usually strepto-coccal, infections, so that through the 1920s the 'toxaemic' conditions combined accounted for between a third and a half of the hospital's mater-nal deaths annually. The hospital collected its statistics erratically, but in 1913–14 did record the number of confinements where the mother had protein in her urine — albuminuria — and produced that appalling figure of 300 out of 1391 deliveries, or 21.5 per cent, double the rate common today. Even allowing for poor laboratory technique, it suggests the degree of chronic kidney disease in the community. As puerperal sepsis from a hospital delivery almost disappeared as a cause of death, sepsis deaths from confinements outside and from incomplete abortion, either induced or spontaneous, held up and even increased. Antenatal care seemed to reduce the incidence of full-blown eclampsia and a fall in the rate of stillbirth registered greater success in the management of the toxaemias of preg-nancy. But over the full range of work in the midwifery wards there was much variation in patterns of intervention. Forceps ranged from 19.6 per cent in 1923–24 back down to 10.6 per cent the following year. That was a good year, the first without a destructive operation since the 1850s, and perforation and craniotomy retreated as the caesarean advanced.

Both the older and the younger generation of obstetricians regretted the decline of the obstetric art. Dr Cairns Lloyd warned the modern obstetrician that 'dramatic and spectacular' as the caesarean operation might be, as well as lucrative and time-saving, it was still a risk to the woman both now and later should she have another child. Any abdominal operation had its dangers, even a relatively easy one like the caesarean, and scarred uteri had ruptured during subsequent labours. Cairns Lloyd had trained at the Rotunda and he was convinced of the value of the conservative approach to pre-eclampsia; he would never rule out surgical removal of foetus from a fitting woman, but there had been cases when even that had not stopped the convulsions.[50] At the same meeting of the BMA in November 1921, Cairns Lloyd's colleague at the Women's, R. H. Morrison, neatly summarised the honorary staff's concept of medicalised childbirth, the dividing line between the natural to the unnatural, and the crucial place of asepsis in that history of medicalisation:

> There is much difference of opinion as to whether or not child-bearing is to be classed as a pathological process. Let us then look on it as a physio-logical function which is very prone to become pathological and which certainly calls for very careful pre-maternity supervision! No one can dis-pute the fact that every case of labour must be treated as a surgical case.

It is to the perfection of asepsis following on the antenatal care that we must look to diminish the mortality, the morbidity and the after-effects of labour. In discussing this subject, the fundamental principle must be kept in mind of endeavouring to have a viable child delivered with the minimum amount of trauma and pain to the mother.[51]

Yet as the decade advanced, despite better control of midwives, more antenatal care and the Maternity Allowance of £5 instituted in 1912 which was intended to pay for the attendance of a doctor and a trained midwife, or for a private or public hospital (the Women's took £2 5s), the maternal death rate around the nation did not fall as it should have. The leaders of the profession knew from the emergencies they received at hospitals and privately that there were many doctors practising in the community whose obstetric skills and judgement, as well as their aseptic technique, were poor. The maternity allowance had also made it lucrative for doctors, midwives and self-styled nurses to open small private maternity hospitals, which too often were unsanitary and understaffed. There was a large section of the population — respectable working class and lower middle class — who could not afford good private hospitals but whose income was too high to permit admission to a public hospital.[52] There was also a stigma against the Women's; it was where 'the unmarried mothers' and 'the abortion cases' went, and so many preferred the small establishments. One young first-time mother from Richmond bitterly regretted her decision to enter the private establishment of a local midwife,

> It was a slaughterhouse. She was a great big horse — she should have been a horse doctor. See in these days they don't let them suffer — they don't! I walked the floor all night in agony. Poor old *Fred* — God love him — he came up and saw me in this intense agony, walking up and down in that room on my own. He said 'I can't sit here and watch you'. I said 'Go home', and he went to the pub and got full. He couldn't stand me. I was thirty-six hours in labour. I was almost unconscious when the doctor came and gave me an anaesthetic and took the baby away because he was a whopper. When I came to he said, 'You've got to be quiet — you've got stitches there'. I didn't know anything.[53]

In eight months of 1926, 1762 women were delivered at the Women's Hospital and of them 909 had had antenatal care (later known as 'booked cases'). Not one of them died. But of the remaining 852 emergency cases ('unbooked'), eleven died. In the small private hospitals the doctor was often called too late so that interference was unavoidable, and poor hygiene and after-care led to infections.[54] Some operators used midwifery as a screen for illegal abortions, and the 1920s saw the blossoming of the entrepreneurial midwife abortionist, the most notorious being Nurse Hannah Mitchell of Richmond, whose court appearances were like celebrity occasions.[55] By the end of the 1920s there were 173 private obstetric hospitals in Melbourne, of which over a third were found by Dr Marshall Allan to be 'poor or bad'. Some had uncertificated nurses; and where the proprietors also did home midwifery, inpatients could be left unattended for hours at a time. Only 5 per cent had a good nursery, most had no means of isolating infectious cases, and often babies were kept in the kitchen or staff dining room. Only 40 per cent were found to possess 'a fairly satisfactory system of sterilisation'.[56] Private hospitals were to remain notorious for their infection rates for decades to come.

But the offenders were also doctors, and the medical students on extern calls for the Women's, full of the hospital's doctrines on good midwifery, often witnessed with horror how things were done 'in private'. In March 1921 R. A. Spence and Sister Pennyquick were called to a para seven, aged thirty-two:

> Received call at 12.20 p.m. and left by tram for South Melbourne. Mother informed me she had been in labour four days and that the membranes had ruptured early that morning and that she had always had chloroform and instruments. Nurse arrived at this juncture. Abdominally either a large single infant or twins, limbs being felt on both sides. Head was not fixed and the presentation probably LOA. PV: Membranes ruptured, os 7/6. Head not fixed.
>
> Mother was having strong pains, but having been chloroform spoilt, did not make good use of them. Rigged up pulley and box from foot of bed and got my knees into her back which gave her good purchase.
>
> Now we were informed that she had a private Doctor engaged but we kept up our attentions in case he should not arrive. However he arrove [*sic*], busted the membranes with a hair pin straight from Sister's head, put on high forceps and gave them to me to pull — no axis traction, no chloroform — an example of 'how we do things in private'. I could not shift the head which was caught on the symphysis. He had a go and after sweat broke out and the woman howled for a little drop of chloroform, I gave her 'chlo and pit' and then hopped round to slip back an anterior lip of cervix and mop up faeces. I took charge again when HOP and delivered some normal babe. The doctor leaving a flood to clean up. I bathed the baby which weighed 16 pounds by the scales in the new bay ie the baby was $12\frac{3}{4}$ pounds.
>
> I never want to see another baby of this size. [He did, twelve days later.] Placenta came away 15 minutes after child. No PPH and patient felt quite comfortable. Home in time for tea.[57]

It was clearly a question of medical education, both of the already qualified practitioners and the doctors of the future, and if the teaching of obstetrics was to have the importance it deserved, it needed a university chair. The moving spirit from 1924 until the appointment of Marshall Allan to the chair in 1929 was Dunbar Hooper, and the chair was named in his honour in 1967. In response to the widely publicised investigations in the USA, Canada, New Zealand and above all that by Dame Janet Campbell in the United Kingdom, in 1924, Hooper moved, as chairman of the Victorian Branch of the BMA, that the branch appoint a Victorian Obstetric Committee. Within three months a questionnaire was sent to all Victorian doctors seeking their support for a chair and, raising the spectre of interstate rivalry, noted that Sydney University now had a professor of obstetrics. At the Women's in October a Medical Faculty Unit

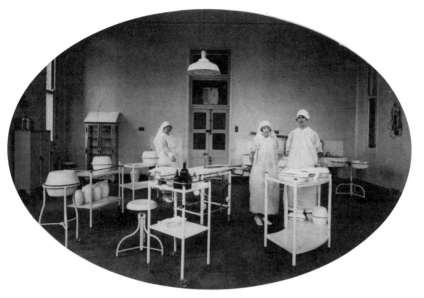

Operating theatre, 1927
RWHA

was established, elevating the next lecturer in obstetrics and gynaecology to be an ex officio honorary and allocating him ten midwifery beds, four antenatal cases and eight gynaecological beds. The honorary staff were also informed that they were to permit teaching to take place in the septic wards.[58] Hooper, who as a young doctor had dragged the Women's into the antiseptic era by conducting case analysis, knew that the future lay with research and science, as well as clinical teaching. But, essentially, all the hospital had was intellectual capital. Since 1921 it had been treating cancers with radium, and had investigated using it for cases of haemorrhage from chronic subinvolution of the uterus.[59] It had a pathology room, but no proper laboratories of any sort: nearly all the pathology was conducted at the university's laboratories or by the 1930s at the Baker Institute. It did not even have the facilities to make its own sterile saline solution, so that every day it was made up in the university and carried over Swanston Street to the hospital. But Dunbar Hooper could envisage a great future,

subinvolution of uterus: failure of the uterus to revert to its normal size during the six weeks following childbirth (*OMD*)

> . . . the day is fast approaching, thanks to the enthusiasm of some of the members of the obstetric staff of the Women's Hospital, when that institution will make full use of the enormous clinical material at its disposal which is said to be the largest in the British Empire. Very soon that institution must be in charge of a master in obstetrics who will be the superintendent and have an enthusiastic, energetic professional staff to work with him so that the annual reports of the Women's Hospital in the near future will show a great diminution in maternal mortality and morbidity and be of such value to the medical profession in Australia as to equal the force and influence of the Rotunda Hospital reports from Dublin.[60]

By early 1925, Dunbar Hooper had secured £10 000 from the Edward Wilson Trust (the *Argus* newspaper) so that a Director of Obstetrical Research could be appointed, and in November Marshall Allan was

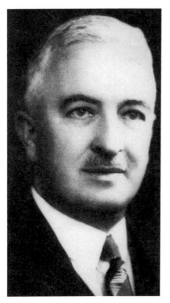

Professor Marshall Allan
RWHA

recruited from Brisbane. The first term of the next academic year, Arthur Wilson was appointed the lecturer under the new conditions while Marshall Allan commenced his designated task of investigating obstetrical practice in the state of Victoria. He inspected every licensed obstetric hospital in the state and interviewed almost every medical practitioner before submitting his final report in 1928. It was a masterly document. It looked at the components of mortality, the patterns of infection, the effects of antenatal care, the impact of criminal abortion on the maternal mortality and morbidity rates between Melbourne and the rest of the state, the differences between the reproductive health of the women of 'the industrial suburbs' and 'the residential suburbs', the quality of hospitals, of services such as ambulances, refuges and the Melbourne District and Bush Nursing associations. Those at greatest risk in childbirth were women under twenty, the single, the older mother with many babies and the poor without antenatal care. The use of doctors for childbirth in the industrial suburbs ranged widely, but too often the doctor was called to an emergency by an incompetent midwife and knew nothing of the patient's history. Whether it was the records of the Women's Hospital showing that 36 per cent of all gynaecological admissions were due to the effect of the previous confinement, to the cranial injuries found in 80 per cent of deaths of breech babies, in 68 per cent of forceps deliveries and only 36 per cent of normal deliveries, much pointed to a poor standard of obstetrical intervention. (Syphilis, to their surprise, was not a major cause of perinatal mortality according to autopsy reports.) There were fascinating class differences in perinatal mortality: deaths from prematurity were more prevalent in the industrial suburbs than in the residential areas, while the reverse was observed as regards birth injuries.[61] In other words, middle-class patients received more clumsy, early intervention; the poor had less but then as charity patients had less 'say'. How much was the excess of intervention driven by the demands of the private consumer?

The long-term solution lay in medical education, and Marshall Allan was appointed the first professor in 1929. Meanwhile Arthur Wilson had borne the full burden of undergraduate teaching at the Women's and his surviving lecture notes reveal a profession very conscious of its duties and shortcomings. Maternal mortality and morbidity in Australia of the 1920s remained an unacceptable scandal and doctors had to take much of the blame, he taught. There were too many preventable deaths from infection and poorly managed eclampsia and haemorrhage. Ninety per cent of confinements were uncomplicated and best left to Nature. The doctor was there to watch, to wait, to ensure care, but only to intervene when clinically, as opposed to socially, necessary:

> The first rule of obstetrics is <u>care</u>
> The second rule is <u>care</u>
> and The third rule is <u>care</u>
> To amplify this 1st care in the antenatal period; the 2nd care in the natal period and the 3rd care in the post-natal period.
> We do not all have the same manual dexterity — neither do we possess in equal degrees that indefinite quality known as 'brains', yet we should have or be able to develop the capacity for being careful with our patients.

Develop an obstetrical conscience. Before embarking on any line of treatment ask yourself would you pursue the same treatment if the patient were one of your own womenfolk. In any obstetrical case the chief persons to be considered are the mother and her child, not yourself. Your time and convenience are as nothing compared to the life and health of your patients. Take a pride in your art. Your profession should mean more to you than a means of making bread and butter.[62]

This was an obstetrical regime which implied the total medicalisation but not the pathologising of reproduction. The modern doctor was there to watch, record and assess, and to respect the processes of Nature, rather than to intervene. His or her task was partly educational: expecting mothers had to be taught about diet, hygiene, exercise, rest and sensible self-care. The continuing dangers of infection, now that its mechanics were better understood, deterred the invasion of childbirth by intervention and returned it to the self-directing biological world. But such purity of practice was difficult outside the public teaching hospital. The working woman, Wilson taught, coped better with labour than the 'delicately nurtured' or the 'athletic', hence it was in private practice that paying patients would demand anaesthesia or narcosis even in the first stage of labour and 'always during the second stage'. It was an appalling obstetrical dilemma: the poor gave birth in pain, but the better off gave birth in greater danger.[63] Doctors were therefore not in control of their practice unless they kept an 'obstetrical conscience', even at the risk of losing private patients. These were high standards and high ideals. Having completed their lectures and conducted deliveries under the supervision of the Labour Ward sisters and the residents, Wilson's young students then went out into the homes of the poor to put his teaching into practice.

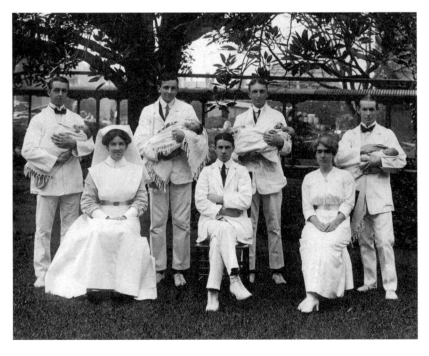

Student group *RWHA*

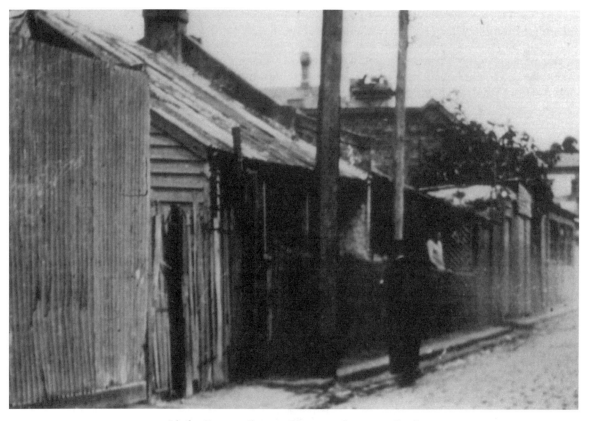

**Little George Street, Fitzroy, photographed
by Oswald Barnett in the 1930s**
Fitzroy Historical Collection

'An Interesting Introduction to the Family Life of the Proletariat' The Extern Midwifery Case Books 1920–1931

9

Found oldest inhabitant, he of bilious mien and rheumy eye, who gave explicit directions: Little George Street is in the centre of Fitzroy's vendetta district, lined with garbage bins and paved with defunct rats. House two-roomed, bed against front door; eldest child in bed in kitchen with measles (my opinion asked and grandma's diagnosis confirmed). Mother sullen, and didn't want doctor. Grandma, also pregnant very truculent. Husband out of work for weeks, gone to look for a job. Auntie aet 9 seemed to have a grip on things. Examination made. Sister gave enema and Quin. Sulph. Sister suggested bath; Mother rather puzzled, always went to Grandma's for those things. However, Sister boiled tin of water and improvised wash tub while I left for breakfast. Arrived back, just in time. Bath had done the trick. Baby born successfully. Mother penitent and apologetic. Bathed baby while Sister cleaned mother. Enjoyed walk through Exhibition Gardens.

An interesting introduction to family life of the Proletariat.[64]

The home deliveries conducted by the medical students were for most their first experience of working-class life. But it was more than an opportunity to cross class lines. They saw the patient in her natural state, not washed, reclothed and subdued as in the hospital. These privileged young university students saw the patient in her own place and at her most vulnerable. Some did not like what they saw of working-class private life. Those with prejudices sought confirmation; those who were quick to condemn, did so. But however much they were prepared by lurid hospital stories and student legend, many were deeply shocked and moved,

Located a dirty single-fronted place in Burnley. Knocked at door and after explaining myself to scared mother through the front window, I entered. Found the mother was the only inhabitant of the house with exception of several sleeping kids. Mother was standing up & coincident with my arrival, the membranes went. Told mother to get into bed whilst I put swabs on [to boil]. Had just found a saucepan with food a good month old still adhered, when a frantic yell sent me scurrying into the bedroom. The mother was still on her feet and the head was out. Hastily helped her on to the bed and managed the rest of the labour with no pretence of asepsis. Perhaps the fact that this was the sixth child in six years accounted for the peri remaining intact. Sister arrived just as I was tying off the cord. Placenta arrived half an hour later. Membranes were incomplete although we waited half an hour to give them a chance to come away properly. Mother and child fixed up and mess straightened out. Left at 11.10 p.m. with Sister after a most hair-raising and strenuous evening.[65]

The character at the centre of the narrative is mostly the student, and the narrative in the case book helped them to cope with their fear, their elation at success, their shock and their distaste. Much of it is crude student humour, but much of it is also a struggle to come to terms with very difficult experiences. Mona Blanch set off on her first case in December 1922, knowing that the midwife could not come until later: 'Imagine my feelings — my first case and no Sister'. She found the house in Napier Street, Fitzroy, where a family of five lived in one room. The husband met her and ushered her into the room without saying a word. She began to prepare, and borrowed a pudding basin for the lysol swabs from the family who lived in the front room: 'the cherries for lunch were tipped out just!'

A few minutes later I caught a glimpse of the head at the vulva, so got her on her side and started putting on my gloves. A yell from the bed brought me over with only one glove on, and I tried to hold the head in, and consequently flex it, with a lysol swab until the pain ended. However, there was no end so I had to deliver the child with only one

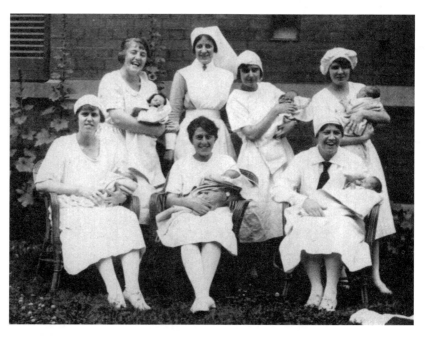

Student group, December 1922
Back: May Anderson, —, Sybil Hawkins, Amanda Liebert
Front: Mona Blanch, Mary Waite, Margaret Playle
Photograph courtesy of Dr Janet Fitzpatrick, daughter of Mary Waite

glove on. The patient wriggled round to such an extent that by the time the head had been born I was sitting on the chest of drawers at the top of the bed. The kid safely out, I got the mother on her back and held the fundus with one hand while I dangled the child by its feet until it yelled lustily. The lady of the cherry bowl then came in and took the fundus while I tied off the cord. The placenta followed some twenty minutes later — the only incident of interest before that being the arrival of a drunk man who chucked the baby under the chin and leered at the mother, not at all abashed by her nakedness, until I could get him out of the room. Sister arrived while I was cleaning up the mother and she bathed the baby while I went on with what I was doing. The baby nearly broke the spring balance, we were very thrilled to see it was 12 lbs. Father buried the placenta, a neighbour took charge of the soiled sheets, I administered 3 drachms ergot and left 3 drachms to be taken at 4 p.m. Sister and I left at 1.20 and I got back to a belated lunch at 1.40 p.m.[66]

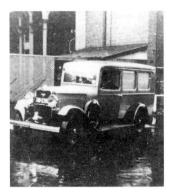

Ambulance in courtyard, 1938 *RWHA*

The Women's Hospital had always maintained an interest in an extern midwifery service. During its past septic crises it had boarded out midwifery patients, but it was not until 1905 that it formalised the service. It began in collaboration with the District Nursing Society, which had been founded in 1885 to provide home care for the sick poor, especially septic and chronic cases which the public hospitals refused to treat indefinitely. In 1894 the District Nursing Society added home midwifery to its services for those unable to use the Women's Hospital. From the beginning the Society had a close relationship with the hospital, permitting students to gain obstetric experience with its midwives, and relying on the hospital to admit emergency cases. There remained tensions, however, over the training of midwives: the hospital insisted that they needed a hospital-based training, while some in the Society looked to the English example where many qualified midwives received all their training in home deliveries. But all trainees did need lectures from doctors as well as from tutor sisters. The hospital made its bid to control both intern and extern midwifery training and practice in January 1918 when it proposed to provide its own midwives for the cases attended by students. The doctors argued that primiparas should not be delivered at home, because they needed attention longer than the two hours the District Nurses were allowed to stay after delivery. They also argued that 'elderly primiparas' — women over thirty having their first baby — needed to be in hospital. Finally it was resolved that the District Nurses still attend the confinements, and the hospital was only to send students out on cases which had been booked three months in advance. The mothers were to pay one shilling if they could afford it, and the taxi fare if the case was at night, although that seems to have been waived in later years. The District Nurse would visit before and after the confinement, and all severe complications were to be sent by ambulance to the Women's Hospital once the Sister had asked the advice of the matron of the Society's Nurses' Home. If instruments were to used, or an anaesthetic needed, or a death certificate for a stillborn child required, a private doctor had to be called.[67]

In practice, it was much harder than this. The poor did not have telephones, public telephones were few and often vandalised, pubs closed at six, and after 10 p.m., when babies are apt to get serious about entering the world, shops were shut, so that often the police station was the only place open with a phone. Poor and drunk people sometimes did not know how to operate a public telephone: a drunken new father in out-lying Fawkner tried to feed one a pound note. (It was a difficult case: 'Mother a neurotic who screamed every time something was done to her, and demanded "chloroform" at frequent intervals"', and father suggested they drown the baby'.)[68] A Richmond woman in premature labour walked half a mile to find a phone: 'damned lucky that she didn't drop the kid on the pavement'.[69] Some phoned after the baby was born. But even if they phoned in good time, during the day the two accoucheurs independently took a tram, or made their way to the railway station, and hoped that each would arrive in time and at the same time. At night they took a taxi or a District Nursing Society car, and later in the 1920s a hired limousine was provided. But once they left the central city area, they entered a world of lanes, and back streets, lit only occasionally by an intact street light globe. Twenty and thirty years after the bringing of electricity to Melbourne, the industrial suburbs were still in darkness, because the poor could not pay the bills and neither could the local councils. In September 1922 Annie Hensley and Sister Arbuckle were called to Little Docker Street, Richmond. It was two in the morning:

> While progressing tentatively up Church Street we encountered a friendly policeman who suggested we should turn at Gipps Street. Slowly up and down we paraded searching for a light till Sister's piercing gaze lit on a male shadow — she jumped down from the taxi and followed the man down a lane nearby. I shouted frantically for the taxi man to follow, which finally he did, to a house with a light. Requested by the male shadow to walk 'right along in', I did so to be greeted by 'Oh nurse — the baby's in the world, the baby's in the world' from an assembly of elderly females — and with Sister gazing fixedly at the most marvellous concoction of mother, liquor, placenta, baby, blankets, coats and blood. I held the lamp in a most professional manner while Sister collected buckets, basins and water from nowhere and gradually extricated mother and baby from the rest. Grandfather carried mother wrapped in the one dry blanket to another room and I bathed the baby while Sister clothed the mother.[70]

Miss Hensley and Sister Arbuckle had come upon an age-old scene, the family birth, attended by women from family and neighbourhood. Around one in ten babies were 'born before arrival' — BBA — and while some families and friends knew what to do, others did not. Most babies survived: one was found under the bedclothes sucking its thumb,[71] but stillbirths were more common if BBA. They failed to reach one Richmond mother in time to save her breech baby: 'I followed Sister inside to be greeted by the sight of mother and a dead baby lying in the bed in a horrible mess'. The child had been delivered by a sister-in-law.[72] Husbands sometimes delivered the baby, aunts and grandmothers often; one poor woman was found lying on the floor with a cyanosed and deformed foetus and only her thirteen-year-old son to help her.[73] And there were often neighbours. In fact home birth was free local entertainment, with an entire street galvanised into attendance, so that the accoucheurs usually found their way to the house by the crowd of 'excited neighbours' gathered outside even late at night. There was no space for privacy:

> Delivered child which cried lustily bringing the people across the lane to their windows. An amusing interlude was the charge of the patient's children to help her when she screamed out when HOP: [head on perineum]. They tumbled down the stairs at a great rate, but were successfully intercepted by nurse at the door.[74]

One Port Melbourne woman's seven-year-old-son watched the full proceedings through a window with his friends looking on.[75]

Certainly there were women with good midwifery skills, but there were also many who thought they knew more than they did. The 'lady across the road' was dreaded for her intrusiveness, and techniques were

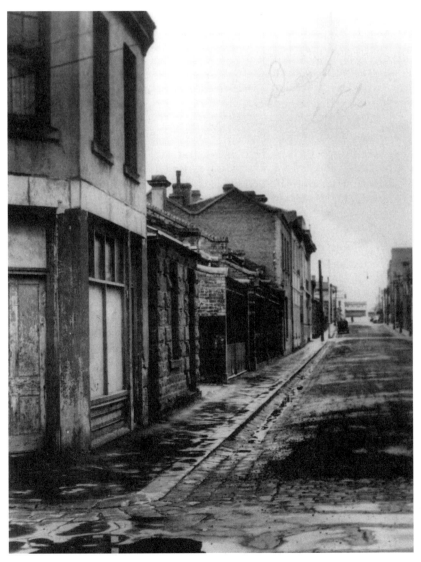

Webb Street, Fitzroy, c.1949, *Herald and Weekly Times Fitzroy Historical Collection*

inevitably primitive: the accoucheurs found cords tied with bits of string or a shoelace, but if alone, they were often thankful for the assistance of a neighbour or relative. In September 1927 Gwen Haines was called to a house in Franklin Street, West Melbourne:

> A truly dreadful business although all went quite normally eventually. On arrival — with no prospect of Sister arriving for about two hours — a really filthy house with no one in it but the mother who could not speak English — no fire alight and no clean saucepans or anything of the kind to boil water. Managed to light a fire and rouse a neighbour — very deaf but fairly useful — and held the fort until about 5 o'clock when Sister arrived. Despite an almost hysterical mother — things progressed quite well.
>
> The result being the most beautiful babe I have ever seen. L.M. $10\frac{1}{2}$ lbs.[76]

Women were often delivered in their ordinary clothes, no matter how unsuitable they might be; one had delivered her eighth baby in nine years, sitting on a kitchen chair, and when the team arrived, she was on the bed surrounded by neighbours, with the placenta half out.[77] J. G. Stoneham entered a South Melbourne house to find 'a tearful neighbour grasping a grinning foetal head which was completely born'.[78] Edward Gault had two consecutive BBAs in 1926, the first in South Melbourne where a neighbour had saved the child's life:

> Congratulated the neighbour who had done the deed and found that pains had been very weak, but waters had suddenly gone, babe's head had come out, and as looked very black, they had pulled child out, tried artificial respiration and tied off cord. I felt that my presence was rather superfluous. As Sister had not arrived I had neighbour hanging on to the fundus — tied off cord, set things out and later completed third stage.
>
> With Sister made the very dirty room look like heaven and bathed babe in front room being watched closely by two mothers and so home to breakfast.[79]

Recovering from his 'strenuous morning' he was called out again during lunch. He took the train to Kensington, where he was met at the station by 'two shy girls, second and seventh of a series'. He was greeted at the door 'by an irate woman who told us that the baby had arrived twenty minutes before and they were trying to stop its cry reaching the children in the backyard as they'd been told the doctor was bringing the babe in his bag'. The baby had been born very quickly, 'pushed out, the neighbour not having the "sang froid" of Mrs C.s friend and had done nothing'.[80]

There were tragedies. Margaret Clark was called to the home of a young first-time mother in South Melbourne:

> Received call at 11.40 and left hospital at 11.53 a.m. Reached destination at 12.20 p.m, being escorted along the street to the house by Father, father's sister aged sixteen and some woman with no sense at all. Nos 1 & 2 informed me that patient was very bad; the third informed me that the baby had been born some time. Arrived in the bedroom to find Mother

in bed covered in bedclothes — turned back clothes and found the baby lying in bed covered with a caul. I tore off the caul at once — Mother said baby had been born half to three quarters of an hour before — so I thought it most likely would be dead. Baby was covered in meconium — evidence of distress — the cord had ceased pulsating — there was no trace of a heartbeat. I clamped cord on mother's side; tied it on baby's and immediately attempted resuscitation — I swung baby for half an hour without the desired result. Then as Mother was beginning to expel placenta, I scrubbed up — got to bed in time to see placenta pass out. I gave mother 2 drachms Ext Ergot liq and was cleaning her up when Nurse arrived; handed Mother over to Nurse and left 2 drachms ergot to be given two hours later.

Melbourne in the 1930s, a five-mile radius of the GPO. Housing and Slum Abolition Board, plan of areas investigated.
VPP, 1937, 2

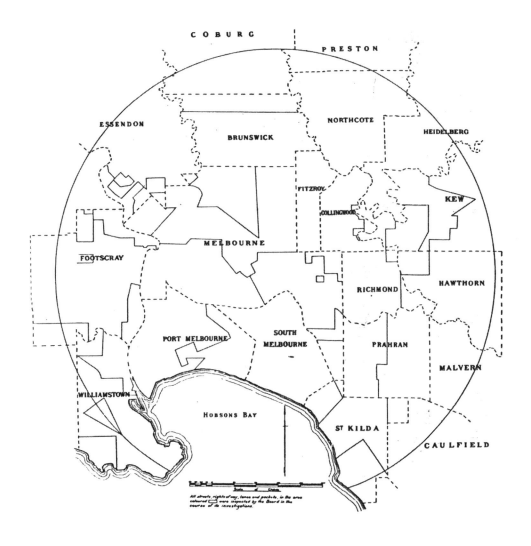

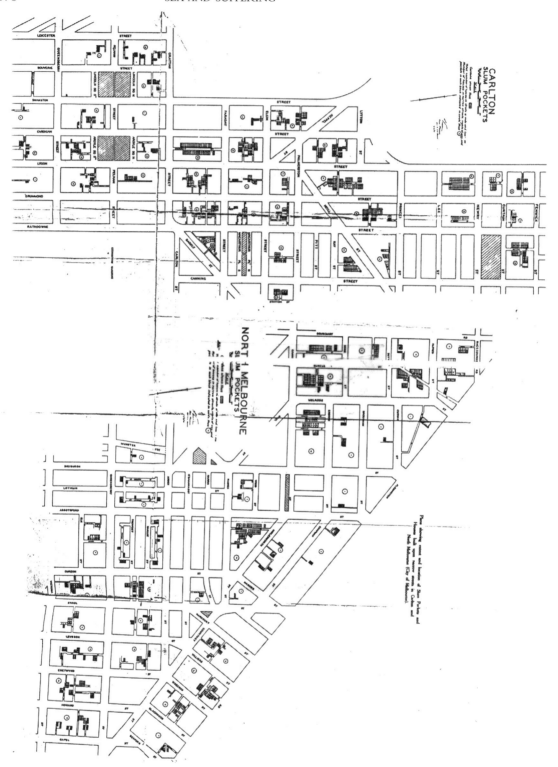

**Carlton and North Melbourne Slum Pockets
investigated by the Housing Investigation and Slum
Abolition Board.** *VPP*, 1937, 2

Had another look at the baby which I forgot to say was in a state of white asphyxia when I pulled the caul off its face.

I tried to console the stricken father and then left, reaching hospital at 2.10 p.m.[81]

The system was flawed. In 1927 a Richmond woman lost her baby because no doctor could be found to manage a suspected transverse presentation. An ambulance was called and the student came in with the mother, holding the baby back. By the time it was born the child was in a state of white asphyxia.[82]

T. L. Tyrer was summoned to the home in Burnley of para nine in January 1924, to a scene he reconstructed as almost Dickensian:

Was met by a woman carrying two poodles — Sister had not arrived so I was escorted into room with large double bed and a cot in which a small infant alternately slept and woke to cry 'Mummie' — to this remark 'mummie' would cleverly reply 'Shut up you little devil'. The lighting consisted of a kerosene lamp with sooted glass. The woman from next door held this for me tilted so that light could come from the top. I looked at the perineum and there appeared to be plenty of time, so started an abdom. exam. At this stage the good woman from next door remarked, 'It's a good job Doctor arrived — we can do without Sister, but not without Doctor'. I was much bucked. A moment later mother said, 'Quick Dr' — Obligingly turned on her side — cocked up her leg and the baby was delivered by a process of walking out. This saved all the trouble of a scrubbing up and a *P.V.* Sister arrived to see the placenta come away.

Whilst I was looking for a mouth gauze the woman next door obliged by lifting up her petticoat and wiping out the kid's mouth with the hem — she was promptly kicked out lest she should spit in the kid's eyes as a substitute for argyrol.[83]

It was not just germ theory that was not understood; much bodily function was a mystery interpreted by old wives' tales, both modern and ancient. One mother feared that her baby would have a deformed mouth 'as she — the mother — had had a couple of teeth extracted when she was about six weeks pregnant'.[84] Another's sister-in-law declared that a baby born with a thick coating of vernix showed that the mother had failed to take proper care of herself in pregnancy. She was quickly disabused of this notion, relieving the young mother of at least one item about which to feel inadequate.[85] Another poor soul was in such a state that she called for attendance even though she was not pregnant, because she had weaned her youngest a few days before, and awoken that morning with a fever, dizziness, headache and a rasping cough. Her neighbour had kindly informed her that this was the result of her breast milk 'going to her head'. The student examined her and heard moist sounds all over her chest, then left her to Sister, who was on her way.[86]

The midwife and the student were bearers of order and cleanliness, but as it was for the 'slum dwellers' themselves, home facilities made order and cleanliness difficult. The women who sought the District Nurse and medical student were those too poor to use a private doctor and nurse

argyrol: (silver) used externally, and to a lesser extent internally, in the form of its salt, nitrate of silver. Argyrol was a compound of silver oxide with albumin. It was a brown powder soluble in water and was much used as an unirritating antiseptic in conjunctivitis and for washing out the bladder in cystitis. (Black) Used routinely in the newborn to prevent ophthalmia neonatorum, 60 per cent of which was gonorrheal.

let alone enter a private hospital. And some had a good reason for not using a public hospital. A home birth made it easier to look after older children, and reduced the danger of a husband clearing out with whatever money there was. Many had a dread of hospitals, and saw two weeks in the Women's Hospital as two weeks of being bossed and bullied, washed and humiliated, subjected to nasty procedures they did not understand, and of numbing loneliness, cut off from family and friends. Only husbands were allowed to visit, and even then they had to pay for the privilege. Moreover the visiting hours were awkward for shift and night workers. For alcoholics, hospital meant a nasty couple of weeks off the grog.

The extern midwifery served the poorest of the poor, those stigmatised as the underclass, the rough, the 'residuum'. Richmond was the most visited suburb, and the cases were mostly in its meanest streets and lanes. The North Melbourne cases were even more conspicuously concentrated in narrow back lanes, in the oldest housing and in the dense enclave known ironically as 'Happy Valley'. These were homes with the lowest rent and the worst facilities. Melbourne may have been a comparatively young city, but it had terrible slums within half a century of its founding. In 1936–37 a survey of 7330 homes by the Housing Investigation and Slum Abolition Board was to find:

14 per cent were in good habitable condition
43 per cent were unfit for habitation without expensive repairs
42 per cent were incapable of being made fit for habitation
28 per cent were without bathrooms
45 per cent were without washing facilities
76 per cent were without kitchen sinks.[87]

If the poor seemed dirty to the affluent, it was not surprising given the logistical difficulties of washing bodies daily and clothes more often than weekly. The very poor often had only one set of clothes: one Richmond woman remembers owning one dress, one pair of underpants and no toothbrush in the Depression: 'We didn't realise that we had to have a change — we washed our underclothes out each morning'.[88] Every rag was precious, so that in some families in the 1930s there was only one to spare for menstruation in a household of menstruating women. Even for those who wanted to be clean, cleanliness was almost impossible. Soap was such a luxury that in one tiny South Richmond street, a bucket of soap suds was shared between the neighbours so they could scrub their floors. Very few had a hot-water heater — all hot water had to be boiled up on the stove or in the copper out the back.

The houses all smelt sour and dirty because most of them had inadequate ventilation, therefore rising damp; and leaking roofs, therefore rotting internal plaster. Floor-boards disintegrated, and their undulations and gaps made sweeping and washing less than satisfactory. The respectable had their own linoleum which they took with them from rented house to rented house. Mice and rats scampered over and under floors and behind walls. The fortunate had a copper in the back yard and enough fuel to boil the family washing in it on Mondays; the less fortunate boiled the washing up in a kerosene tin on the one-fire stove. Fleas,

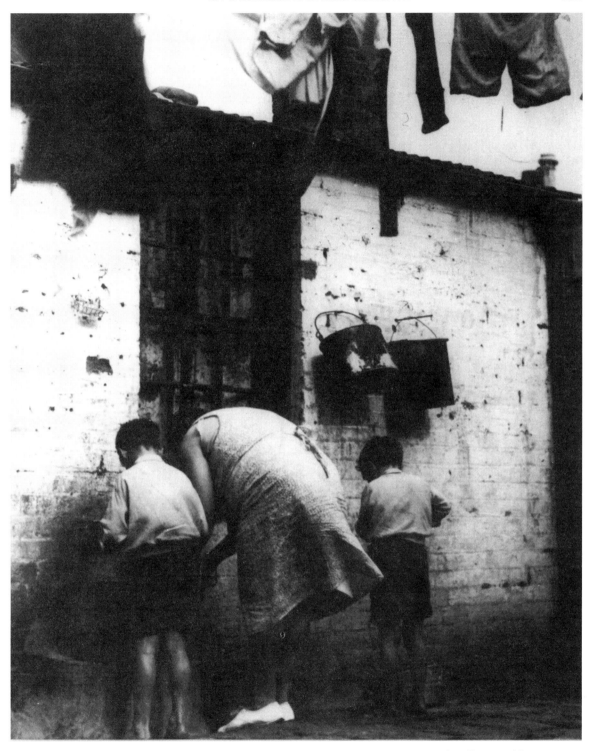

A family's washing facilities
Herald and Weekly Times

lice and bedbugs attacked the sleeping, and shared beds and scratched bites assisted epidemics of impetigo — 'school sores'. Most children suffered a 'winter cough' or chronic ear infections, leaving many slightly deaf and unable to learn in a large, restless, scratching, coughing class. Among the most destitute, children older than babies shared their parents' bed: J. W. Kenny was appalled by the sleeping arrangements of an extended family in Windsor: 'I then discovered that the family consisted of grand-father and mother, husband, two sisters and children who all slept in the one double bed that night — what a tight fit — not even a flea could get in as well, so they came in to us'.[89] But the particular horror of Australian home life was flies. They were everywhere, breeding in the food waste left in the street gutters by door-to-door fruit and vegetable sellers, and even fishmongers, and in the animal droppings on the roads and lanes. Until fly-wire screens began to appear in the 1920s, the Sunday roast would be black with flies within minutes of being put on to the table for carving. Flies crawled all over babies' eyes and mouths and runny noses. The horror of a BBA in North Melbourne was made worse by entering the bedroom to find the flies crawling all over the mother's vulva and the baby. Another in Station Street, North Carlton, was 'a filthy hovel, busy with flies . . . only with great difficulty was the window coaxed open . . . and the atmosphere was nearly solid'.[90]

In the worst cases, a squalor existed which was scarcely imaginable, and in fact almost a remnant of another age, before the great changes in private life that came even to the working class in the second half of the nineteenth century. The instances which survived into the 1920s and 1930s were the consequence of psychiatric illness, intellectual handicap, alcoholism or very occasionally plain ignorance. In Abbotsford Street, North Melbourne, during 1924, the student and nurse were called to the second confinement of a young woman with a concealed accidental haemorrhage which required that she be admitted to hospital. But first she was assessed at home:

> Sister and I left the house, not, however, without observing the poverty-stricken appearance and filthy condition of the house and contents. Sister was certain it was the filthiest house she had ever been in. The house consisted of two rooms, the front room containing the mother, while the back room served as a kitchen. The floor covering was 'conspicuous by its absence', and consisted of bare boards covered with dirt over which two small sea-grass mats, 2' by 4' had been placed in parts. There were no sheets at all on the mother's bed, and the blanket present was absolutely black with dirt and grime. The mother herself presented a very unkempt appearance, her hair was unkempt and tangled, her face, hands, in fact her whole body was filthy dirty which gave Sister the opportunity of bathing her, a job which the Sister did not seem to relish, and which was exceed-ingly difficult as the patient absolutely refused to turn over onto her stomach owing to the pain.
>
> In the kitchen there was a hole in the floor, in which a man's no. 8 boot could easily have lost itself. The gas for a small gas stove had been cut off, as evidenced by the blocked piece of lead tubing leading from a penny-in-the-slot meter. The water needed in case was boiled on an open

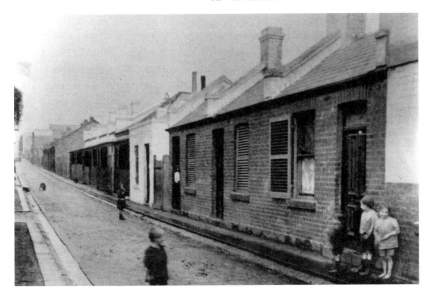

Little Napier Street, Fitzroy, *c.* 1905
Fitzroy Historical Collection

fire which was the only means of heating in the house. The husband was a Maltese who could speak very little English, while the Mother came from Bendigo. The mother admitted to us that she could not understand what her husband was saying when she married him. The child of the house was a bright little youngster of two or three years of age, who certainly did not get his good looks from either his father or mother.[91]

The patients were expected to have everything ready for the confinement, and some did have the room neat and clean, with supplies of cotton wool, towels, napkins, lysol, cooled boiled water and boiling water on the stove. Others had only baby clothes, and some not even those. But most had done something, and when houses were particularly clean, the case notes recorded these triumphs over despair and ever-invading dirt. A Jewish mother of eleven in Carlton presented an 'exceeding clean and tidy household', and in Wood Street, on North Melbourne's more respectable Hotham Hill, 'the seat of the operations was spotless, with everything prepared, and good supplies of hot water, lysol and cotton wool'. Waiting there during a protracted labour, the student enjoyed a long, if sometimes incomprehensible conversation with 'an old Scotch lady' who

> chattered away like a cage of monkeys, every now and then lapsing into the broadest Scotch. She was very experienced I fancy, for she was quite ready to help me if Sister did not arrive, which by the way, I had made up my mind would happen. At the grand denouement we were given tea and biscuits, both excellent and welcome.[92]

On entering the house, the first task of the midwife or the student was to heat water to boil up swabs and gloves. Some homes had only fire stoves and fireplaces, with no fire going and no fuel, although it was rare for it to be impossible to boil water. The District Nurses always carried a penny for the gas meter if needed. Water often came only from a tap in the back yard, and in some parts of Richmond the mains pressure was so bad that it took twenty minutes to fill a bucket, while in Dryburgh Street, North Melbourne, it took half an hour to fill the kettle. Then there needed to be saucepans or kettles, basins and buckets, but often they were hard pressed to find enough and neighbours had to be asked to help. Next came the bed. Were there clean linen and towels and rags? If there were not, then newspaper was spread over the bed and on to the floor. The bed itself often occupied almost the entire room and sagged in the middle which made the accoucheur's job much more difficult and gave the patient little purchase for pushing. Some men students provided support with their back to give her something to push against; the bed-post was often a useful anchor; or sheets could be wound around the bed head to provide a grip. The patient had to be 'prepped' — washed, shaved and clothed appropriately except that some homes had no razor and some patients no other clothes. When that was completed, the mid-wife and the student, wearing aprons and sterilised gloves, made their *per vaginam* and abdominal examinations to assess how close the patient was to full dilatation. If it was night-time the lighting in the house often was

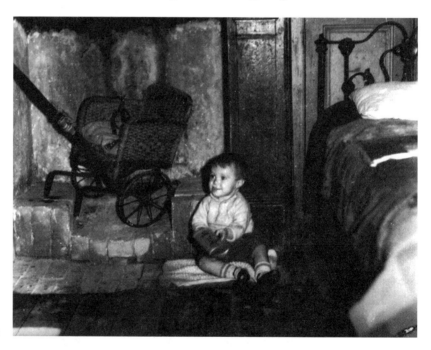

Herald and Weekly Times

quite inadequate because many of the very poor used candles or oil and kerosene lamps; one student had to light matches to perform a *p.v.* in North Melbourne.

　　If there was a long way to go, they might leave her and return later, or if that was unwise or too inconvenient, they would stay and resort to various techniques of accelerating labour. There was the time-old practice of 'walking the floor' (one energetic East Brunswick para six challenged young Edward Hurley to a running race along the hall, 'but with effort remembered I was a "Dr" and declined to accept the challenge').[93] Another old favourite was the enema, as well as inserting a catheter to empty the bladder. It was almost routine in the 1920s to administer quinine sulphate to irritate the uterus into stronger contractions, and there was no hesitation in rupturing the membranes.

The enema was crucial because a loaded rectum, as well as a distended bladder, can impede the passage of the head. Even worse, a loaded rectum may empty itself during delivery. One of the nastiest nursing problems in home births were the involuntary bowel actions of the labouring mother. Obviously asepsis was impossible, but it was not a rare occurrence and the most frequent 'offenders' were grand multiparas who, out of long experience, had dosed themselves with purgatives the night before to bring on labour: 'Arrived just in time to scrub up and deliver the baby; the room was filthy — the bed literally soaked in faeces resulting from three laxettes taken the evening before'.[94] A para fourteen overdosed herself with castor oil in 1927. Also that year 'Two bells rang just after breakfast and proceeded to the wilds of West Brunswick renowned for the Brunswick tip and numerous flies. Bright young thing of eighteen summers and scantily clad greeted me kindly at door, and brought me to mum who was groaning sorrowfully but defecating cheerfully into the bed'.[95] Sometimes Sister's enema was too good, as in the case of a constipated East Melbourne woman: 'The good lady had one long action from the beginning of the accouchement to the end, with the result strict asepsis was not quite possible'.[96] As student G. G. Price noted in August that same year: 'Asepsis, management, luck — these three, and the greatest of these is luck'.[97]

While the preparations were being made, a history was to be taken by the student. The District Nursing service was meant to have collected a history antenatally since the patient had booked in three months before, but from the case notes it looks as though many accoucheurs went in 'cold', and certainly if the student arrived first, the history was taken for the first time. The quality of the histories varied enormously: some were careless and frivolous; others models of care and conscientiousness. And the very best were taken by students who later rose to eminence in the profession, especially obstetrics. The screening by the District Nurse and the regulations that the Hospital would not attend single mothers or primiparas, did not eliminate all potential problem cases. The full histories reveal a daunting case load of high risk patients, especially of grand multiparas. Sister Grey's first case was made easier because it was the mother's sixteenth: she was 'very hefty' and the baby took after mum at 11 pounds. ('Sister quite a good sort', noted the student, R. J. Farnbach.)[98] They found women with tuberculosis and heart disease. They found alcoholics 'away with the fairies'. They found the obese, but seemed only to measure blood pressure if the woman 'looked eclamptic' and her urine was to be sent to the Hospital for analysis. They delivered women under treatment for syphilis and sometimes did not know until afterwards: one student had a Collingwood patient's membranes burst into his face, then

Just as we were about to leave — my face still smelly with liquor, Sister said 'Oh yes, a nice baby, and she has been attending the VD clinic for six months'. 'Oh yes', I said and requested some Argyrol to be instilled into my conjunctiva'.

The situation was confirmed by father who brought in the other child for doctor to see. A beautiful child with haemoglobin about 15 per cent and an elbow joint and forearm which I at once remember seeing at the Children's Hospital operated on for gummatous osteitis. More Argyrol at W.H. All's well that ends well (so far).[99]

If it was to be a long wait, then much more could be learnt by either 'side' about each other. The sister often waited by the bedside while the student waited in another room or out the back. The male students mostly passed the time by smoking, reading the paper, and chatting; nurses did not smoke in public, but knitted and talked. In 1927 Eileen Murphy and Sister Monteith, in between 'counting the pains eagerly' during a tedious labour: 'admired the view from the front door, which opened on to the pavement and did our best to look the part of strong, silent women of mystery for the benefit of interested neighbours'.[100] Very few read books, and the enforced intimacy with the patient and her family was often the first occasion that these university students had ever had a prolonged conversation with the very poor. Many complained of its tiresomeness: they found husbands too taciturn or too talkative, especially if they were 'political sorts' and lectured them about the Labor Party and trade union-ism. Sport provided a lingua franca. Many families were very welcoming and hospitable; some were frankly frightening. John Freedman delivered a young red-head in the heart of Fitzroy:

When I took the placenta wrapped in paper to the back yard, a big burly brute of about 6'3" and sixteen stone, who turned out to be the husband, told me, 'Put it near the copper doctor'. I felt as big as sixpence beside him, and made a mental note not to give him back answers. As the woman with fourteen kids [a neighbour] told me that the husband and wife lived on charity, that the husband never worked, and that any money they earned was spent on beer, and as I learned after leaving the house, that Mahoney Street was the place where all the shooting vendettas took place, I was extremely relieved when I left the neighbourhood, which I did, as soon as possible after seeing Sister to her tram and carrying her bag for her, and arrived back at the W.H. in time to stop the interns from finishing all the tea.[101]

Some used these occasions to learn more about their patients' lives and past health; many had thrust upon them the patients' previous con-finements, as well as the 'bad times' of all the other females attending the birth. They found themselves examining other members of the family and dispensing medical advice, and some of these young people, still virgins most of them, were asked by desperate couples for advice on birth control or infertility. One 'chatty', 'bright soul' having her sixth at age thirty, 'Threatened to clear out if Dad got up to tricks again'. She also remarked to Sister Burgess that '"You sisters don't ever seem to have children — I suppose you know too much". I enjoyed watching Sister's face in the mirror opposite'. Later the father took the student aside: 'Was also asked to "give a few hints on contraception". Not knowing any, I couldn't enlighten him'.[102] A Kew couple had more luck with their student:

After a cup of tea and cake, the father returned to the drawing room and gently closed the door. He then explained that this last baby had been a mistake and wished for some advice against further accidents. After a brief survey of the methods which I had personally found least unreliable, I referred him to the local practitioner.[103]

(Despite great opposition in 1934 Dr George Simpson succeeded in opening on behalf of the District Nursing Society Melbourne's first birth control clinic.[104])

Sometimes a real rapport occurred. G. Raleigh Weigall came from a distinguished Melbourne professional family, but he chatted away to working-class patients and neighbours who 'were particularly pleasant and intelligent group' and was sorry to say goodbye. At another case in South Melbourne he found:

> ...a very clean little house with an enormous population, mostly temporary, of very pregnant women from the neighbouring houses. They were all very willing to help and quite enthusiastic about doing the most menial tasks. Also they showed a most welcome tendency to ask me questions instead of telling me about it as I was afraid they would. They must have all been primiparae I think. Besides having good experience in obstetrics in this case, I got some good general surgery in too. The kid had a double inguinal hernia and was referred to the C.H.; the others had various degrees of disease and deformity — including the father, who had ruptured a few fibres of his rectus femoris and had a good subcutaneous haematoma; also psoriasis all over the place — appropriate treatment prescribed in all cases.[105]

Reg Worcester was to become medical superintendent and later an honorary at the Women's Hospital, with a particular commitment to the care of septic abortion patients. On 4 February 1927 he had a not untypical case where all sorts of things could have gone wrong, but did not. It was in West Melbourne, the mother was forty-four years old, and facing her eighteenth confinement. She had only eight living children out of the seventeen, the oldest being twenty:

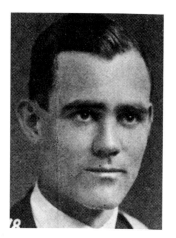

Dr Reg Worcester *RWHA*

> In no more than 15 minutes I arrived and to my pleasant surprise a District nurse got off the same tram. We soon found the place. Aunty was waiting at the gate. I left Sister to the expectant mother while I boiled up some swabs in the kitchen. The house was moderately clean and the eldest daughter not too bad. Going back, Sister said all ready so our *PV*... head hard to palpate and I felt I'd rather depend on the abdom. palp... Sister agreed... gave quinine sulph. ten grains, rescued my *Herald* from father, and sat on the verandah to read the news. At 7 p.m. gave another dose quin. sulph. After Sister had a cup of tea, I was invited to do the same. Sitting at the family table I had a cup of tea and was not unwillingly pressed to have a couple of fried eggs. Feeling quite OK now that my appetite was satisfied, I again went to the bedroom. Again *PV* and this time... the head pushed the membranes and in less than half an hour I brought into the world a LM 8½ lbs.

Leaving at 9 p.m. the father insisted on us having a taxi ride home.

Quite unlike my predecessors (I believe). I merely talked to the nice Sister on the way home.[106]

More than two thirds of the deliveries went well, despite the unpromising environment and the potential complications in a cohort of ill-fed, overworked multiparas. In the 227 deliveries conducted between December 1920 and October 1921, no mother died during or straight after delivery, although we have no idea how many later developed a post-partum infection or suffered other postnatal complications. The live births included five sets of surviving twins, and over all there were only four stillbirths. Thirteen cases, or just under 6 per cent, were sent in to the hospital because of complications. There was only one threatened eclampsia, but then under 5 per cent were primiparas. In fact one of the particular uses of the home birth cases is that they were multiparas attended by the hospital, at a time when single primiparas were still overrepresented among the inpatients. Only twice were private doctors summoned to deliver with forceps, even though, if the scales were roughly accurate, the babies were big. Just over 10 per cent were born before arrival, and of the mere nine women who needed sutures to tears of the perineum, three, including the worst, were BBA. Another seventeen only had small mucous tears which required no stitches. It was a most creditable performance by both midwives and students, but the patients' multiparity reduced the risk of tears enormously. When tears did occur, the student had to return the next day and insert sutures, usually silver wire, using cocaine as local anaesthetic.

The gravest obstetric risk faced by these multiparous women was postpartum haemorrhage, when their tired uteri could not contract strongly enough after separation of the placenta. Miraculously only six of these 227 women in 1921 had a haemorrhage, and all were saved. Of the over 7000 home deliveries conducted by the District Nursing Society between 1930 and 1948 there were just four deaths, three of them from haemorrhage.[107] In 1927 Norman Solomon encountered one in Collingwood, a mother of two aged thirty-five. Her waters ruptured and the head began to show:

> Got mother to edge of bed, donned gloves and apron, and proceeded to deliver infant with mother's right leg slung around my neck and trying hard to push my face into the bed. Delivered infant with difficulty as in the process mother slid into the centre of the bed and almost disappeared from view. Then cut the cord and pitched infant into a clothes basket ready for its reception and proceeded to wait for the placenta.
>
> The cord lengthened after about twenty minutes. However before I got properly to work the placenta shot out of the vagina and with it a deluge of blood with a continuous stream of blood behind it. My heart stopped for about 10 minutes, but finally picked up courage and expressed the rest of the placenta as quickly as possible, although this did not stop the bleeding. By this time I had wind up properly and began to think of funerals and murder trials. Kept rubbing the fundus and injected 1cc pit and 1cc ergot, but did not seem to act very quickly. Was on the point of sending for a doctor when Sister arrived and whether it was her presence

or my good management I don't know, but the bleeding stopped and the uterus contracted up.

Pulse around 120. My own about 450 or thereabouts.

Arrived home in time for tea, which I found great difficulty in eating.[108]

Amanda Liebert's left hand shook for a day after she had held on to the bleeding fundus of a para eight in Hawthorn.[109]

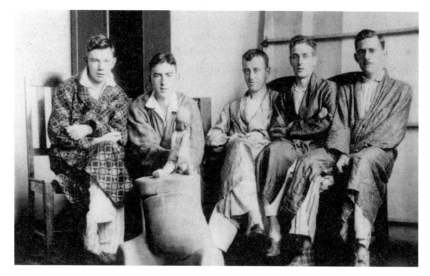

Medical students in their dressing gowns, with obstetric teaching dummy

These students had been well trained — John Freedman did sixty deliveries during his time as a student in 1924 — and even the larrikins and casual types who wrote the most perfunctory notes, came good in an emergency. And in some you can sense the doctor they were to become. Albert Coates, who was to conduct the most extraordinary makeshift surgery on his fellow prisoners of war in Changi, was confronted on his first extern case with a breech and footling presentation, membranes descending, meconium streaming everywhere and a prolapsed cord. It was too late to send the mother to the hospital, and when he rang a local doctor he was told to 'carry on' for the same reason. While he was ringing, the redoubtable Sister Burgess had done just that: catheterised the patient and delivered the child. Coates then took the baby, a nine pound female with 'Asphyxia Livida', and 'vigorously handled [her] and by use of mucus catheter and cutaneous stimulation, the child began to gasp'. Later he recorded: 'The Lord preserve us from such another case on extern' and then he underlined, 'It was a thrilling experience!'[110] Ian Wood did not feel any thrill with a case of adherent placenta he attended in Fitzroy in 1926, and he also took the time to record what happened to the patient once she was admitted to the hospital. The case started colourfully. He was given a lift to George Street by a local doctor: 'Conversation was poorly until he confided that one Nurse Mitchell, a lady of low cunning and a large ?obstetrical practice, was acting in a curtain-raiser to "The Vanishing Race" a movie at the Capitol'. This was the patient's fourth confinement, two of her children were living and in her last two deliveries the third stage had been delayed and the placenta had had to be expressed by Credé's method. To make things worse, ten months before she had aborted herself by syringing her uterus with castor oil and ergot: 'Result — patient was blown up like a balloon and an incomplete abort was curetted at the WH for four hours [*sic*]'. Wood delivered her of a 7¼ lb daughter, but was unable to make progress in the third stage:

> Husband sent out at 1.15 a.m. for doctor — at 2 p.m. had tried four doctors with no result — Pulse gone from 80 to 108 — patient restless — increasing anaemia — so ambulance called and journey undertaken with me hanging anxiously on to the fundus.
>
> <u>Hospital</u> On arrival in ward a very passionate credé was performed by Sister which nearly brought on syncope — patient very shocked. Hot packs — foot of bed raised — pulse 120. At 4 p.m. patient looking better — placenta removed by Resident by vigorous credé and traction on cord. Patient had lost c. 3 kidney dishes in all — very shocked after final removal. Rectal saline. Placenta was dense, fibrous and ragged.

Two days later he checked on her: 'Mother and baby both OK'.[111]

Among those who stood out was George Simpson. He was called to his first case in Vere Street, Collingwood, on 26 March 1921:

> Received call at 11.35 p.m. just after returning. Told to hurry and catch last train. This I did and found home without trouble in the heart of the slums. Arrived at 12 Midnight to find fairly clean though small and dilapidated house with four rooms. Husband was aquiver with excitement as it was his first — having married a widow. A married friend of mother's was also waiting. As nurse had not arrived I obtained the history — pains started at 11 p.m. yesterday. Show during night. Membranes not ruptured. Last period June — five previous pregnancies [included three miscarriages] — instrumental last five years ago. Was wondering what to do next when Nurse arrived.
>
> Nurse got busy and prepared for a *PV* while I had a warm in front of kitchen fire. When ready I made an examination. Abdominal palpation LOA, head fixed, flexed and well down. Fetal heart 140. Maternal 80 (Mother had inevitable 'weak heart'. *PV* showed Cx 7/6 taking well up except anterior lip. LOA. Membranes intact but not bulging. Ordered Quin. Sulph gr x and went back to fire. Case progressing slowly but mother had good pains and behaved well. At 2 a.m. nurse did *PV* which showed slight progress of head and ant lip of cervix still in the road — put on a tight abdominal binder which helped things a little. At 2.50 a.m. mother began to tire, pulse was 96, fetal heart 136. I prepared for another examination and the psychical [*sic*] influence brought the head on the perineum, so instead of doing a *PV* I delivered the child. Delivery was easy and the child was delivered as the Town Hall clock struck three. Cord round neck. Membranes had to be ruptured with scissors and I found no trace of liquor. Tied off child and put in a safe place. Turned mother on her back. Nurse gave a heave on the fundus and placenta was born by Schultz's process. The retroplacental clot was large. I spilt it on the bed and later Nurse spilt it on the floor. Fundus contracted down very firmly. Washed baby while Nurse fixed up mother and hubby ordered our taxi.

Credé's method: a technique for expelling the placenta from the uterus. With the uterus contracted downward, pressure is applied to it through the abdominal wall in the direction of the birth canal. (*OMD*)

Gave mother ergot 2 drachms and left 2 drachms to be taken at 6 am.

Baby was a tiny thing weighing only 8 pounds. Head showed fairly extensive moulding and slight caput. The one kerosene lamp in home had nearly burnt out so was glad to get out into the moonlight. Arrived per taxi at Nurses' Home, where we parted at 4 a.m.[112]

It was a textbook case, and already the set phrases, like 'put baby in a safe place', indicate the mastery of procedure and instant, almost automatic response. Most telling was his delight in the baby 'a tiny thing weighing only eight pounds': this was not irony, but wonder at the frailty of new babies. In his next case he was aggrieved when a complication in the third stage required him to attend to the mother and Nurse had the pleasure of bathing the baby. George Simpson had fallen in love with newborn babies and midwifery. He was to become the doctor to the District Nursing Society and have a long, illustrious career at the Women's Hospital. And at the Australian Medical Congress in 1948 he would defend home births as 'safer, happier and more comfortable' for the patient and cheaper for the state: 'childbirth should be a normal physiological event, not a major surgical crisis, which confinement in hospital suggested and often implied'.[113]

And there was Kate Campbell, who as a medical student sounded already like the great doctor she was to become. It was 1921 and she was called to a house of a para four in Auburn:

Call came at 9.5 a.m. and I left WH at 9.35. I had some difficulty in locating the house and did not get there till 11 a.m. where I found Nurse waiting at the door to meet me. I scrubbed up immediately as she said the head was arriving. I waited for about 7 minutes and as affairs were remaining stationary and had been so for about an hour (so Nurse told me) I did a *p.v.* and found the head well down the vagina, with a very slight caput, and in the LOA position. We waited another 5 minutes and liquor containing meconium began draining away. I began to get apprehensive of foetal distress and as I was washed up, was about to ask Nurse to time the foetal heart, when much to our relief the head began to appear at the vulva. Mother's pains were not very effective in expelling the head which was very large, but I was able to ease the perineum over it after some manipulation. The head resituated but I experienced difficulty in extracting the shoulders, owing to the large size of the child. The cord was also over the anterior shoulder but after pushing the cord back and pulling forcibly, the anterior shoulder was disengaged and the rest of the child followed easily. Baby was rather pallid but quickly responded to artificial respiration and was soon crying vigorously. I attended to Mother and was glad to see an intact perineum, the placenta having been previously expelled with a very large amount of blood clot about ten minutes after the birth of the child.[114]

The baby weighed 11 pounds.

Now it was time for Kate Campbell and Sister Nolan to show 'the baby to the rest of the family, aunts, cousins and interested neighbours'. While some babies were unwelcome as just another mouth to feed, many big families were still overjoyed. Understandably, when after seven girls, a North Fitzroy mother bore her first son, 'a long unbroken line of sisters rejoiced in a 9 lb brother and a father bade us good morning in a deliriously delighted fashion'.[115] Another had a second girl after two sons and a daughter, and 'Frantic delight exhibited by Grandma who on learning of the arrival of a live [female] commenced frisking around throwing cushions up like the proverbial two-year-old'.[116] A para three's safe delivery of an eleven-pound boy was awaited by a houseful of aunts and uncles, as well as granny and husband: 'Exhibited babe to proud father and grateful granny, who gave us tea and hot buttered toast which we much enjoyed'. They were then 'seen off by the entire family': it was Boxing Day.[117]

And yet in all these stories, despite their startling intimacy, there is an astounding silence — the mothers' pain. None of the female accoucheurs (apart from Ethel Osborne, wife of Professor Osborne and mature-age student) would have themselves experienced the pain of childbirth; and the young men had never accompanied a partner through birth of their own children. They really had no idea how much it hurt. Indeed you could be excused for thinking that all these confinements were painless, while many were in fact excruciating. Some of the procedures — the manipulations, the manual expression of placentae, the labours delayed by prolapses, the big babies — could be agonising. But those who booked themselves a 'District' home delivery knew that this meant they would get no chloroform. Occasionally it is recorded that a woman yelled for it, but most knew they had no hope of relief. 'Good' patients endured it in silence, pushed when told and 'used their pains'; bad patients screamed, resisted and refused to do as they were told. Some were hysterical and received careful reassurance, but women medical students were more likely to attend to the feelings of the patient and her family than were the men, who left that 'women's business' to the nurse. Certainly, a patient out of control at delivery was in danger:

> Mother was very bad patient and despite loud barracking from both sister and myself, every time a pain came she threw herself all over the bed. Finally we got her in the left lateral position, but she immediately rolled out of it. I then applied a perfect crutch hold and body press while sister applied an arm and toe hold . . . and I managed to keep the head flexed and the baby was born.[118]

It had been easy to find the house 'as yells which could be heard 50 yards away were issuing from it'. The good doctor and the good nurse were required to be controlled, calm and emotionally neutral. They acquired a 'clinical voice': they could not afford to react to patients according to how they felt about them, because they were required to attend to patients whom under normal circumstances, they might not like at all. They could not afford, like Norman Solomon, to start thinking of funeral parlours and murder trials; they were trained to react quickly, clearly and confidently, and in obstetrics they had to react fast if something was amiss.

But they were also being taught by their lecturer in obstetrics, Arthur Wilson, that while all midwifery patients were to receive the same care

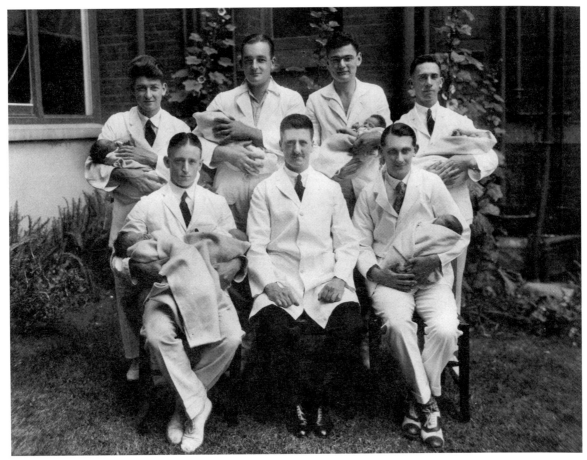

Medical students
with babies
Back: J. W. Johnstone,
N. G. Row, H. T. Tisdall,
J. D. Hagger
Front: R. W. Dungan,
Dr W. P. Heslop,
G. C. V. Thompson *RWHA*

as they would give their own mothers and sisters, only private patients were routinely given anaesthesia and analgesia. The working woman was a tougher breed than the lady: she felt less pain and she popped out babies like shelling peas from the pod. Alongside 'savages', she had not yet partaken of the moral benefits and reproductive deficits of modern civilisation. Hers was a world apart and below. But there were medical personnel who did not see it that way: some chastised their fellow students for their 'unethical' comments on patients, and the 'Extern Case Book' as a literary genre, petered out after the Great Depression.

The good doctor and good nurse were to see only the patient's body and to shut out the environment around her. But in doing that there could also be losses, because the patient isolated from her context was no longer a whole person. Those who went out on the extern cases before the 1950s were often much affected, however disgusted or fearful they might have been. Whatever the bravado of the case books, most students took with them into later life a trope of poverty gleaned from their extern experiences: the family with only one tea cup, Sister's penny for the gas meter, the home with no food, the father found washing the BBA baby in the gully trap in the backyard.[119] And such experiences did much to develop that distinctive social conscience of doctors: they deplored poverty and saw more of it than most, but they saw no acceptable general solution to it and so applied themselves to relieving the individuals who came under their immediate care. The 1930s Depression, however, did elict a new social compassion. The Depression was different because many of the 'deserving poor' were workless, through no fault of their own, unlike the boozers and gamblers and 'dirty poor'. The plight of unemployed returned soldiers particularly touched them. But the Depression also made its impression medically: the midwives were reporting more prolonged labours in malnourished women.[120] It all quite overwhelmed G. M. Oxer on Armistice Day in 1930, while attending a family in Windsor where the father had been out of work for a year:

> Sister said it was the most poverty-stricken place she'd visited. There were two kids outside in a miserable back yard — nice kids but with very dirty faces. The father said they found it difficult to get enough to eat. The mother had had no breakfast that morning. He said they only get 7 shillings from the Council.
>
> This unemployment is very demoralising. Of the four places I have seen the husbands in three of the cases were unemployed — 14, 6 and 12 months respectively. In all cases the people seemed quite decent, this last one of the four being the only one in which the habits of the people seemed somewhat slatternly. The influences causing unemployment — economic conditions, parliament, the Trades Hall, or what not — have a lot to answer for.[121]

At least the deserving poor were not to blame, even if their trade unions and Labor governments were. But these medical students, along with many other middle-class people, were shaken out of their class prejudice by the disasters of the 1930s.

V

'Enormous Clinical Material'
1932–1960

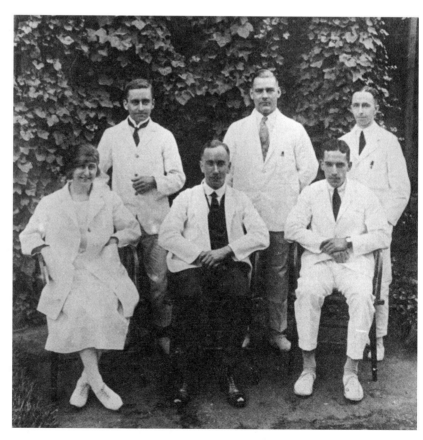

Resident medical staff,
1924–1925
Back: Drs R. E. Street,
F. J. White, M. C. Patrick,
Front: Drs Kate
Campbell, W. D. Saltau
(Medical Superintendent),
A. W. Bayley *RWHA*

Poverty and Pain

10

In February 1936 Lorna Lloyd Green commenced her year as a resident medical officer at the Women's Hospital. Sixty years later, the most vivid impression still fixed in her mind was of the labour ward:

> My memories take me straight back to labour ward — of a big ward with a row of beds on either side with a high ceiling, radiators in the centre which were steam heaters, over which there was a slab of marble that was used as a bench for all sorts of things. There we would be called at night to listen to people like 'Bung' Hill talking. He had a propensity for arriving at 9 o'clock at night and we were called out to hear what he had to say and it was always worthwhile, so we'd always turn up.[1]

There was no question now that the Women's offered a world-class training, as many of the young doctors were to confirm when they later went overseas. At their disposal was the 'enormous clinical material' that Dunbar Hooper had extolled. Every conceivable obstetric emergency and gynaecological condition passed through the wards: eight thousand admissions a year by the mid-1930s, with more than 3000 babies delivered annually and almost as many gynaecological admissions. The hospital would now claim that it maintained the biggest maternity service in the British Empire. As in the 1890s, the Great Depression brought a new class of patient, respectable and temporarily impoverished, and there appeared more former private patients whose complications or conditions could not be treated elsewhere.[2] As women suddenly found themselves unable to afford a private doctor, they flocked to the Outpatients Department, where attendances for gynaecology outstripped antenatal visits for the first time and continued to do so until almost the end of the decade. These were patients with whom middle-class medical and nursing staff could more readily identify and sympathise. And some of the worst things they saw could not be dismissed as the wages of sin, but instead were

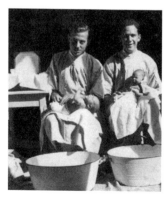

Bathing babies, old style, 1929 *RWHA*

private tragedies for which history and society had to take some blame.

The intellectual energy of the hospital was coming now from a younger generation: a number of the newer honorary staff, like Arthur Wilson, John S. Green, Edward White, George Simpson, Ivon Hayes and Professor Marshall Allan; and a succession of outstanding medical superintendents who were to remain forever 'Women's men': R. G. Worcester, J. W. ('Hoppy') Johnstone, Arthur Machen ('Bung') Hill, Donald ('Blue') Lawson and Ronald Rome. World War II would bring Margaret (Alison) Mackie, the first and only woman to be made medical superintendent. Clinically and educationally, the medical superintendent exerted considerable power, but the dominant figure in a cast of very able young doctors was 'Bung' Hill, a man of many gifts and a wicked wit. He was unpunctual, mischievous, eloquent, charming and brilliant. He loved women and women adored him. He deplored the sufferings of sex, and is remembered for often saying: 'Oh, I've just been tidying-up Mrs So-and-So', doing the little extra repairs to a body battered and torn by too many babies and not enough care. He was an extraordinary clinician and he was later to remember the 1930s as 'those old, colourful, rich, warm, deadly days of clinical medicine at their worst and their best'.[3]

The residency was intensive and exhilarating. It started with six months gynaecology, which included the septic wards, then followed with six months obstetrics, building up experience until the last two months when the resident took all the cases. Frank Hayden was there in 1934:

> And that was where Bung Hill was so good. You had all the primary breeches, for instance. Bung would be there with you if you wanted him. He never took a case off you. We all got great experience, and as a resident at the Women's you got more gynaecological and obstetrical experience in your year than a general practitioner would have had in fifty years.[4]

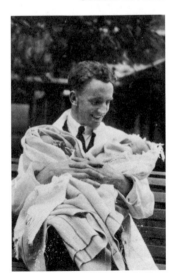

A Resident Medical Officer *RWHA*

Ronald Rome remembers likewise:

> It was dramatic. In those last two months as senior resident you rarely went to bed. It was the only hospital in the whole of Victoria coping with all types of midwifery abnormalities. If a patient had a ruptured uterus or something really dramatic in Warrnambool, you went down and came back with the patient in the ambulance and you had to set up a drip and get blood in Melbourne.
>
> You can die from a post-partum haemorrhage in seven to eight minutes. You turn on the tap, and oh cripes, you've no idea. And the worst ones were just horrible. And I suppose the two most serious conditions we were called out for — especially to places on the verge of Melbourne — were post-partum haemorrhage and eclampsia.[5]

It was still difficult for female medical graduates to be accepted as resident medical officers. Kate Campbell never quite forgave the Children's Hospital for its prolonged misogyny, and in 1924 she had been forced to do her residency at the slightly more welcoming Women's despite her commitment to paediatrics:

They had had women before, and had been pleased with them. It was a happy place and we worked very hard there. I remember a particularly heavy day in the labour ward working alongside a male colleague, when he 'flaked out'. I suggested that he lie down and I would get him some brandy. His masculine pride was stung to the quick, he sat bolt upright and shouted 'You'll not get me brandy. You look like three halfp'worth of God help us, and you're as tough as an old boot'.[6]

The Women's was still, however, a male preserve. Lorna Lloyd Green:

Ella Macknight had preceded me by six or so years at the Women's and it was very interesting to see how different people reacted to female resident medical officers. The nursing staff were marvellous and the honoraries on the whole very good, but there was one who made life difficult. And yet when I got my membership and my mother came to the first presentation of certificates, he just fell all over her as though I'd been the most marvellous person in the world and I thought 'You hypocrite'. When he told me to hold a retractor one way, the next time I'd do it that way and he'd tell me it was the wrong way, until the anaesthetist who ultimately became a psychiatrist, said to me, 'Unless you stand up to him he's only going to continue to do this'. So I said to him one day, 'Sir, that's the way you told me to hold it last time' and I didn't hear any more.

But it was the patients who affected her most:

The lack of privacy of those women in labour. Very frequently they delivered in the open ward — it depended on who was doing it, but the screens were not always used. And those well-intentioned, in many ways marvellous midwives, coping with very great difficulty. Patients without any training whatsoever in what childbirth was going to be about — with tremendous fears. And all they could do was scream quite often. They were just told to keep quiet. And they were told that they were not to do this or do that — they'd affect their baby. Which was always horrifying to us because we knew they were not going to hurt their babies, they were going to hurt themselves more. We weren't going to let them hurt their babies.

And the other thing that horrified me was the amount of energy that the sisters put into putting binders on them. It was considered important in those days that you got pressure on the abdomen, which aided expulsion of the foetus as it were, and even initiated labour. So if you were starting them off and doing an induction of labour, you would always bind their abdomens very tightly. So tightly in fact that I have known patients to have these huge safety pins put through their skin.

It's a wonder to me that they didn't complain, but they were very, very uncomplaining. I think it was still the Christian ethic that in childbirth you shall have lots of pain. They weren't looking for sedation and help that people are today, so they just bore it. I don't know how they coped, I really don't, especially with the long labours.

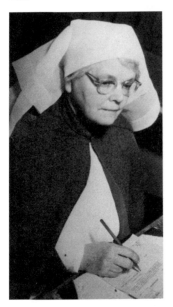

**Miss M. E. McDonald,
matron 1927–1947**
RWHA

The other revelation was to see how male middle-class doctors failed
to identify with working-class female patients:

> What used to worry me no end at the Women's, especially with one
> obstetrician was: I would say — it's just terrible that she's lost that baby
> — we should have been able to do something about it. And he'd reply,
> 'She'll have another' and I would get mad — 'How do you know that
> she'll have another? We have no idea that she will have another'.
> Psychologically and physically there was everything against her.

And yet even the most sensitive could scarcely guess at the difficulty
of their patients' lives. Now aged over ninety, 'Ina' remembers having her
first baby at the Women's in 1928. A dyslexic, she did not learn to read
until she was sixty. Her husband had a tiny back-yard dairy which he
lost in the Depression, driving him to a nervous breakdown. But when
she had her daughter in 1928, it went quite well:

> I had a shower and went up to the ward and that's all I remember.
> They must have given me a dose of something. Her birth was quite
> good evidently. We were in a ward with two other ladies. I saw very
> little of her. I never had a bonding with 'Dorothy' at all when in
> hospital. I was there a whole fortnight. She was brought to me, loved
> and cuddled and I talked to her, then she had a full meal. We stayed in
> bed to wash and had a pan always. I expressed milk. I had enough to
> feed two prem babies as well.
>   No visitors. My husband used to stand down in the hospital
> grounds and hold up a card board with 'I LOVE YOU BOTH' written
> on it. The nurse would hold 'Dorothy' up to the window to see. That
> must have been the only time I stood on the floor. After about two
> weeks being shut in the ward, I needed oxygen. I asked three nurses all
> day if I could have the windows open. They said you must think of the
> other mothers. That night 'Dorothy' used all my milk. When the nurse
> came to express my milk I said, 'I'm sorry, I've only got enough for my
> own baby tonight. You wouldn't open the windows all day, and that's
> it. They let me go home the next day. We went home in the milk
> cart.[7]

Home with her baby, the local Baby Health Centre sister told her that
she needed all her teeth extracted for periodontal disease:

> I pushed the baby a mile in her pram to the dentist. He removed all
> the top ones. Then I wheeled the pram home across the paddocks.
> The next time I went back I said, 'If you don't take the lot out I won't
> come back'. So he did and he put me and the pram out on the streets.
> Mum wasn't with me this time. When I walked home again, pushing
> the pram, I was bleeding badly. Mum got the doctor who couldn't find
> which hole to stop the bleeding, so he said, 'Here, get to the chemist
> and get this made up. If it doesn't work, don't call me, I can't help
> you'. My sister gave me a cup of cold water and that stopped it to a
> degree. My young brother went to the chemist and that did stop the

bleeding. I was without teeth for years as there was no money to spare
for such a big job.

Many new mothers were much younger and less experienced. 'Phyllis'
became pregnant at fifteen and married with her mother's special
permission. It was 1932 and the Depression was at its worst:

> My husband, who was a musician, had to pay off his banjo before we
> could get married so I was four and a half months. We were married in
> a manse and all that jazz, and of course we got a bedsitter and we were
> very lucky, we were never evicted. We always had that ten bob and the
> 2/6 for his fares. And every now and then he got a ball and got three
> quid. The thing is when I was eight months pregnant, he had to go on
> susso. We had no food, only digestic meal. We had to wait a week.
> We got a card for ten shillings and had to spend it at the grocer's.
> I couldn't stand it. After two days I go down. Of course my husband
> really took to me. I was a bad wife. I only had to speak out of turn
> and I'd get a smack on the mouth. It actually taught me to live on
> practically nothing. This week I'd get a pound of rice and the next
> sago. I had it all worked out. When I had the baby we'd get an extra
> 1/6. If you went to the Health Centre and showed your susso card,
> you'd get this little bit of paper that gave you a shilling's worth of fruit
> and vegies. And down I went every week, religiously — apple juice,
> pears, plums, whatever was in. Much to my husband's horror. He
> wasn't very happy showing the susso card. But it was ridiculous. His
> was pride; mine was absolute need.[8]

She knew to take advantage of the antenatal clinic at the Women's,
and that too was an experience:

> I went to the Women's — I must have been six months pregnant — and
> the sister said, 'They're all coming today', then 'Bloomers and corsets
> off. You'll have to sit round there. Get around there.' That's how she
> spoke. I sat there and sat there and sat there. Eventually she comes back
> and says 'And what are you doing here?' I says, 'You told me to sit
> here'. She says, 'But everything's gone back'. Then in comes all these
> different girls and then a very well dressed woman. 'What are you in
> here for?' 'You're here for the same bloody thing we are — V.D.'
> I didn't even know what V.D. was. They spoke to us like absolute dogs.

When 'Phyllis' went into labour, there were more shocks. They didn't
have the fares so she walked the three or more miles from Richmond,
'running up lanes having wees and all that jazz':

> We eventually got there, and they said, 'Wait for her clothes, say
> goodbye to her'. I kissed myself goodbye. Then the very first
> unforgivable thing they did, they made me have a bath and they tipped
> Phenol water over me. I screamed out, 'What do you mean, phenol, we
> clean out the lavatory with that!' 'Just in case you're lousy.' I thought —
> isn't that the last gasp!. Then up to the ward. There it was raining

mothers. There used to be eight or sixteen. This little sister said, 'Are you married?' 'Of course I am' — I didn't realise how young I looked. The gowns were open down the back and turned over, and the sister said, 'No modesty' and kept tucking us in.

I pluck up courage late through the night. I have visions of cutting open. 'How is the baby going to get out?' She says, 'The same way it got in.' I had never connected sex with babies.

'As for you', the sister said as she left at six in the morning, 'You'll have your baby this afternoon'. Of course I was nearly collapsing at the thought of this going on for ever. He was born at 8.10 AM.

The food never worried me, I ate what was going. The thing that absolutely horrified me was the 'Get over there, Do this, Weigh yourself, Do that'.

'The most vivid memory I have of my time in this hospital as a student is of a great battleaxe of a Labour Ward sister slapping a woman hard across the buttocks and shouting: "Come on Mother! Put your bum over here or you'll never have your bloody baby".' *James Smibert*

It was not just the hospital. Every institution, every professional encounter was soured with authoritarianism: 'If you were working-class they just thought you were idiots. They don't tell you anything; you just learn the hard way. I'm very proud that I'm working-class'.

But the sheer injustice of the Depression and the plight of the unemployed could not be denied by even the most hardened staff. As in the 1870s and the 1890s, the hospital saw victims of the Depression every day in the wards, women reduced to seeking charity who once had no need of it. And again there was a fall in mean birth weight which corresponded with the known trajectory of the Depression. The decline was of 0.2 lb (~100g), which is about one third of the decline in the mean birth weight in the Dutch famine, or equivalent to that caused by smoking in Australia in the 1990s.[9] It is still grave, and it is particularly significant because the general indicators of public health — infant, child

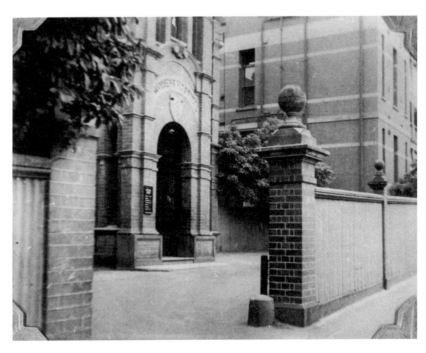

Entrance to Midwifery department, 1938 *RWHA*

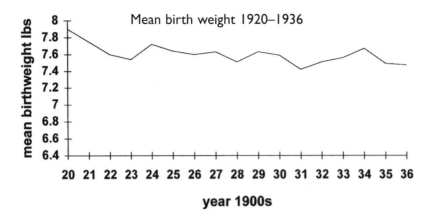

and maternal mortality, tuberculosis deaths, child morbidity and growth reported by school medical inspections — all indicate, as F. B. Smith shows in an unpublished paper, an improvement in the health and well-being of the Australian people despite the Depression.[10] Even though the material standard of living improved for those who stayed in work or profitably in business as they benefited from falling prices, the afflictions of the one third of the population overall in 1931 hit by unemployment do not show as you might expect in the public health record.

This is not to minimise the sufferings of the unemployed but rather to specify them. The Depression came at a time when social and medical interventions were beginning to make a real difference: to diarrhoea, to streptococcal infections of all sorts, to childbirth and abortion mortality, and to infections aggravated by personal dirtiness and poor diet. School milk and dinners made a big difference to working-class children; infant welfare centres, bossy as they were, did assist to reduce infant morbidity and hence, mortality. Even tuberculosis mortality continued its fall through the 1920s and 1930s, registering its fastest decline — amazingly — in the worst years of the Depression. The Depression produced some paradoxical benefits: alcohol consumption fell dramatically: spirits by 50 per cent and beer by 20 per cent in the early 1930s.

But if sustenance was keeping men and children fed, some mothers were still sacrificing their own health and that of their unborn children for the sake of the family. The Women's Hospital mean birth weights establish that some women were very hungry, so that even if the official statistics we do have of unemployment and destitution do not fully support the recollections of deprivation that have echoed down the years, these Women's Hospital figures suggest that hunger was real for some. Sustenance payments, furthermore, were commonly made to wives rather than husbands in the belief that working-class husbands could not be trusted to keep out of the pub. Women were usually in control of house-hold budgets and the distribution of food, therefore they chose to sacrifice themselves for the sake of their families. As in the previous two severe Depressions, the proportion of married women delivering in the mid-wifery wards rose as the mean birth weight fell. Unlike before, however, these women were receiving antenatal care and supervision, for by 1931, 80 per cent of those delivering were recorded as previous attenders of

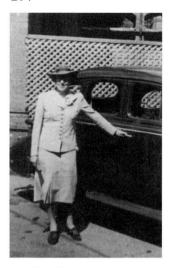

Miss K. Jacob, almoner, with her car, 1938 *RWHA*

the Women's antenatal clinic. By 1938, also, Professor Marshall Allan noted that the worst years of the Depression had seen an increase in uterine inertia and post-partum haemorrhage in women weakened by malnutrition.[11]

The disease afflicting the patients above all was poverty, and by 1933 the Women's Hospital's treasurer could no longer resist the Board members' demand to employ a medical almoner. Medical social work was a new discipline in Australia, brought first to the Melbourne Hospital in 1929 by an English almoner from St Thomas' Hospital, London, whose other task was to be Directress of Training for the new Victorian Institute of Hospital Almoners.[12] By 1934, when the Women's Hospital finally found the money to employ Miss Marion Urquhart, eight other hospitals, including the Geelong Hospital, had already established positions. The almoner's first role was to assess the patient's capacity to pay, and next to maximise her benefit from hospital treatment, but it at once involved the almoner in difficult and tragic lives. And it took time for the rest of the hospital to integrate the almoner into daily patient care:

> Mrs T. had not seen the Almoner before her confinement mainly because she did not attend antenatally — perhaps she felt it superfluous as this was her seventh confinement. She was delivered of twins, and although her mental outlook was poor she was still not referred from the ward to the Almoner. Only after she was transferred to the After-Care Hospital did the Matron there ring to ask what she could do, as she felt the patient was incapable of caring for the babies. When given the bottle to feed one of the babies, she took the top off and drank the milk herself. The report runs — 'The Almoner contacted the husband, a very worn man struggling to make a living under very difficult home conditions, his eldest boy helping him in the shop and the eldest girl did the washing for the six children and two adults.
>
> 'He agreed that the Almoner should try to arrange for the twins to be placed in a Mothercraft Home for a time and for his wife to be referred to the Welfare Clinic with the doctor's consent.
>
> 'The Matron of the After-Care Hospital was most grateful for the arrangements made and told the Almoner that the husband said that if he had had anyone to advise him in this way before, he would have been able to avoid much of the trouble in his family.[13]

Providing supplementary charity help, finding clothes and layettes, organising child care, negotiating with sustenance offices, arranging adoptions, all were part of the almoner's work. The almoners also argued against the universal charging of a £3 midwifery fee and sought to exempt the destitute. But immense efforts were also required to persuade women to accept treatment, especially the near one half of antenatal patients who were referred annually for dental care: in 1935–36, 941 midwifery patients were referred to the dentist and seventy two-dentures were eventually fitted.[14] As with the sacrifice of their diet in pregnancy, women exhibiting 'a tendency to do without treatment', both out of fear and 'maternal martyrdom'.

But the work of the hospital which was to become emblematic for the Depression, and cruelly stigmatising for the institution itself, was septic abortion. Women were now determined to control their fertility, yet at every turn the medical profession, the churches, governments and hospitals refused to assist people, especially the poor, to practise safe birth control. Doctors condemned rather than helped the sexually active unmarried and often intimidated the married who asked to be fitted for a diaphragm or cervical cap. Condoms were expensive and many men were too embarrassed to ask for them in a pharmacy. In some country towns there was no way at all of buying contraceptives other than by mail order in plain brown wrapping (until the federal Labor Government banned the advertising and sale of contraceptives by post in 1942). In 1934 Dr George Simpson and Dr (later Dame) Mary Herring wanted to establish a family planning clinic, and when Dr Herring sought the advice of an obstetrician at the Women's Hospital under whom she had trained: 'He expressed his disgust with what she had in mind and had shown her out of his office; "And he a Women's Hospital man!"' Dr Margaret Anderson had been 'allowed' to establish a birth control clinic at the Queen Victoria Hospital. George Simpson, by arguing the case for the woman for whom another pregnancy would be a death sentence, finally received the backing of the District Nursing Society, and the clinic's first session was conducted in October 1934. The clinic was scrupulous in reporting the medical conditions which justified the giving of contraceptive advice: by 1936 130 had been counselled, their average age thirty-three and their average number of children being six. (The clinic ran until 1940, operating from the Society's After-Care Hospital in Victoria Parade).[15] Thus it was that still the only method of birth control which was easy for women to find out about was criminal abortion.

People were otherwise controlling their fertility largely by abstinence and infrequent intercourse and, as the Depression deepened, more and more couples 'did without' sexually as well as materially. The birth rate fell, but there were still 'accidents' and the solution was abortion. There were some private doctors who performed abortions: some broken-down members of the profession, others in the inner suburbs, motivated by a desire to help women. Dr Albert Bretherton, one of a country policeman's thirteen children, had never forgotten his own mother's distress at a late unwanted and dangerous pregnancy. Through the Depression he aborted the poor without fee and aborted the rich to pay for it. He never lost a patient from septicaemia but he was made a scapegoat for less able practitioners' poor work, as well as for the dying women who found their way to his surgery. He died from a stomach haemorrhage while operating on a patient who would have died if he had stopped the operation, and a vast crowd of grateful women brought Prahran to a standstill at his funeral in 1937.[16] Shurlee Swain found only four doctors' names emerging from her research into the single mother during the inter-war years; far more numerous were the chemists and the midwives, ranging from the true backyarders to the well-organised and well-disguised operators of nursing homes.[17] But the women admitted to Wards 3 and 6 at the Women's Hospital had overwhelmingly induced the abortion themselves. And most were married and already mothers.

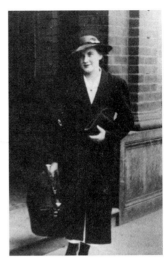

Visiting nurse service, 1938 *RWHA*

Almoner at work, 1938 *RWHA*

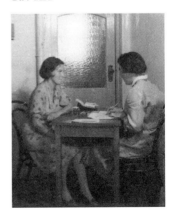

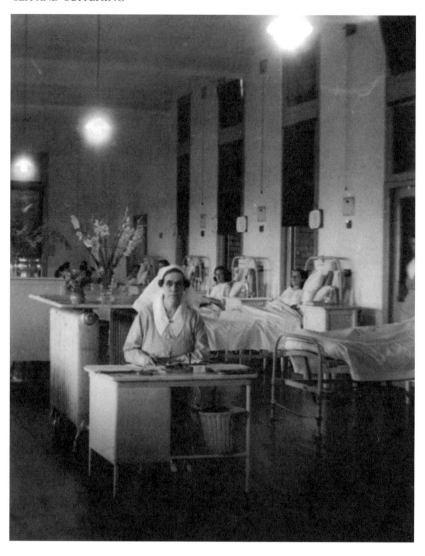

**Ward 6 with Sister
Rankin** *RWHA*

It is impossible now, as it was at the time, to put any accurate figure on the incidence of induced abortion. R. W. Worcester, in a paper to the National Health and Medical Research Council in 1938, quoted the Women's Hospital' admissions for 'abortion' since 1900 and showed that the ratio of 'abortions' to deliveries rose from 8 to 1 to 5 to 1 in 1910 and 2 to 1 in 1920, a ratio which remained fairly constant until 1935. This figure of course included spontaneous miscarriages which were incomplete, threatened or inevitable, the medical terminology of 'abortion' meaning both spontaneous and induced. And this has perhaps confused later historians and caused them to exaggerate the incidence of deliberate termination of pregnancy.[18] It became precautionary practice at the Women's to assume that all 'miscarriages' that became septic were the result of interference, even though this was not invariably the case. It was an unfortunate assumption and many women with septic spontaneous abortions found themselves stigmatised. None the less, the increased admission of women to the midwifery wards with incomplete, threatened or inevitable abortions from the 1890s suggests a rise in the practice of induced abortion as well as changing attitudes to hospital care for miscarriage.

The puerperal sepsis cases in the wards were still too numerous, but they did not reflect so much on the hospital's own obstetrical practices as on the work in private hospitals and homes. Lorna Lloyd Green:

> We had an epidemic of puerperal sepsis in a small hospital down the line, and these patients all came into the Women's. And would run the most amazingly swinging temperatures — terribly, terribly ill. Most of them formed abscesses all over the place and most of them died. And what could we do? Even towards the end in my time on that ward we got M and B 693, but after all it didn't do much good. Got them too late. I can remember very well the bed where I gave the first transfusion and I knew that this patient was going to die — but what could I do? I hoped that the transfusion might help — I don't know if I said white cells in those days — we didn't know much about immunity — but it might back up her immunity a bit. She ultimately died after weeks and weeks. It was an awful way to die, and morphia was the only thing we gave them, and it had side effects too with nausea and vomiting, and constipation, drowsiness and loss of alertness.

M and B 693: first sulphonamide (sulpha drug). 'In 1935 a German chemist Domagk announced the effect of protonsil on streptococci. It was later found that this action was due to the conversion in the body of protonsil to sulphonamide, which acts by inhibiting the growth of various bacteria, especially the ubiquitous and dangerous *Streptococcus hæmolyticus.*' (Black)

After a dreadful thirty-one deaths from puerperal sepsis in 1927–28, the toll began to fall smartly, with only a swing upwards in 1934–35.

Improvements in prevention and treatment — to some extent the result

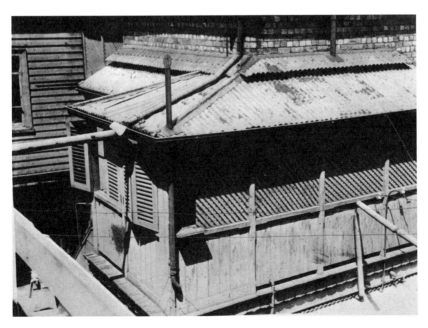

Ward 4 toilets, 1930
RWHA

of the Marshall Allan report and its wide publicity among the profession
— were working despite the domestic privations of the decade. But not
so with septic abortion: deaths rose steadily and the manner of those deaths
aroused a new horror. The dominant figure both in the Women's Hospital
and soon around the nation in the treatment and understanding of
puerperal and post-abortal infection was 'Bung' Hill. Hill later remembered the hospital of the 1930s:

> Common in the wards were sweats and rigors, high fever and tachycardia,
> pallor and collapse, jaundice and cyanosis, distension and dyspnoea, foul
> and purulent discharges, anuria, incontinence, delirium, and the muffled
> movements of the mortuary trolley. The heavy burdens of nursing and
> medical care, often without hope, would appal the many who today move
> quietly about the wards in their scheduled span.[19]

There were others without whom the work could never have been done,
for the hospital and the medical research infrastructure of Melbourne,
its university and public hospitals, while still small and poverty-stricken,
now had enough intellectual critical mass to make good clinical research
possible.

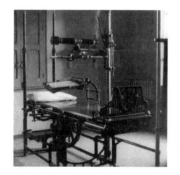

X-ray machine, 1938
RWHA

World War I had seen the foundation of both the Walter and Eliza
Hall Institute in the grounds of the Melbourne Hospital and the
Commonwealth Serum Laboratories, and the Alfred Hospital's Baker
Institute began in 1926.[20] These three as well as the laboratories at the
university all contributed to the clinical work of the Women's Hospital
in the 1930s. It was an exciting time in the bacteriological investigations
of infection, and puerperal infections in particular, and it was work which
both in England and Australia included a number of women. Dr Lucy
Bryce at the Walter and Eliza Hall Institute in 1928 traced a fatal epidemic
of streptococcal septicaemia in a private hospital to a nurse with an antrum
infected with the same bacterium, and began an intensive study of the
bacterial flora of the genital passages of pregnant and parturient women.[21]
One of the Women's Hospital's two most important laboratory scientists,
Miss Vera Krieger of the university's Biochemistry Department, in the
same year published her first collaborative paper, observations on the
chemistry of blood and urine in toxaemias of pregnancy, with the honorary Dr John S. Green.[22] That year she became officially the hospital biochemist, but her position was still insecure. The other was a bacteriologist,
Miss Hildred Butler of the Baker Institute, who began doing investigations
of infections for the hospital in 1931. The Women's was on the threshold
of its first world-class research achievements but it still did not have a
laboratory of its own. Specimens were carried over to the university or
sent down to Hildred Butler in Prahran. The value of intravenous saline
and glucose was being realised in the 1930s and the techniques of
transfusion were improving, but the hospital could not even produce its
own sterile solutions and Vera Krieger had to organise the staff of the
biochemistry department at the university to 'cook it up' each day and
walk it over. In 1934–35 they produced 500 units; in 1946 the hospital
was to use 15 000.[23]

The Women's Hospital might be a good clinical school setting the

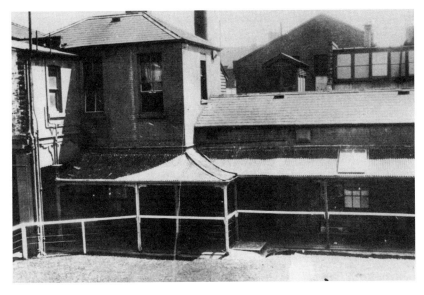

Old store and kitchen, 1935, later demolished to make room for the Pathology block *RWHA*

standards for obstetric practice for the state of Victoria and graced by distinguished consultants, but it was still a pauper's infirmary. It might be at the scientific frontier of research into infection, but the ward instruments and transfusion equipment were still boiled in the same steriliser as the bedpans. The public hospitals' chronic financial problems continued to grow, as did the community's demand for public beds for those too well off to qualify as charity patients, but too poor for good private care.[24] The Women's Hospital survived the Depression with ferocious cost cutting, reducing the cost per bed from £197 to £164 between 1930 and 1932. Falling prices of food and fuel helped, as did the 10 per cent cut in all government wages and salaries, but food was further reduced so that patients received only one hot meal a day, and if relatives or friends could not bring an egg for supper, you had just bread and butter. Some patients do remember being hungry; others had been hungry for so long that the plain fare at the hospital seemed like a feast, and consumed other patients' leftovers as well as every scrap of their own meals.[25] Betty Lawson would one day be matron of the Women's Hospital, and she is still angry at its impoverishment in the 1930s. After training at the Melbourne Hospital under the great Jane Bell, she went to the Women's in 1937 to do her midwifery:

> It was terrible. The people at the Women's would dispute what I say, but they had nothing like the equipment we had at the Melbourne. The Women's didn't have anything — you had to go scratching for everything.
>
> I used to go back from my days off at Eaglemont and take vegetables for the diabetics because we had to cook the diabetics' meals ourselves and we could never get enough variation in vegetables. I used to take back chemist's bottles, all sizes — little ones we used to feed the premature babies with. And Ponds Cream jars because they became nipple bowls — one for the swabs and one for the water — never enough of those. All these kind of things you had to provide

yourself because the dispensary supply was limited. We had to have
needle and thread to sew the binders on — there were never enough
needles or anything, so I used to have my own needles and cotton.
We used to have pockets in our uniforms and I would buy little tins of
Brasso at Coles to clean the brass with. We had to use our own money
and I only got 4s 8d at the Women's because 4d was deducted for
unemployment tax.[26]

And yet, the research was possible, in a way, precisely because it was a
paupers' infirmary. The 'clinical material' was richer than ever before.
Despite the growing reputation of the Queen Victoria Hospital, the
Women's drew most of the complications, and the hospital's growing
expertise in puerperal and post-abortal sepsis saw patients admitted to
the septic wards as emergency cases who were not charity patients. 'Mavis'
had her baby in a private hospital in a nice suburb in 1938. It was a forceps
delivery, and after fourteen days at home and 'in extreme pain', her
husband took her to the Women's:

> When I went they didn't admit me for at least two and a half hours.
> I went into casualty dept. I sat down on a form in a lobby. I was
> breastfeeding and my husband asked if we could have a cup of tea.
> They said no, there weren't any facilities. My husband had to run next
> door to a cafe for a tray of afternoon tea. It was a gruelling experience.
>
> They put me in a huge ward, sixteen people. They put me under a
> sort of canopy, they had all light globes in it, a heating thing for half
> and hour or so. I was feeling pretty rotten by this time, cold and
> miserable from sitting on that form for two hours and nursing the
> baby. I found it a great relief, warm, secure, comfortable. After that it
> was wonderful.
>
> They used to bring the baby in to me to feed it. Then I wasn't too
> well — my temperature was 105 degrees. I should have been dead.
> They said the baby would have to go home. I cried and carried on and
> got blood pressure, so they said perhaps it would be better, even
> though he'd have to be on the bottle, it would be nice for me to have
> him so they let him stay. I fed him the bottle — my milk had started to
> dry up.
>
> There were all sorts of treatments. I used to have metal things
> pushed into me. By this time they decided I had infected fallopian
> tubes. They were trying to get rid of the infection, trying to break a
> boil apparently — they put a metal rod in through the vagina. They did
> bring away a lot of pus-y stuff and everything.
>
> There was a medical conference on so they decided to give me
> [Protonsil], a forerunner of sulphur drugs. They wanted to see what
> effect they would have. They cured me. I was there for about six
> weeks. I used to have mustard plasters on my stomach. The doctors
> really didn't tell you anything. Years later when I was still having these
> pains, they decided I'd better be X-rayed.
>
> The nurses were wonderful, they really were. I didn't have one
> cross word. They were so lovely to the baby. The medical staff, the
> doctors were beautiful, they really were trying so hard, they were so
> sympathetic. I couldn't speak highly enough of them.

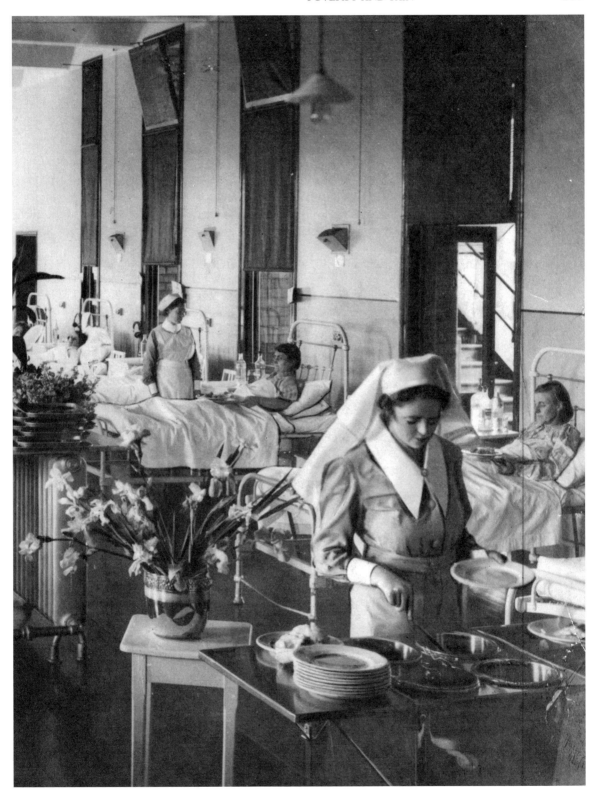

Ward 4 with Sister Hannah RWHA

My husband was only allowed to come on the regular hours, after 6:00 o'clock, some ridiculous time. I had other visitors — the girls from work came. The meals weren't that much. The girl next to me was from the poorer classes, and she used to eat everything I left. There were really poor people round in 1938, 39. My mother and sister used to bring me in tasty bits of food. I've always been a fussy eater. My husband did too if I fancied anything. I wasn't interested in the food. All I was doing was existing. I think they gave us porridge for breakfast. They were very good with cups of tea.

I didn't have any injections. I didn't care for the baby, didn't even change his nappy. I've never had the care of a small baby. I used to be feeding him his bottle. We missed out on his babyhood. Later we tried to adopt but the doctor said he didn't advise it if you had one of your own because you're inclined to lean to your own. So we didn't, we just battled on.

I had sponge baths. One terrible thing — I came home with nits in my hair. I shared a locker with the girl in the next bed. She really was a funny girl. She used to amuse me, not that I was the 'upper classes', but she had a different view of life from what I had. She wasn't rough, she was just common. I read quite a lot when I was there. I suppose I was pretty sick.

It was an experience. I'd never been sick and I'd led a pretty sheltered life. I found that I encountered people that were the best people I could have had. You were assessed money-wise. My husband was getting five pounds a week and we used to have to pay half our wages to the Women's. It wasn't free — you had to pay what you could afford. We managed all right. I don't think I'd be here now if it hadn't been for the Women's. It was a bit primitive, but you really got wonderful treatment. They seemed to be very professional.[27]

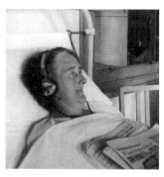

Patients' wireless service donated by the ABC, 1938
RWHA

'Mavis' was never able to have another child and in 1942 returned to the Women's with pelvic inflammatory disease. At eighty-four she still gets pain in her side.

There was now a sufficient volume of cases passing through to be able to notice the unusual and the new. Between 1930 and 1933 inclusive, the hospital treated 4424 women for abortion, of whom a massive 1069 were septic.[28] In the two years of 1933 and 1934, 3049 were admitted suffering from abortion, of whom 678 were infected on admission. In each year twenty-five of the women died, but they were dying in increasing numbers in a new and terrifying way — from gas gangrene caused by the bacillus *Clostridium welchii*.[29]

One was a twenty-three-year-old married woman from North Fitzroy, who was admitted at 5 a.m. on 12 November 1934.[30] Before him the resident saw 'a sallow woman, inclined to vomit'. Her temperature was 103°, her pulse 90 and of poor volume. She was eight weeks pregnant and close to aborting. She admitted to using a gas taper two days before to induce an abortion; she already had a four-year-old and had suffered 'only two' miscarriages, the last three years ago. She had shivers, was bleeding slightly, had lower abdominal pains and diarrhoea. She was ordered rest, medical stimulation and pituitrin.

At eleven that morning she was seen by Dr Hill, who although Medical Superintendent, was also in charge of grave septic cases. He noticed that she was jaundiced and her pallor out of proportion to her blood loss. He ordered a vaginal smear, which found no gonococci but many other bacilli. Blood was sent for culture to Miss Butler at the Baker Institute, but that would take three days. She had bad pyorrhoea in her gums, he noted and her lochia was 'somewhat offensive'. Blood and bile were to be examined and any blood was to be kept. He had his suspicions as to what was wrong, because once alone, she told him that she had also syringed herself with a Higginson syringe, which she assured him was newly bought. He knew that to wait three days for the pathology report on the blood culture was too long, and ordered that she be given 40 000 units of anti-gas-gangrene serum.

Hill saw her again at 7.15 that evening: 'This patient is now <u>bronzed</u>', her conjunctivae were chocolate coloured, and there was deep bruising at the sites of hypodermic injections in her arms. 'Obviously B *welchii*

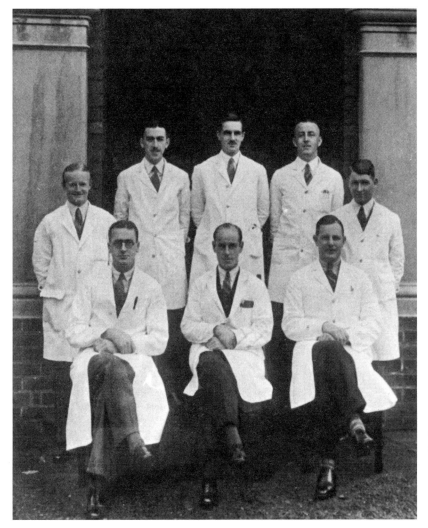

Resident medical staff, 1934
Back: Drs R. Warden, F. J. Hayden, J. G. Bonnin, J. G. O'Donoghue, J. W. Johnstone
Front: Drs G. R. Stoneham (N.Z.), A. M. Hill (Medical Superintendent), R. B. Charlton *RWHA*

progressing fast'. He was angry that he had not been told that at midday she had passed 4 ccs of 'bloody, deep mahogany, burgundy coloured urine'. She was now an 'urgent case of B *welchii* septicaemia' and he ordered immediate action: curettage under ethylene and oxygen, intravenous anti-gas-gangrene serum, and saline and glucose, quantitative blood cultures, intra-uterine aerobic and anaerobic cultures, including one to be sent to the Commonwealth Serum Laboratories. She was to have sub-mammary infusions of sodium bicarbonate. Sodium citrate and fluids with sodium bicarbonate as for a diabetic coma were ordered. Finally linseed poultices were to be applied to her loins.

By 8 o'clock, the curettage was under way. She vomited badly during the induction and the whole general anaesthetic had to be stopped and restarted. Hill began the curette:

> An offensive dark placenta was visible. Removed with sponge forceps; typically soft (rather like Cheddar cheese the way it scrapes off the uterine wall), necrotic-smelling, grey-dull red colour, adheres to the curette in a sticky, pasty fashion.
>
> In middle of curette, patient stopped breathing & pulse ceased, & she was to all intents and purposes dead, yellow and blue, with fixed dilated pupils. After artificial respiration and two coramine injections she came round, and the curettage was completed without further anaesthesia. Uterus cleaned out with iodine and plain gauze, and glycerine gauze left in for twelve hours.

coramine: a proprietary name for nictinic acid diethylamide, a drug which is a strong heart and respiratory stimulant (Black).

He saw her again at 10.15 that night and ordered two pints of continuous sub-mammary saline to be given.

Hill returned at 9 the next morning. She had had 40 000 units of anti-gas-gangrene serum intramuscularly at 4.30 a.m. The bronzing of her skin was even deeper and there now was definite cyanosis of the fingers. Her haemoglobin was 50 per cent. He ordered a blood transfusion and blood was taken from her husband and she was given 22 ounces. By the afternoon she was a bronze mahogany colour. Gas was heard exploding in her abdominal cavity while an intra-uterine glycerine injection was being given.

The next day, two after admission, her colour deepened and she developed rapid, grunting respirations with signs of congestion at bases of both lungs. She was placed in a carbogen tent to assist her breathing and injections of atropine and coramine were given alternately every two hours. Her urine was still acid and full of broken-down haemoglobin, so Hill, after consultation with Dr Kellaway, ordered a continuation of alkalis in her fluids. Her abdomen was now distended and slightly tender, but needling in three places yielded little microscopically. Her vaginal discharge had begun to smell necrotic and Hill confessed 'Prognosis now, from being 98 per cent, has become 100 per cent hopeless—quite impossible'.

The next day, 15 November, she had clinically improved although her colour had not: 'Nails cyanosed and slate-grey, fingers dusky bronze, palms have violent pink erythema'. Her serum showed less blood pigment but she still excreted only 3 ounces of urine for the day. She was puffing out with oedema and the necrotic smell was worse, 'suggesting that whole uterus, through muscular wall and (from abdo. and P.V. exam) probably to peritoneum is necrotic and rotting'. Yet by 5 p.m. she was still 'holding her own and astonishingly fit'. Hill confessed to being 'in a quandary as to whether it was wise or unwise to continue intravenous therapy. But will desist for present; her serum contains blood pigment, but seems rather better than yesterday'. The therapy included four-hourly rectal salines containing brandy; bi-daily sub-mammary salines 40 ounces; one intramuscular injection of 10 cc of 10 per cent of calcium gluconate; and 80 000 units of *Cl. welchii* anti-toxin intramuscularly in two injections separated by fourteen hours.

By the 16th, however, Hill was completely pessimistic. Her heart was still strong but her kidneys had begun to fail and her liver probably also: 'Regard prognosis as still ultimately fatal'. She was given more blood from her husband and by the afternoon she was sleeping and apparently improving. Hill thought that by now her blood was sterile, but she was becoming increasingly uraemic.

On the 17th she had severe abdominal pain. Abdominal needling produced straw-coloured fluid which yielded 'vast numbers of organisms with the morphology of *Cl. welchii* and streptococci'. She was immediately operated upon under local anaesthetic in her bed—a bilateral iliac, muscle-splitting laparotomy to drain the abdominal cavity: 'considerable quantities of brown-yellow, slightly faecal-smelling fluid containing lymph escaped'. Her urine by now smelled 'horribly offensive and necrotic—as though passed from a gangrenous bladder; penetrating odour through cotton wool stopper of test tube'.

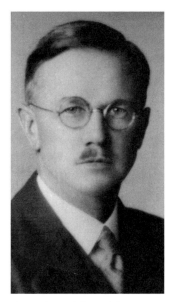

Dr Edward R. White
RWHA

The next day she was opened up under local anaesthetic again for drainage. Now the twitchings were fairly frequent and she had bouts of air hunger, and 'she wanders in her speech at times'. By the 19th she was 'semi-conscious, and though rousable is confused and quite disorientated, talks to herself a little and quite inconsequentially and sinks off into apparent stupor again'. Hill saw her again at 3 p.m.:

> Going downhill pretty rapidly now. Pulse poor tension; rate 100. Looks a terrible colour—mixture of deep jaundice, mahogany and a suggestion of an underlying greyish hue; though for the last three days has not been cyanosed.
>
> Is crying out a good deal; not saying anything or enunciating actual words. Is otherwise unconscious. Will die in a very few hours.

An hour and forty minutes later she died.

When Hill saw her at 6 p.m. he found that she had not been given the serum he had ordered because the hospital had run out. The day before M. B, single, aged twenty-eight, from Port Melbourne, had arrived in a moribund condition, perfectly conscious, but blotchily deeply jaundiced, bronzed to mahogany. At first she only admitted to taking beer and Epsom salts, but when interviewed alone by Dr Hill without any nurses present and told of the seriousness of her state, she said that she had syringed herself four days before with Lifebuoy Soap using a Higginson syringe. She confessed to having induced four miscarriages in the past, and died

Most common suburban addresses of 170 women admitted for septic abortion between 1 July and 31 December 1934 in descending order, excluding 49 which were single entries.

Suburb	No.
Carlton	21
Brunswick	16
Fitzroy	12
South Melbourne	10
Richmond	9
Collingwood	7
Northcote	6
East Melbourne	5
Footscray	4
North & West Melb.	4
St Kilda	4
Windsor	4
Prahran	4
South Yarra	3
Port Melbourne	3
Albert Park	3
Coburg	2
Hawthorn	2
North Brighton	2

four hours after admission. Two other septic abortions were admitted that day: one a married woman with a history of diphtheria, scarlet fever and rectal abscess, who had had a stillborn child many years before and who now had also a lacerated cervix, and denied any interference. And there was a twenty-eight-year-old single waitress from Carlton who had had a catheter 'passed by a nurse' seven days before. She had lost the foetus but a full five days elapsed before the 'nurse' removed the placenta. Hers was not a *Cl. welchii* infection and she did not die. Over the next five days there were five more septic abortion admissions, none fatal. Then on the 24th there were four in one day, two of them *Cl. welchii*, A. R. was eighteen, single and a machinist from Brunswick. For two months she had been taking medicine and 'black pills' from the chemist until she finally used a 'new' Higginson syringe with water. By the time she was admitted she was already deeply jaundiced and bronzed almost to mahogany. She died that day.[31] E. C. was a twenty-seven-year-old married woman whose only child was just eight months old. She lived in a small pocket of working-class South Yarra where three near neighbours were also admitted to the septic wards in 1934, suggesting a local source of dirty interference or shared equipment. Two months before she had syringed herself to no avail, and had been 'taking pills' ever since. She denied interference and died six days later of kidney failure. The post-mortem revealed a haemorrhagic mass in her left fallopian tube — a possible burst ectopic pregnancy.[32] By the end of the day, the staff were so anxious that they immediately gave E. S., a young married woman, anti-gas-gangrene serum even though the pathology later showed no sign of *Cl. welchii*.[33] That November eleven women died of septic abortion in Wards 3 and 6.

World wide, gas gangrene post-abortal and post-partum infections were in fact rare. When Hill went to write up his Women's Hospital series, he could find only eighty-four recorded cases in the international literature. But between April 1933 and February 1935 the Women's Hospital had thirty two cases, thirty of whom were treated by Hill and documented in what has remained the largest series of clinically observed cases on record.[34] (His paper in the *Journal of Obstetrics & Gynaecology of the British Empire* won the Katherine Harman Bishop Prize for Obstetrics in England and earned him an international reputation.) It was an epidemic and the impact on the medical and nursing staff who witnessed it was devastating. No one who saw a woman die of *Cl. welchii* infection ever forgot the horror of it, and few without strong religious sanctions against terminations of pregnancy, did not have their moral values changed. In the history of the Women's Hospital, the medical and nursing profession, and the birth control and pro-abortion movement, it was a defining moment.

It was one of the hospital's finest hours and one of its most stigmatising. The Women's was the place where 'all the abortions went', where 'they all died from gangrene'. The smell of the septic ward was notorious: all public hospitals had stinking gangrene wards, but only the Women's was talked about. The Queen Victoria Hospital treated septic abortions also, but its image was always more ladylike and respectable.[35] The abortion victims were all assumed to be 'tarts' or unmarried girls who had been tragically seduced; but most were married women who could not afford either financially or personally to have another baby. The women came from all over Melbourne and the country, but most from the inner suburbs. They were of all religions, but Catholics were under-represented compared to their numbers in the midwifery wards. Evil back-yard butchers were depicted as the perpetrators, but most women aborted themselves. Knitting needles and sharp instruments were assumed to be the most common culprits in the deaths, but in the 1930s it was the Higginson syringe, sold by the hospital itself for many years and by chemists everywhere, and used in respectable families for enemas and douching after intercourse. And perhaps it was the prevalence of syringing which seemed to earn for Melbourne, along with Chile and a few other places around the world, the stigma of 'Welch City'.

The aetiology of these infections remains unclear. *Clostridium welchii* lives in the bowel and some form of contamination had obviously taken place. In the post-abortal infections it was assumed that one cause was from a syringe already contaminated after being used for an enema. However, all the women who admitted to using a syringe in Hill's study claimed that the syringe was new.[36] Dirty mechanical interference, induction of labour by rectal tube, and contamination from a delivery where an enema had not been given, were clearly implicated in the puerperal cases. Many of the post-abortal cases had been taking so many pills of various kinds to stimulate contractions, that many must have had diarrhoea. Finally we do not know how many syringed the vagina after the cervix had opened and did not report that to medical personnel.

The common home methods of inducing an abortion show how easy it was for something to go wrong. E. C. from Footscray, a Presbyterian whose husband had been on the land, was just twenty-seven, had already been pregnant seven times, and delivered four children. This time she had been taking aperient pills and when her subsequent incomplete abortion became septic, she nearly died before she was curetted.[37] Abortion was clearly 'birth control' for another young Presbyterian wife: married just five months, she did not want a baby yet and so had been syringing herself and taking quinine until she aborted and became septic.[38] Another, and more cynical, patient was in fact admitted for the second time that year for a septic abortion. M. R. from Collingwood, had an Irish-Catholic name and at her first admission put down her religion as 'Methodist' and the second time as 'Presbyterian', probably to deter a pastoral visit. Her husband's occupation changed too in the eight months from 'seaman' to 'boilermaker'. She had taken 'three pills' the night before.[39] An Anglican wife of a shop hand from West Melbourne, with three children already, combined the old with the new and fell down some stairs, then three days later syringed herself with lysol.[40] None of these four had *Cl. welchii* infections and none died. One who also escaped death was a nineteen-year-old single girl from Princes Hill, a Methodist, who had had influenza and diarrhoea before her abortion began (or was induced). She had a triple septicaemia of *Cl. welchii*, a streptococcus and a staphylococcus. She was in hospital for ninety-seven days: the anti-gas-gangrene serum killed off the *Cl. welchii* and, they believed, blood transfusions had helped her fight off the streptococci, 'showing the therapeutic value of blood in

Religions of 860 admissions to septic wards between 28 December 1933 and 31 December 1934

Religion	No.	per cent
RC	216	25.1
C of E	420	48.8
Meth.	67	7.8
Pres.	100	11.6
Baptist	19	2.2
Other Prot.	17	2.0
Jewish	8	1.0
Unknown	13	1.5
Total	860	100

Religions of 170 admissions for septic abortion between 1 July and 31 December 1934

Religion	No.	per cent
RC	43	25.3
C of E	89	52.3
Meth.	10	5.9
Pres.	23	13.5
Baptist	1	0.6
Other Prot.	3	1.8
None	1	0.6
Total	170	100

Marital status of 170 women admitted for septic abortion between 1 July and 31 December 1934

Married	138
Widowed	3
Single	29

haemolytic: causing, associated with, or resulting from destruction of red blood cells. Sudden and rapid destruction of red blood cells causes acute renal failure partly due to obstruction of small arteries in the kidneys. (*OMD*)

sepsis'. The staphylococcus moved around her body for months, breaking out in gross abscesses. She survived, but her kidneys would have been severely damaged.[41] Frank Hayden was a resident on her ward in 1934 and remembered her sixty years later. Renal failure was finally the killer of those severely infected with bacteria which had a haemolytic capacity: 'Ones we thought were getting better — we'd be very proud of them, but then they would die in a week or two of renal failure from the jaundice. Nowadays with dialysis they'd keep them going'.

The septic wards were both tragic and exciting — 'terrible days' for Lorna Lloyd Green; for Ronald Rome, who followed her as a resident and then became Medical Superintendent, they were tragic but also 'really exciting'. Clinically they were challenging, and they took these young professionals into a world they had hitherto only read about in the tabloids. Dr Rome:

> One of the interesting things that took place was that if a lady had had an illegal abortion and she came in and we thought she was going to die, she was asked unfortunately, would she like to make a dying deposition. In many cases the answer was yes. Now we had to ring up the CIB and two of them would come up and very nicely and quietly talk to this girl about the circumstances. We, as doctors and nurses, wouldn't wait for that — that was secret. But the police would ask them pertinent questions, realising that at any moment the patient was likely to roll over and die. And they had all the well-known abortionists fairly well taped. We were bound to do this otherwise you became a party to the offence and we built up a remarkably good relationship with the Victoria Police.

In one patient's record in November 1934 it was noted that her septic abortion had been induced by 'Dr Bretherton', one of the instances where he was falsely accused.[42]

It was emotionally very difficult for all staff. The sisters who stayed on in the septic wards are remembered by Dr Rome as 'magnificent': older women who lived in the hospital for years, and rarely seemed to go off duty, 'always coming back to see how Mrs So-n-so was'. Gynaecological nursing attracted those who relished the intensive care required — maternity nursing gave you too little to do for the patient. Frank Hayden remembers Dolly Gray fondly, who had two canaries called 'D' and 'C' and was a prodigious gambler. But most nurses were passing through on their training, and few were prepared for what they saw. Most were sexually innocent and had no idea that women 'got rid of babies' in sordid and dangerous ways, and that the 'romance of motherhood' was tainted. Therefore while many felt acutely sorry for their patients, others were shocked to the point of repulsion. Patients could find themselves snarled at by one nurse, and tenderly cared for by the next.

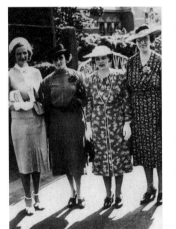

Sisters Rae, Kinnear, Gray and Rankin off to the races, late 1940s
RWHA

Many with the strongest ethical convictions against induced abortion, like Frank Hayden, still regarded the victims with compassion: 'You'd have the greatest sympathy for these poor unfortunate people who were so desperate and the things which really motivated them were the social disgrace or poverty'. But the sheer volume of cases, the epidemic of

induced abortion, combined with the poverty and tough efficiency of
the hospital, coarsened it as an institution. Many staff dealt with the
awfulness of it all by depersonalising patients and using a language which
removed abortion and its consequences from normal human experience.
The conditions and atmosphere were always punitive. And it hurt.
Shortage of money was always the excuse, but many straightforward
curettes for incomplete abortion on 'scrape day' were conducted without
any anaesthetic until well after the war. Kate Picouleau was seventeen

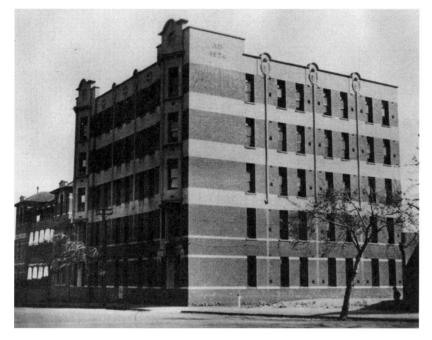

**Nurses Home, Cardigan
Street, 1934** *RWHA*

and working as an assistant in the Pathology Laboratory in 1947, while
she waited to enter nursing at the Melbourne Hospital:

> My knowledge of the world was restricted to a plain, ordinary,
> middle-class respectable upbringing. And I suppose I knew about
> abortions — I must have read about them. But my first experience of
> them was in a part of the Women's Hospital which has been knocked
> down now. There were six old-fashioned wards with verandas and long
> rows of beds. And going about getting blood samples for Pathology,
> there were days of the week when there was a lot a traffic — trolleys,
> lots of rushing about and people being rushed in. And I went back to
> Pathology and asked what was going on there.
>   — Oh it's scrape day.
>   Which didn't mean anything to me. They were all very refined
> ladies — you didn't talk about those sort of things socially.
>   — What do you mean by that?
>   — Oh they do the curettes — they're usually people who get into
> some trouble and they have to come into hospital to have curettes.
>   And I remember thinking at the time how terribly primitive it was.
> At times it was very cold and women were in a walkway, lined up on

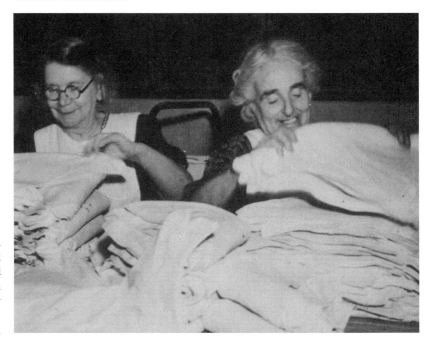

Laundry workers: Mrs N. Williams who had worked at the hospital for twenty-five years and Mrs M. Steele, sixteen years, photographed by *Women's Weekly*, 8 April 1944, *RWHA*

trolleys. There was no dignity, no privacy. Anyone could have walked past and seen what was happening. A feeling of haste — of something not quite nice about it all. I remember being quite shocked — not morally, but by the way the women were being handled.

And then she saw more:

I used to go to the wards to take samples and one woman I can remember had *Cl. welchii*. This woman was dying, she was very jaundiced, she looked ill but she wasn't unconscious and I had to take a specimen of blood. And I can remember her face — fifty years later — she had found herself in this big public ward, very ill, dying, and it was all somehow something that she hadn't quite understood. And she did die in fact a few days later and that aroused my curiosity and I asked more questions. And it all tended to be 'Oh we don't talk about those sort of things' and it always remained in my memory.

Later on I talked to colleagues and other nurses — they'd all had the same impression that I did — that this was something that shouldn't have been allowed to happen.[43]

The *Cl. welchii* epidemic in Melbourne intensified the crisis of conscience over induced abortion and birth control, and permanently changed the hospital's culture. The fear of it hung over the emergency department and the septic wards into the 1960s, and it remains the most common memory for those working at the hospital between the 1930s and the 1970s. Between 1931 and 1960, 147 women died of *Cl. welchii* infections, 136 post-abortal and 11 puerperal, compared to 101 (54 post-abortal and 47 puerperal) from haemolytic streptococcal infection which was the greatest bacterial killer of women in puerperal and post-abortal infections around the world.[44] In just four and a half years to early 1937 there were seventy-seven cases with forty-nine deaths.[45] The last woman to die this way was in 1970, twelve hours after admission, for it remained a danger well into the antibiotic age. But if the death toll was appalling, the legacy of lifelong sickness was even worse. One in fifteen died of the 4027 septic abortions treated at the Women's between 1931 and 1940, but Hill would later remind his colleagues:

> Death rates, of course, tell only part of the story. They give no idea of the sum total of human suffering, of the countless numbers who recovered only after long or debilitating illness, or who became disabled or died later elsewhere. They also tell nothing of the still common danger of obstinate or irrevocable sterility due to blockage from low-grade infection after apparently successful abortion from which the patient suffers little or no inconvenience. The legacy of these women, so many very young, is almost certain unhappiness.[46]

V.E. Day at the Women's
Hospital: Sister Morrison
and Deputy Matron
Richmond with a group
of pupil midwives *RWHA*

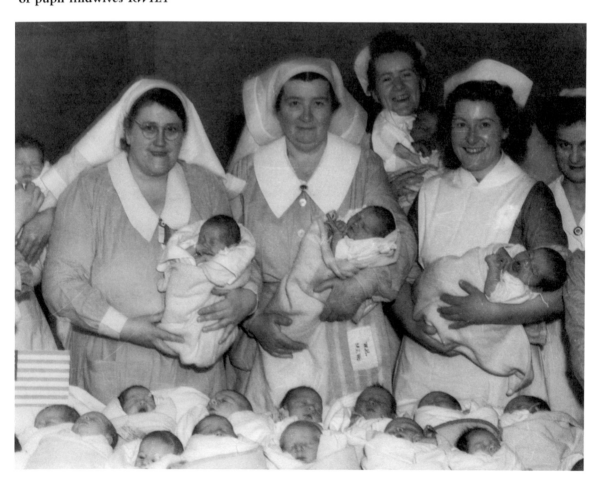

Watersheds　　　　　　　　　　　*11*

From the late 1920s through to the 1960s medical science transformed the biological life chances of women. The control of puerperal and pelvic infection, the better management of eclampsia, the storage and transfusion of safe blood, and finally the discovery of the oral contraceptive, changed everything for women. On an evolutionary scale, these advances, achieved within a span of just twenty-five years, were the most dramatic in our biological history. Their social and economic consequences remain to this day, uncertain and still unabsorbed by human societies everywhere. They were technologies, and as such depended on individual and collective will as to whether they were to be extended to all women or only to a fortunate minority. But potentially for the first time in the human story, they liberated women from their reproductive burden.

Used correctly and wisely, the technologies gave women choice over when to conceive and protection against the potential disabilities of childbearing. Healthy women could expect to have a baby and return to full health afterwards. Risks still existed but they were vastly reduced. It was a biological liberation which could underwrite a social liberation. The advances came from a marriage of clinical practice and laboratory science, and the great teaching hospitals, with their ample 'clinical material' and intellectual capital, provided the ideal environment. Clinicians and scientists belonged to the same institution, and while some medical doctors found it difficult to recognise scientific doctors as their peers, the most able among them seized the opportunity for collaboration. And a handful revealed themselves to be both excellent clinicians and good scientists.

Infection

The medical revolution began with the assault on infection. 'Bung' Hill had initiated three projects in the 1930s: first the determination of the bacterial pattern of obstetric infections in the hospital; second the clari-

fication of the problem of *Clostridium welchii* infections; and third, the
introduction of a bacterial smear test for rapid diagnosis. Hildred Butler
was the key player in all three projects. Since the pathology room and
its part-time staff would be useless for twenty-four-hour clinical diagnosis, in 1931 the hospital enlisted the support of the Baker Institute,
and already by the next year Hildred Butler, in collaboration with the
director, Dr W. J. Penfold, had published findings which showed anaerobic
streptococci to be the most frequent culprits in the hospital's obstetric
infections. By 1937 they knew that the problem of serious infection in
the hospital was largely that of four bacteria: the anaerobic streptococci,
the haemolytic streptococci, *Staphylococcus pyogenes* and *Cl. welchii*. Less
important were *Bacillus coli*, anaerobic gram-negative bacilli and aerobic
non-haemolytic streptococci. That same year Lancefield's serological
typing of haemolytic streptococci was established and their identity as
of groups A, B, C and G were routinely reported. Hill was frank about
their limitations, however, revealing that in 36 per cent of the deaths
believed to have been caused by infection, the bacterial cause was either
not sought or not found.[47]

The *Clostridium welchii* project did not begin properly until 1933. Prior
to 1931, genital tract infection with *Cl. welchii* had never been diagnosed
at the Women's, but as the death rate from criminal abortion rose in the
1920s, some deaths were attributed to unspecified poisoning from abortifacients. Occasionally the toxicologist could detect lead or carbolic acid,
but there were many unexplained cases of women dying horribly with
deep jaundice and blood in the urine. Hill initiated the full investigation
in 1933 and it was carried out at the clinical, bacteriological, biochemical,
haematological, toxicological and pathological levels. The clinician (usually
Hill) attended the autopsy, studied the findings and took away tissue and
fluid specimens for examination by the bacteriologist, the pathologist and
sometimes the Government Analyst. Both Hildred Butler at the Baker
Institute and Dr Charles Adey at the Commonwealth Serum Laboratories
were involved, and once the *Cl. welchii* was isolated and identified, Adey
developed an anti-gas-gangrene serum. Clinically the infection was complex and took a number of forms. It was clear that the only hope of
saving a patient lay in early diagnosis both for the administration of
anti-gas-gangrene serum and for the removal of the uterus to halt
the gangrene. Typically, the *Cl. welchii* infection did not present obvious
symptoms on admission, and thus the need for rapid clinical diagnosis
drove the third project, the diagnostic bacterial smear test.[48]

This was Hildred Butler's finest achievement. In 1939, trying to find
a fast method of diagnosis, she began to examine direct smears from the
vagina and cervical canal of patients who had had swabs for bacterial
cultures. She taught staff, both nursing and medical, to take swabs in the
ward and immediately smear them on to a glass slide before applying
them on to an agar plate for culture, rather than preserve them in jelly
for transport to the laboratory. This not only saved valuable time, it
produced specimens which were untainted by jelly and therefore easier
to read. She found that 'each type of genital tract infection has a charac-
teristic smear pattern derived from the number and the morphology of
the bacteria and the nature of the local leucocytic response'. By 1941 an

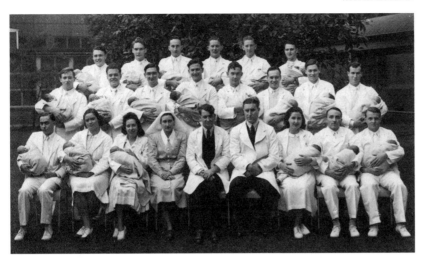

accurate direct-smear diagnosis of *Cl. welchii* infection could be made in twenty to thirty minutes; by 1946 of group A haemolytic streptococci and their potential virulence; and of other bacterial causes by 1950. By 1945 this technique provided a swift and accurate diagnosis of 90 per cent of the hospital's infections. It became routine to examine the smears from all abortion patients on admission and of all midwifery patients with a vaginal discharge suspected of being infected, as well as all those whose membranes had been ruptured for more than 24 hours or who were in prolonged labour. And it was also used to monitor therapy.[49] By the early 1960s the Pathology Department was dealing with between 5000 and 7000 smears annually, and Hill later estimated that in her thirty-three years at the hospital, Hildred Butler had investigated some 250 000 women with infection during childbirth and 64 000 who had aborted.[50] Butler herself, although not medically trained, became a superb clinician, somewhat feared by younger staff; and she would come at any hour of the day or night to see a woman suspected of *Cl. welchii* infection. Those who followed in her footsteps always found stressful the responsibility of deciding on the identity of the bug at the bedside while the clinical staff waited. (The hospital still practises this rare bedside pathology for genital infection, and it remains a world leader in the diagnosis of sexually transmissible diseases and of post-abortal and puerperal infections.)[51]

Hill's success in London in 1936, combined with the desperate situation in the septic wards in Melbourne, strengthened the hospital's case for a proper pathology department, and by 1938, after a generous private donation from the Connibere family, it was built. The Hospital's Pathology department had been recognised for the first time as 'an approved research institution' in 1937 and as such it needed a proper director. Vera Krieger was to be awarded a DSc in September 1939, but the hospital doctors would not admit her to the doctors' dining room because she was 'not a real doctor'. Hildred Butler was recruited as the bacteriologist in 1938 on £350 a year, after she had refused their first offer of £325. She was to take out her DSc in 1946. At the Children's Hospital, the great Reginald Webster was being paid £800 a year and being permitted the right of private practice. The new director needed to be medically qualified so

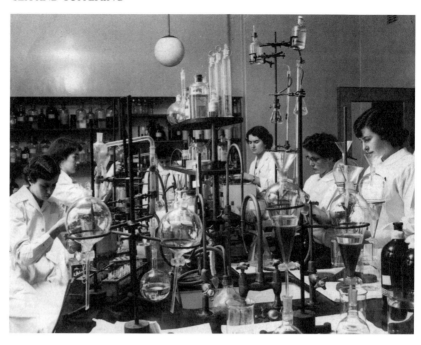

**Pathology laboratory,
1947** *RWHA*

in 1938 the search was on for a suitable man to head Pathology at the Women's. Dr Hans Bettinger, a German refugee from Nazism, was recruited from the University of Sydney on a salary of £1000 a year. Bettinger was a fine anatomical pathologist, and he brought invaluable scientific and linguistic skills to the position. His most important work was in the pathological diagnosis of cancer and he raised the standards of hospital reporting and pathology throughout Melbourne's hospital system.[52]

Leonard Colebrook's pioneering work on the 'strep-throat' carrier in the 1930s revolutionised the supervision and clothing of attendants in the labour ward. Recent sufferers from tonsillitis or infected sinuses, along with asymptomatic carriers of the bacteria, were shown to be the principal source of this form of puerperal infection. Lucy Bryce and Phyllis Tewsley of the Walter and Eliza Hall Institute and the Queen Victoria Hospital were asked to investigate an outbreak of puerperal sepsis in the intermediate wards of a community hospital in 1937, and the incidence of Group A streptococci carriers among the midwifery workers in contact with the three sick women was found after swabbing to be 22 per cent. Night staff were particularly implicated. A control sample of doctors and nurses who had not been known to have been recently in contact with Group A carriers was 3 per cent and 6.7 per cent respectively.[53] These were the infections against which the first antibiotics, the sulphonamides, were most effective, but in the Women's patients, the Group A haemolytic streptococci, *Escherichia coli* and the anaerobic gram-negative bacilli were responsible for fewer than 10 per cent of their infections. By 1937, when supplies of sulphonamides improved, their efficacy against the severe and life-threatening group A streptococcal infections became apparent. None the less, most infections remained resistant.[54]

The war brought shortages of staff, drugs and equipment, although

Hill remained a civilian and the women carried on. The number of deliveries and abortions fell, the admissions in 1942 being the lowest in a decade, yet the incidence of *Cl. welchii* infections rose again, with fourteen deaths in both 1941 and 1943. These were difficult years: one wartime midwife recalls a tragic night when each of the five babies delivered was dead by the morning: 'and I sank down behind the autoclave and wept'.[55] One in five maternity admissions were emergency ('unbooked') cases and the toll of exhausted multiparas and neglected young women in a severely dislocated society remained high. The hospital, however, had never been so professional. As medical superintendent from 1938 until he went to the war, Ronald Rome initiated the first annual clinical report — a massive document which analysed every part of the hospital's clinical work. (He received his first copy while on active (medical) service at Tobruk.) And Hill and Butler continued their investigations. Hill established for the first time that the Group B streptococcus could cause fatal infection, but he and Butler continued their work on the most prevalent and insidious of the infections, the anaerobic streptococci. These they found to be responsible for 80 per cent of Melbourne's puerperal infections, and 50 per cent of the post-abortal infections. They were normal inhabitants of the vagina of around half the patients at term. They were complex in their clinical manifestations and widely damaging. Their bacteriological success depended on the weakened immunity of the woman, in particular from blood loss, less often from fatigue or tissue damage. And they needed the opportunity to ascend into the normally sterile uterus. (The 'success' of the Group A haemolytic streptococcus, and of *Cl. welchii,* depended on the intrinsic virulence of the strain, not so much on the state of the woman's resistance.) The prevention of these anaerobic infections required, first, the avoidance of haemorrhage and trauma; and second, the early and repeated use of blood transfusions.[56] In August 1946 Hill and Butler gave a joint paper to the Victorian Branch of the British Medical Association which drew together all their wartime work. They had established that the anaerobic infections, which were by far the most prevalent, were not infectious between patients; and that the

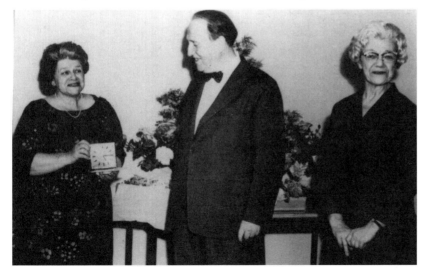

**Drs Vera Krieger,
Hans Bettinger and
Hildred Butler**
RWHA

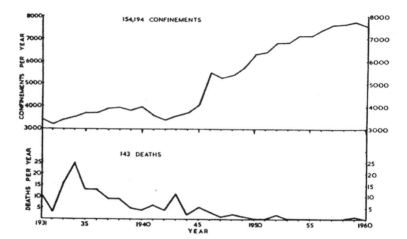

**Puerperal infection
deaths 1931–1960**
Hill, 'Why be morbid?',
MJA, *25 January 1964,*
pp. 104–11

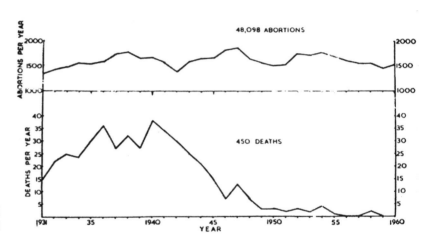

**Deaths from infected
abortions 1931–1960** *Hill*

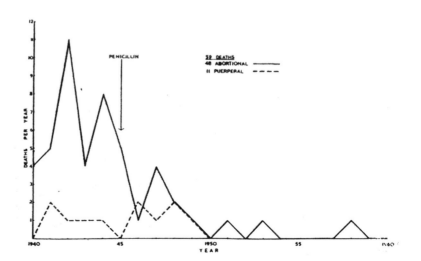

**Deaths from anaerobic
streptococcal infection
1940–1960** *Hill*

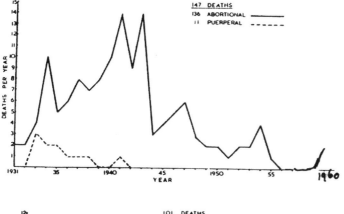

Deaths from *Clostridium welchii* infection 1931–1960 *Hill*

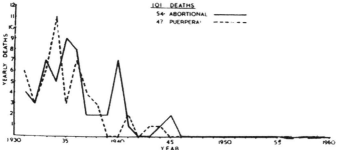

Deaths from haemolytic streptococcal infection 1931–1960 (from 1937 Group A only) *Hill*

two that were, Group A streptococcus and *Staphylococcus pyogenes,* were transmitted by droplet, dust and contact in the former, and only by dust, objects and person-to-person contact in the latter. So much of the conflict and fear which had clouded the hospital's management of infection was shown in retrospect to have been unnecessary. The prevention of infection had proved to be far more complex than isolation and asepsis: management of labour and lying-in were also significant, and avoidance of haemorrhage critical. In 1941 the Victorian Midwives' Act had been amended accordingly.[57]

The war produced what Hill was to describe as 'two of the greatest medical advances of our time': the development of blood transfusion and resuscitation services, and penicillin. Penicillin proved equally effective against the anaerobic streptococci, the Group A streptococci and *Cl. welchii*, once it became available in 1945. Deaths from both puerperal and post-abortal infection fell at once, however supplies were not sufficient until 1947 for all patients with suspected infection to be given a five-day course. This led to a fall in puerperal morbidity, from 5.2 per cent in 1947 to less than 1 per cent in 1949. As Hill later wrote:

These then were wonderful years, years when there was as much romance in infection as there was infection in romance. At that time, in the course of a single day, one might meet in reality each of the images described with imaginative power and graphic brevity by William Blake a century and a half earlier:

> To see a world in a grain of sand,
> And a heaven in a wild flower,
> Hold infinity in the palm of your hand,
> And eternity in an hour.

The bacterial world which had decimated women was very much smaller than a grain of sand. With penicillin had come the heaven in a wildflower, for no bloom which delights the senses has brought such peace and solace to mankind as this humble fungus with its stumpy stems and simple spores. For the first time the clinician, face to face with desperate infection, held that power which is infinity in the palm of the hand. But as human frailty is never far away, there was always the occasional patient who had been wrongly treated, or admitted to hospital too late to be saved, and for her it was eternity in an hour.[58]

But it could not last. The Women's was conservative in its use of anti-biotics, but it was using them preventively as well as therapeutically. Like hospitals and practitioners everywhere, however, it unconsciously relaxed. In 1956 there was an increase in staphylococcal cross-infection in the hospital. In Hill's words: 'The staphylococci in the hospital environment were becoming resistant to tetracycline, the choice of broad-spectrum antibiotics by the medical staff was haphazard and operating theatre disci-plines were not sufficiently taut'.[59] The most alarming problem developed in a premature nursery, where the repeated prophylactic use of tetracy-cline increased the proportion of tetracycline-resistant staphylococci from 10 per cent to 90 per cent in three months. An Infection Control Subcommittee was formed, a phase-typing laboratory established, disci-pline over aseptic technique and behaviour tightened in theatre, and the staff was forced to accept the principle of unified control of hospital chemotherapy. Again, infection changed the culture of the hospital. All 773 staff were swabbed: 27 per cent of nurses (among them the matron) were found to be nasal carriers; 19 per cent of all other staff, including doctors, likewise. Since nurses were the greatest 'culprits', they had to touch patients, especially babies, as little as possible. Modified rooming-in commenced and all babies were fed 'at a distance'. Babies were not to be cuddled, and premature babies most of all, were not to feel the caress of a carer, let alone of their mother. Visitors to the premature nurs-ery were banned.[60] Peggy Taylor was a staff nurse then charge sister of the premature nursery from 1958 until 1971:

> I still have terrible guilt feelings at how many problems I must have caused about mothers and babies being together, because we kept them totally separate when they were in prems. There weren't any visitors.
>
> In fact the thing that convinced me that it was absolutely the wrong thing to do was that we had one baby in an isolette which was dying, and the mother was not allowed into the nursery at all. And she stood at the window and she was crying, she was hysterical and tears were streaming. She was wanting to touch that baby, to hold it, to cuddle it, and she couldn't. And we were so cruel to do that.[61]

Marlene Kavanagh once helped a patient who had delivered her first live child after fourteen miscarriages to sneak a five-minute cuddle in the premature nursery: 'And I had the most horrific worries for the rest of that baby's stay that somehow if it got an infection, it was all my fault because I'd let the mother nurse the baby'.[62] Finally the best solution

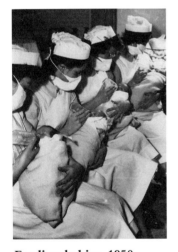

Feeding babies, 1950s
RWHA

was found in the routine use of hexachlorophane emulsion on the skin of newborn babies and on women before labour or surgery. Thus the Women's Hospital coped with another 'septic crisis', but the impact on its culture outlived the microbiological threat.

Eclampsia

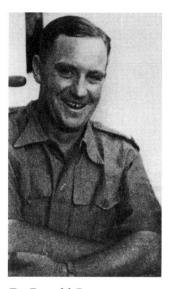

Dr Ronald Rome on active service in the Sudan *RWHA*

In 1938, as the new Pathology Block was being built, the hospital had committed itself, at the behest of the Federal Health and Medical Research Council, to two major projects combining laboratory science and clinical medicine. One was the study of obstetric infection by Hill and Butler; the other was toxaemia of pregnancy under the recently appointed biochemist, Vera Krieger, and Dr Ronald Rome, the then Medical Superintendent.[63] Krieger had already begun to publish, producing in 1938 two major papers on laboratory tests for renal function.[64] Krieger and Rome's first paper did not appear until May 1941, by which time Rome was in the army. It was a large study of 651 pregnancies, looking at both the primary cases of toxaemia and their subsequent pregnancies, with special attention to renal function. The results were disturbing, revealing a wastage of foetal life a young country could not afford; and there was evidence of permanent renal damage from the initial toxaemia. As a result of their findings, the Women's Hospital had changed its policy so that a woman with albuminuria who failed to respond to treatment would have her pregnancy terminated within five days instead of three weeks.[65] The war brought the project to a halt, but when Rome returned after army medical service at Tobruk and El Alamein, followed by a near-fatal car accident on his way to his next posting, he discovered that the incidence of eclampsia at the Women's Hospital had begun to rise, reaching a record level of 55 cases in 1942. Between 1939 and 1943, 48 of the 92 patients who were admitted before delivery and who subsequently died, had died of eclampsia, pre-eclampsia or chronic nephritis. As death from infection retreated, death from eclamptic conditions assumed the mantle of the greatest threat to women in childbirth. Yet no one knew what it really was and what caused it. It was clinically described and methods of treatment appeared to have some effect. The Women's had treated 1174 women with eclampsia between 1912 and 1943: the mortality rate for the years prior to 1921 had been 20.5 per cent, while during the last decade, it had been 13.4 per cent. Rome noted that the world's best figures for a similar series was 10.2 per cent, so that the Women's was doing well considering the role it served in the community.[66]

Some women had lucky escapes. 'Vera' was twenty-two and visiting hospital for a check-up, when she had a fit:

> They said I had fourteen eclamptic fits that day. I didn't go there to be put into hospital — it was just by chance I was there. I don't remember anything about my labour. I woke with all this awful feeling I was above myself, looking down. They were saying 'We're losing her', and decided I'd better get down there on that bed. I remember them

saying 'You've got a baby girl' and I didn't know I had a baby.[67]

Her next pregnancy was terminated at the Queen Victoria Hospital, but she did have a baby safely at the Women's five years after her first. She then had two miscarriages. She was lucky to be alive at all after fourteen eclamptic fits. 'Win' had twins and eclampsia for her first pregnancy and all three had nearly died: 'My mother wanted to give a donation to the Women's because they'd saved her daughter and her grandchildren'. It was two years before she regained her strength and then she became pregnant again. The risk was too great so her husband's aunt induced an abortion at twelve weeks, again of twins, with castor oil and a syringe.[68]

The warning signs of rising blood pressure and increasing oedema were being heeded by more and more doctors. 'Marion', herself a midwife who had trained at the Women's during the war, was finding her early years of marriage difficult. They were living in a single room, and she had just miscarried her first pregnancy, when she conceived again. Her blood pressure began to rise until her doctor ordered her to hospital. Unable to afford a long stay in the private hospital she had booked for the birth, she spent eight weeks in the antenatal ward at the Women's:

> I was admitted, put into a ward, a six bed ward, all curtained off from the next lot of cubicles. I couldn't fault the staff; I thought the day-time staff were very nice. I felt quite well; I didn't know why I couldn't get out of bed. I didn't have headaches; I felt why am I here? I knew why, of course, I had pre-eclampsia, I had high blood pressure, my kidneys weren't too good. The young medical students always came around with pans asking for specimens etc, testing them, taking my blood pressure. Of course it was a training hospital, but you don't like it when you're the victim. This went on for eight weeks. When I felt well and when the curtains were drawn, I used to get out of bed and run around the bed.
>
> The day before I was to be induced, the waters broke. I had labour pains. I would ring the bell. The nurse would come and she wouldn't even come over to me. 'Why are you ringing the bell Mrs 'Atkins'?' I said, 'The pains are getting stronger.' 'Stop ringing the bell', she said. This went on for a number of hours, and I had no sedative at all. Finally, I knew I was second-staging. Another patient rang the bell for me. The nurse just stood there and said, 'Stop ringing the bell, Mrs 'Atkins'. The sister-in-charge on her rounds looked at me and said to that nurse, 'Get Mrs 'Atkins' on to a trolley.' They bundled me on to a trolley. I looked back and the bed was a sea of blood. They got me into a labour ward and two contractions later, out popped Jennifer. They brought her over for me to see and asked what I was going to name her. That's the last I remember. When I woke up I thought, 'I'm in the b & d room.' The doctor was there and he said, 'She's gone, there's no pulse.' I was screaming at the top of my voice, 'I'm not dead!', but I don't suppose they could hear me because I wasn't making a sound. I don't think they notified my husband until I was conscious. I had transfusions from Friday till Sunday.
>
> The baby had to stay behind in hospital until she was six pounds.

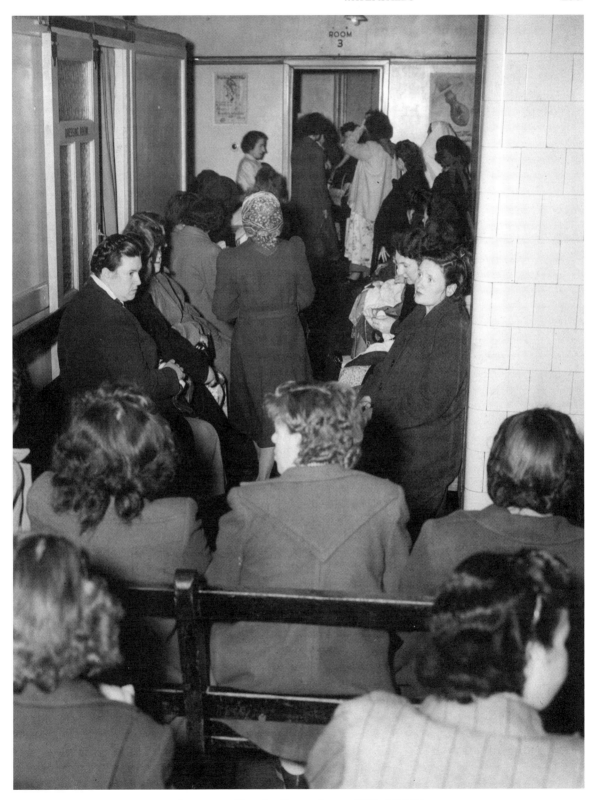

Overcrowding in Outpatients, 1953 *RWHA*

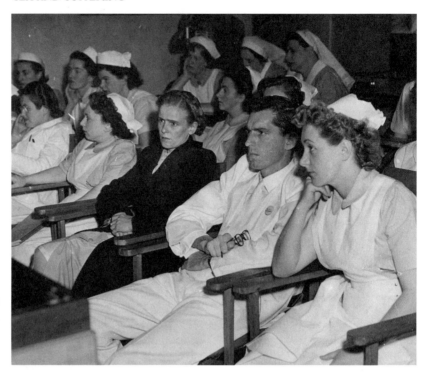

**Viewing the first
screening of a
closed-circuit televised
operation in Australia,
1950** *RWHA*

I didn't touch her until I took her home. They actually let her come
home before she was six pounds because I was a nurse. I used to take
in milk every day, but because I didn't have any stimulation, I didn't
have much, so she had to be bottle-fed at the same time. I looked in
the window to see her. One day, I held up the placard with her name
on it and they held up the wrong baby. I don't know whether they
showed me how to bathe her, it was a long time ago.

The food wasn't all that great. Breakfast was porridge and then they
came along with scrambled eggs and dob it on your plate. I think it
was powdered eggs, which is why most of the women didn't like it.
I felt I had to have some protein so I ate it. The sister-in-charge
shouted to all the women in the ward: 'Mrs 'Atkins' is the only one
who will eat the eggs. She is the only one who is thinking of the
baby.' I don't think I was too popular with the other ladies.

In the evenings you were only allowed to have two visitors and you
could have visitors two afternoons a week. My husband came in the
evenings, my mother in the afternoons. I read and knitted, I exercised
in bed. We had a lovely day nurse and she used to talk to me a lot.
I suppose I really didn't mind the students.[69]

By the end of the 1940s eclampsia was responsible for a third of
Australia's maternal deaths. Those who survived were known to suffer
permanent kidney damage, to be at risk from another pregnancy, and
even to have suffered brain damage from a cerebral haemorrhage.
Prevention by long antenatal stays in hospital was very expensive, and
treatment of eclampsia labour intensive and costly with patients confined
to a darkened room with a nurse constantly in attendance while heavy

sedation and diuretics were used to reduce the condition. Eclampsia also endangered babies' lives, and of those who survived, too many were premature or small, and that was dangerous, traumatic and expensive. Prevention had to be the answer.

The senior medical staff of the Women's Hospital, Crown Street Sydney ('Crown Street'), led by T. Dixon Hughes, had focused on blood pressure as an early sign of pre-eclampsia. In 1948 the hospital began a strict regime of antenatal care: forcing all booked patients (to the extent of sending the local police after visit evaders) to attend the antenatal clinic regularly, for they had found the eclamptics to have been the worst attenders in the past. Next they gave them lectures, delivered by a recent mother with a baby in her arms, to allay fears about hospital care and childbirth, and to persuade women of the importance of antenatal care and of diet. Third, they organised antenatal visits for country women in their homes. Fourth they co-ordinated their campaign with local antenatal clinics. The fifth, sixth and seventh strategies were the crucial clinical practices: careful monitoring of blood pressure, watching for signs of retained fluid oedema in the fingers and the strict control of weight gain in mid-pregnancy by dieting. They argued that albuminuria was too late a sign of trouble to be used diagnostically, whereas if a young primipara with a low initial blood pressure gained more than eight pounds in weight between the twentieth and thirtieth weeks of pregnancy, she would in all probability develop pre-eclampsia or even eclampsia. The diet had to be high in protein and vitamins, and low in carbohydrate: except for the vitamins, almost the reverse of the diet recommended to prevent pre-eclampsia when it was thought to be a toxic state caused or aggravated by an excess of animal protein. And it endorsed the theories of Dr Mary De Garis who had been a lone voice in the late 1920s calling for high-protein diets in pregnancy.[70]

The results at first looked spectacular. Crown Street went from having an eclampsia rate of 1 in 350 among its booked patients from 1935 to 1947, to having none at all by 1950–51. Dixon Hughes gave a paper at

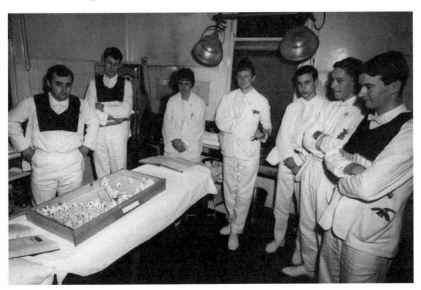

Student life: medical students with display of the Battle of Trafalgar
RWHA

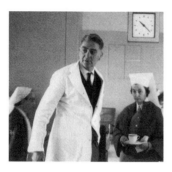

Dr John Laver, Medical Superintendent *RWHA*

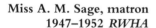

Miss A. M. Sage, matron 1947–1952 *RWHA*

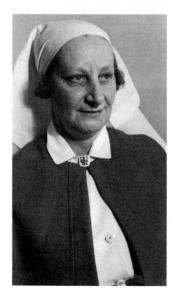

the first Australian conference of Fellows and Members of the Royal College of Obstetricians and Gynaecologists in April 1951, but it did not appear in the *Medical Journal of Australia* until the last issue of the year.[71] The international limelight was stolen somewhat by Crown Street's young medical superintendent, R. H. J. Hamlin, who published an exultant paper in the *Lancet* two weeks later. In a generous footnote he acknowledged that while the conclusions were his own, the successful results confirmed the views held for many years by Dixon Hughes.[72] It seemed an extraordinary achievement for preventive social medicine, and Hamlin was justifiably proud, because above all it had depended on the discipline and attention to detail of the hospital, and that had depended on the dedication and drive of the medical superintendent.

The Melbourne Women's Hospital had the right man in the job at the right time. John Laver was a new breed of medical superintendent: hospital administration was his career and the superintendency was not a stepping stone to senior private practice. He was in office from 1951 to 1969. He towered over his staff, quite literally, being 6 feet 7 inches tall, and many can remember him driving his very large car with a baby between his legs as he transferred a small patient between the hospital and its convalescent home, the Henry Pride Wing. He was the last of the 'hands on' medical superintendents: he knew what was happening in every corner of the hospital. Every day he came to the postnatal ward, looked at the bed list and the temperature list, and then told the charge sister who was going to Henry Pride that day. He was utterly dedicated to the hospital, patients and staff; he was eccentric and a law unto himself when the need arose, 'but nice'. Again, as after World War I, the immediate war service of the medical and nursing staff coloured their professional culture. Laver had had a big war; Miss A. M. Sage, who was matron from 1947 to 1952, had been Matron-in-Chief of the Army Nursing Service; Matron Betty Lawson had a distinguished war record, as had Deputy Matron, Jean Crameri. The hospital became busier and bigger: it was by now one of the largest women's hospitals in the world, and the sheer weight of daily organisation made military discipline almost inevitable. And if the hospital was to turn around such a massive medical-social problem as pre-eclampsia and eclampsia among the most resistant section of the population, the very poor of the inner city, then rigid discipline and a determination to hunt down every evader and over-eater would be needed. The new dietary regimen was going to conflict with age-old maxims about pregnancy: women were *not* to 'eat for two'; they were *not* to indulge in the traditional 'strengthening diet' of refined carbohydrates; they were going to have to give themselves the meat protein that in times of acute poverty they reserved for the working men of the family; they were going to have to forgo all the indulgences of cakes and sweet puddings that made an otherwise dreary menu and stressful daily life more pleasurable. There would have to be an immense act of public education, but as the Women's Hospital in Melbourne was finding, that was going to be difficult because more and more of their patients after 1947 could not speak English.

Yet the hospital was there above all to save lives, and if it was going to have to be cruel to be kind, then so be it. Laver had been following the Crown Street experiment for some time, and had sent on a study visit to Sydney an able young doctor, Frank Forster, who was not set in his ways as were the senior medical staff. Once the *Lancet* article appeared, the case was easier to make and in late March the Honorary Obstetrical Staff issued, through Laver, a regime based on the Crown Street model. It was going to be a massive task: all patients would be educated on diet; all patients over 10 stone (140 lbs) were to be referred to the Dietitian at their first visit; total weight gain was not to exceed 21 lbs; weight gain and blood pressure were to be strictly monitored, especially in the mid-trimester; and if their blood pressure rose, they were to be referred at once to a specialist obstetrician who might admit them to hospital or who might require that they attend Outpatients weekly; finally the medical superintendent himself would be responsible for each patient's ante-natal card to ensure that she kept all her appointments.[73] Between 1952 and 1954 the eclampsia rate among booked patients halved at the Women's and by 1960 the hospital had dramatically improved the prognosis of women with high blood pressure.[74] The new regime may have affected the babies' weights: Ivon Hayes compared just over seven thousand babies born in 1955 with a similar batch born in 1943–45 and in 1955 there were nearly 30 per cent fewer children weighing eight pounds and over than in the previous period.[75] Although this coincided with a marked increase in smoking among the hospital's patients.

It transformed antenatal care into a time of anxiety and guilt for many women, while, both inside hospitals and outside in private practice, pregnancy itself became a more medicalised and potentially pathological condition. Medical and nursing staff, overworked and conscious always of the horror and tragedy of eclampsia, were sometimes impatient and intolerant of the weak-willed, the ignorant and the cussed. Weight-watching became an obstetrical religion which turned the expectancy of motherhood into a nightmare of worries. With a rigid weight-gain limit of 21 lbs, nearly all women were doomed to 'fail' and each ante-natal visit became a test and a trial. 'Fat' became bad, and motherhood was no longer associated with the ample figure it nearly always produced in the healthy. Thinness, which once betokened anaemia and infertility, now represented desirable femininity. Pathological thinness — emaciation

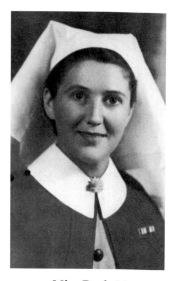

Miss Ruth Meaney, matron 1952–1955 *RWHA*

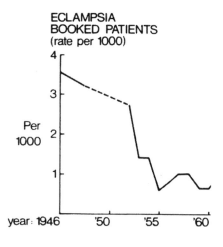

ECLAMPSIA
BOOKED PATIENTS
(rate per 1000)

Per 1000

year: 1946   '50   '55   '60

Incidence of eclampsia at Royal Women's Hospital, 1946–1960 *J. Smibert, 'Fifty Years of Obstetrics', Newsletter of Monash Medical Graduates Inc, 13.2, July 1991*

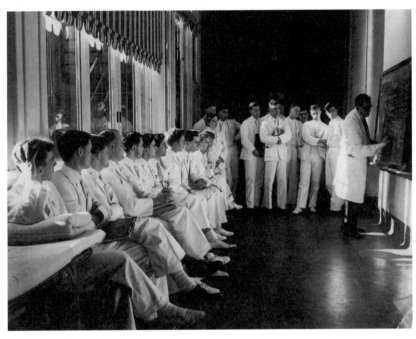

Dr Frank Forster
lecturing to medical
students in the corridor
of Labour Ward 30
RWHA

— in the young, which in the nineteenth century had signified tuberculosis or involuntary starvation, had disappeared. Fleshiness was the enemy
of good motherhood; the anorexic age had begun.

But perhaps it was the migrants who suffered most. Liliana Ferrara
was the hospital interpreter from 1955:

> They were very, very strict with the diet. Every patient who came for
> the first time had to see the dietitian. I was with them — I was so busy
> to see the dietitian, it was unreal. And we used to say, 'You must eat
> this, this, this, and this', and they used to weigh them. And as soon as
> she was half a kilo heavier — oh terrible — must diet! But it was just
> fluid retention I suppose — but no: no pasta, no bread, no potato, no
> minestrone . . . no, no, no, no. Everything was salad and grilled meat.
> They were supposed to lose weight and they'd say, 'You still haven't
> lost weight. And if you don't lose weight you'll have to be admitted'.
> So they were terrified. And it was really dangerous — they could not
> lose more.[76]

Then in 1955 the rate of eclampsia among booked patients at the
Women's began to rise again. Overseas, criticism mounted of Hamlin's
claims, a group from Aberdeen pointing out in 1957 that his paper had
been strong on assertion and weak on evidence. And it turned out that
others around the world had been there before him: in fact weight control
and reduction as a preventative against eclampsia had been first suggested
in the USA in 1923 and disproved before the Americans entered the
war. Yet it also partially worked and so many obstetricians clung to their
faith in reduction diets in mid-trimester, while others abandoned them.
It became a fierce controversy everywhere.[77] When James Smibert abolished reduction diets from his unit at the Women's, the medical super-

intendent asked if he had a £100 000 policy with Lloyds of London because 'he doubted whether the hospital's policy would cover a man flying in the face of accepted medical opinion'.[78] It was not until 1980 that the National Health and Medical Research Council recommended that reduction diets should not be used in pregnancy.

Saving Foetuses

As the major threats to mothers' lives in childbirth retreated, more attention could be paid to those who were losing their babies — either dying in utero or born fatally sick. The causes were perhaps illness in the mother, such as diabetes, or some sort of incompatibility between mother and foetus which was biochemical. The biochemistry of human blood was still far from understood. Patients died in the 1930s from blood transfusions and doctors tended to transfuse blood only as a last resort. The uncertainty of blood transfusions made obstetricians think twice about performing a caesarean and kept haemorrhage as an obstetric disaster to be avoided at all costs. The typing of blood had begun in 1901, but there were still many factors to be discovered before compatibility could be assured. And there were problems of supply. Still in the 1930s, remembers Ronald Rome, 'If you wanted a pint of blood for a patient who was haemorrhaging furiously, you rang Ormond College, and a suitable donor would be sent to the hospital in a City Motor Company transport'. The donor was paid and was scarred for life (Ronald Rome has seven such scars), but by 1939 the Red Cross Blood Bank in Melbourne had succeeded in storing blood safely for later use and the Blood Transfusion Service began in July 1946.[79] The war brought world-wide advances in fluid and blood replacement techniques which dramatically reduced the dangers of all surgery, but blood transfusion remained difficult until the coming of plastics in the early 1960s.[80] Until then, blood was held in milk bottles and delivered via rubber tubing which was not only hard to sterilise, it was difficult to insert into a vein. Kevin McCaul, who became the Women's Director of Anaesthesia, admits: 'A lot of people were not very good at intravenous work — the only people who were very good at it were the anaesthetists. I was particularly adept — I could get into non-existent veins, I just happened to have that ability'.[81] Plastics, for McCaul, revolutionised medicine, and in Melbourne the Alfred Hospital and its Baker Institute were world leaders in plastic infusion techniques.

At the Women's Hans Bettinger, the Director of Pathology, realised in 1941 that the newly discovered rhesus factor in blood was of particular significance in obstetrics. Vera Krieger the following year developed a technique for routinely testing all women for this factor. Where the mother lacked the Rh-factor but her baby had inherited Rh-positive blood from its father, the baby's blood set up an immunological reaction in the mother's blood, which would reject any subsequent foetus whose blood was also Rh-positive. The antibodies would affect the foetus so severely that it would die in utero and abort in the first half of the pregnancy; or be stillborn, bloated with oedema; or be born normal only to develop severe jaundice and probably die; or be born normal but anaemic.

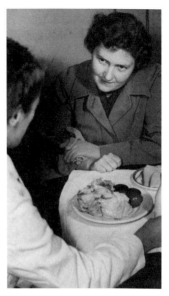

Dietetic service instituted, 1952 *RWHA*

Incidence and mortality of caesarean section, Royal Women's Hospital, 1919–1949 *J. W. Johnstone, 'The Changing Place of Caesarean Section', MJA, 3 February 1951, pp. 188–92*

Period of Five Years	Deliveries	Caesarean Sections	Incidence	Maternal Deaths	Mortality Rate
1919 to 1924	11,840	164	1.4%	10	6.1%
1925 to 1929	16,560	135	0.8%	3	2.2%
1930 to 1934	18,379	212	1.1%	17	8.0%
1935 to 1939	20,590	285	1.4%	19	6.7%
1940 to 1944	19,681	284	1.4%	7	2.5%
1945 to 1949	24,174	638	2.6%	8	1.2%
1919 to 1949 (thirty years)	111,224	1718	1.5%	64	3.7%

Period of Five Years	Caesarean Sections	Foetal Deaths (Stillbirths and Neonatal Deaths)	Incidence
1919 to 1924	164	43	26.2%
1925 to 1929	135	19	14.1%
1930 to 1934	212	25	11.8%
1935 to 1939	285	44	15.4%
1940 to 1944	284	55	19.4%
1945 to 1949	638	79	12.4%
1919 to 1949 (thirty years)	1718	265	15.4%

Foetal wastage, 1919–1949 *Johnstone*

Main Indication	1919 to 1924	1925 to 1929	1930 to 1934	1935 to 1939	1940 to 1944	1945 to 1949
Disproportion, mechanical reasons, dystocia	69	61	79	72	97	206
Failure of powers	1	–	2	5	4	17
'Repeat'	18	39	57	71	81	142
Soft tissue obstruction	6	8	12	15	11	16
Malpresentation	5	1	4	15	6	16
Placenta praevia	12	9	15	51	54	125
Accidental haemorrhage	4	7	4	1	–	3
Albuminuric toxaemia, eclampsia	39	7	17	13	9	71
Liver toxaemia, vomiting	–	–	2	3	1	6
Intercurrent maternal disease	6	–	13	25	19	19
To deliver live child	–	–	2	4	–	6
Miscellaneous	4	3	5	10	3	11
Total	164	135	212	285	285	638

Indications for caesarean section, 1919–1949 *Johnstone*

'Tess' began her childbearing in 1940 and eventually had eleven pregnancies. She started with three normal babies before suffering two miscarriages in 1947, after which she was referred to the Women's antenatal clinic for Rh-negative:

> You had an appointment. They called us in three at a time. You took your specimen of urine. They weighed us. In the 1950s the migrants came in and it was not uncommon for the doctor to come into the waiting room and ask, 'Does anyone here speak Italian?' There were no interpreters then.
>
> About halfway through my pregnancies they brought in exercises. By the time I got the others to school and got over there on public transport, I didn't want to stay for the exercises. I'd shoot through. But

they barred the door and I had to stay and do the exercises which I thought was a lot of garbage.

I had a lift to the hospital for the labour. I was shaved, enema, bath. Once I was real crook at them, because I'd had a shower before I left home. That was the bane of my life, those enemas. They'd get you by the middle — to loosen you up, I hated that. And the war nurses. If you were blind and deaf and dumb I could pick a war nurse. Oh they were rough. One of the women had a husband who'd been to Changi. They said to her, 'You're lucky to be having a baby.' The nurse told me that so many of the men from Changi were sterile.

When I had the first miscarriage in August 1947, I was out on the balcony. It was freezing. Four or five hot water bottles. You were frozen. With the second miscarriage, I was terribly worried. They asked me, not in a rude way, not to upset me. It worried me immensely. The head nurse — I called her Starchy, she seemed to be starch from top to bottom — she was lovely. She could see that I was very upset. She let the doctor come and talk to me by himself. That wasn't done usually.

The postnatal ward was big, six or eight beds. The babies at first were kept in the nurseries and later beside the beds. We were not taught baby care. The food was all right — I never had any complaints. You had to write down anything you wanted your husband to get you or you'd forget in the half hour visiting time. That was really sad, poor fellas coming in straight from work. The children never came in to see me — didn't believe in it. When my husband had to give blood for the last baby, they had to bring a doctor. It's a wonder he didn't keel over.

There were a couple of chaps, medical students who were really good. The nurses used to have fun with them. I used to hear them talking. With my last baby, another woman over forty was having her first baby, and her husband dropped dead that morning. They were lovely to her. The professor said to his students, 'We must see this baby arrive'. Then he turned to the rest of us and said, 'that doesn't mean we're not looking after you ladies'. She had a little girl.

With my last baby who was Rh- positive, I was in all day. They induced the labour with a drip. There was a doctor there all the afternoon. A couple of days later the baby had an exchange transfusion. I had her baptised first. Afterwards she was in the humidicrib. She was jaundiced. The doctor was Glyn White. I had to take her back to the clinic for twelve months. They took blood from her heel.[82]

'Tess's' baby was saved by an exchange transfusion, and at its peak in the 1960s the hospital was performing up to six a day. Vera Krieger was not allowed to devote all her time to serology until 1959. Then in 1964 she was asked to take part in assessing the efficacy of anti-D gamma globulin in preventing rhesus immunisation. With this desensitising vaccine, the exchange transfusion which had been extended to antenatal transfusions in utero faded from practice. Krieger continued this work after her retirement.[83]

Another age-old threat to mother and foetus was excessive vomiting in pregnancy. Women had always died of it and still did so in the 1940s. In 1940 a twenty-seven-year-old para 3 was admitted eight weeks pregnant with a history of vomiting for five weeks, persistent for five days. The medical report continued:

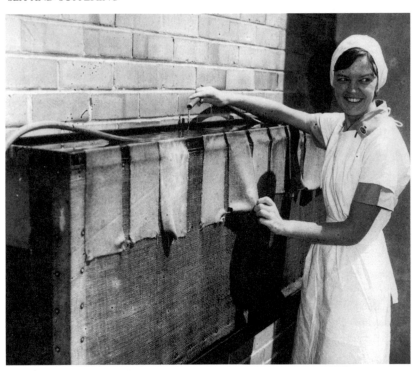

Coolgardie safe for cooling nursery, 1950s
RWHA

Rapidly improved with sedatives, and was discharged in five days. Readmitted three weeks later with history of vague ill-health since discharge from hospital, rapidly becoming worse in preceding three days. Patient was semi-conscious, markedly dehydrated and showing signs of acidosis. Slightly improved with intravenous saline, but became jaundiced, and condition gradually became worse until death on fourth day after admission. Died undelivered.[84]

Freudian explanations of women fleeing motherhood and vomiting up the baby were attractive,[85] and since it was all psychological, vomiters were not to be encouraged so that they were forbidden receptacles for vomitus such as kidney dishes. Doctors dealt in the theories and gave the orders, but it was nurses who had to withstand the pleading eyes and clean up the mess from the floor and change the bed. 'Helen', expecting her second child, had hyperemesis:

> I was brought into the Women's very weak, my husband carried me in from the car. They waived the rule that you had to have a bath on admission. I think they thought it was wrong that I hadn't had that special bath where they really scrubbed you up. I was put in a big ward and curtained off immediately. I heard the other women but I didn't see anyone for ten or twelve days. The other women all seemed happy and chatty except for one. She was in the bed opposite. The priest and her husband refused permission for the doctors to terminate her pregnancy and she died. The women were all in for high blood pressure and kidney problems. There were no migrants.
> My husband and I thought they were going to terminate my

pregnancy because my husband had to sign that they could do it. A sister said, 'You don't want this baby do you — you're being sick because you don't want it'. That upset me greatly. Very tearfully I said, 'We're going to make arrangements to adopt straight away; of course I want the baby'. Just her attitude I suppose, but I was vulnerable at the time.

They kept me closeted because I had to be fed intravenously. It was in my arm, but it thrombosed so they moved to my ankle. That thrombosed. I was still vomiting. They were taking acid off my stomach every two hours so I had a tube down my stomach. Then they put the drip in my anus. I probably didn't look too good. I had no flowers, no visitors, no messages. I was absolutely cut off from civilisation. My mother insisted on coming — she was so calm she just sat there for two hours knitting. That was comforting. One of the nurses came once and told me that the most magnificent bunch of flowers had arrived for me.

The New Zealand doctor had my case — he was charming. He said, 'You're going to be written up'. One night he sneaked in, literally, and gave me a little book of short stories and put it under my pillow. He said, 'For God's sake, don't let matron see it or I'll be in trouble. He was quite in awe of the staff nurse. That helped my six weeks there.

When they opened up the curtains, the other girls said, 'Oh we wondered what you looked like — we couldn't ever hear your voice'. The injections they gave me every day (the girls said it was my forty-second) caused me to grow long black hairs on my arms and legs and my hair went almost titian. I was taking vitamin B-6 which was very new at the time. I didn't ask questions and they didn't volunteer any information. I had a transfusion.

The Women's was the only hospital that had the equipment to look after me. The Women's was so different and I was so ill there and I was closeted — it wasn't very nice for me.

I was upset terribly to think that they thought I was unmarried (because my wedding ring had fallen off due to loss of weight) and that I didn't want the baby. The staff were hard, harsh, some of them. But the New Zealand doctor I had was very nice. The treatment that I had to have was necessary, but when they had to force the tubes down it wasn't very pleasant, I wasn't able to relax. I suppose they were cross with me.

It was another world for me to be in there. I could hear the patients' conversations but half the time I had no idea what they were talking about. It was another language. They had been brought up differently. I suppose I was jolly well protected. I was young at the time. I was naive and far too sensitive. I would be able to accept all that now.[86]

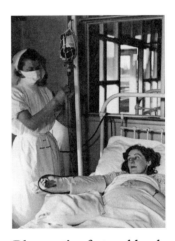

Rh-negative factor: blood transfusion 1947: note the glass bottle and chamber, rubber tubing, no curtains; patient in Ward 14, antenatal, Kumm Stephens Wing *RWHA*

Then the medical profession decided that hyperemesis was not psychological but physiological and the women got their kidney dishes back: some nurses are still bitter about such overnight changes, because if they had appeared strict and unyielding to their patients, they had been required to carry out orders no matter what they privately thought of them. The drug Debendox made an enormous difference to both hyper-emesis and nausea in early pregnancy. Its later discrediting and ban as a possible cause of birth abnormalities was much regretted.

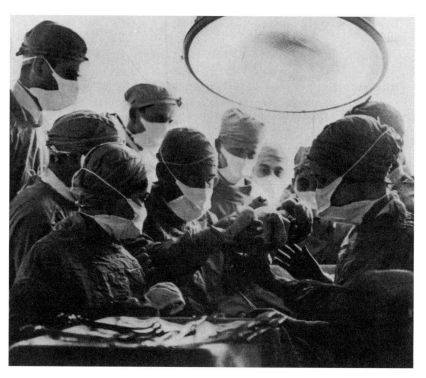

Theatre scene during a caesarean section: the surgeon is Dr W. M. Lemmon, handing baby to sister
RWHA

Saving Babies

The focus of medical attention on to the yet unborn and the newborn shifted the balance in the medicine of childbirth. From the mid 1930s interest in saving sickly or premature infants grew with the advances in clinical science and from 1938 the hospital had been permitted to count premature infants as full patients. There had been 191 that year, and numbers rose rapidly. The medicine of neonatology, as the new specialism came to be known, was highly scientific. Newborns could not tell doctors and nurses how they felt and the things that went wrong with their lungs and brains and digestive systems had to be deduced from careful obser-vation and scientific analysis. And the doctor who stood out in Melbourne in just this combination of clinical observation and scientific insight was Kate Campbell. She was paediatrician to the Queen Victoria Hospital from 1928 and neonatal paediatrician at the Women's Hospital from 1944 until she retired from both positions in 1965. And from 1929 she lectured on the care of the newborn at the University of Melbourne. By the end of her career she was credited with having changed the face of neonatal paediatrics in Victoria from the late 1920s through to the 1950s.

She was fascinated by newborn babies. Every baby, no matter how premature and immature, was to her a full human being. Peggy Taylor, as charge sister of the premature nursery, never tired of watching her examine a newborn baby:

She knew more about babies than anyone I've ever known. And the most wonderful thing was to see her examine a baby. She looked at a baby as a human being and each baby was an individual to her. She had the most gentle hands of any woman. And she would talk away to those babies while she was examining them. She was a wonderful woman — she was first with the best, she had a wonderful open mind, she was a researcher.

She always wore a hat — always the lady. And she was another woman who worked twenty-four hours a day — you could always get hold of Dr Campbell if you were worried about a baby. No problems. You got on the phone and got her. Glyn White was the same.

They were both willing to listen to the nursing staff. They really relied on the nursing staff and they respected your expertise, which quite a few of the registrars and young residents didn't — but they soon learned. In Neonatology Dr Campbell and Dr White treated senior nurses as respected colleagues and taught other doctors to do the same.

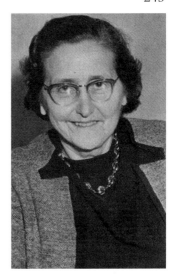

Dr (later Dame) Kate Campbell *RWHA*

Known to all behind her back as Auntie Kate, she was eccentric, tolerant and endowed with a keen sense of humour. Hundreds of doctors remember as a highlight of their medical education Kate Campbell's lectures on the newborn where she imitated their cries and squeaks, grimaces and movements, all of which told the observer much about this tiny, inarticulate human being. She enjoyed the adult human comedy also. One of her favourite stories was of the mother of a baby with glorious red hair: 'Does baby get his red hair from his father?', asked Dr Campbell, 'Dunno' came the reply, 'I never saw him with his hat off'. Kate Campbell believed in watching babies, and many nurses were mystified by this strange woman who would come into the premature nursery at 1 a.m. and ask them to stand with her and simply watch a baby for half an hour. She had an extraordinary gift of diagnosis which sometimes infuriated colleagues because she could not explain how she knew what was really wrong with a baby: 'As well as being persons, my patients are all "Agatha Christie mysteries". You have the clues and you have to find the solutions'.[87] The range of her work was wide, enough for a number of distinguished careers, and it was between 1948 and the early 1950s that she was at her most productive. She published on intracranial injuries in childbirth, their diagnosis, treatment and prevention; on Rh-negative isoimmunisation; on maternal diet in pregnancy; on the care of the newborn, both full term and premature; and most famously, on the role of oxygen in causing blindness — retrolental fibroplasia — in premature infants. This last discovery, in Professor Harold Attwood's estimation, took 'enormous courage', for oxygen was 'good' and surely never 'malign'.[88] The research involved sending questionnaires to scores of mothers of premature babies and following them up with clinical assessment.

The concern for frail and premature babies was fuelled not just by compassion, but by national anxieties over the birth rate and the injunction to populate or perish. The greatest achievement of antenatal care had been in the reduction of 'foetal wastage', and by 1948 the Women's Hospital could report a 50 per cent decline in foetal losses over the pre-

Premature baby *RWHA*

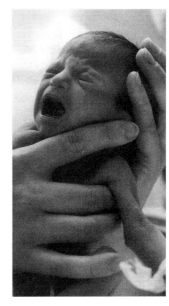

ceding thirty years since the commencement of the antenatal clinic.[89] Community and government pressure was intense. The National Health and Medical Research Council in 1944 dedicated the nation's leading maternity hospitals to the establishment of sterility clinics, and the Women's Hospital, Melbourne, and that at Crown Street, Sydney, to a long-term investigation 'to determine those factors associated with the wastage of potential children due to losses after conception'.[90] If women were to persist in practising birth control and to delay childbearing, then the nation that either populated or perished had a duty to prevent as many neo-natal deaths as possible. But the aim was babies who would be undamaged and therefore assets rather than liabilities to the community. Birth injuries were to be avoided as their seriousness was becoming ever more apparent. The caesarean section was quite quickly

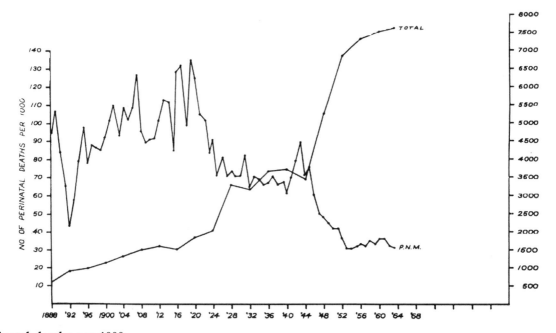

Perinatal deaths per 1000 deliveries, Royal Women's Hospital 1888–1968
J. Smibert, 'Quo Vadis', unpublished paper

changing from being an operation with known dangers, only to be taken when there was no alternative and dooming a woman to having no more children, to a safer choice that did not necessarily preclude future pregnancies. The risk of maternal and foetal mortality was still quite high in the early 1930s, but in the later 1940s the risks fell with antibiotics, better blood transfusions and the wider practice of the lower segment incision. The classical incision, a vertical incision in the uterus through the major muscles, produced a greater risk of rupture of the uterus in a later labour; the lower segment caesarean was less dangerous later but harder to perform, especially when the child had an impacted head or shoulders. The obstetricians at the Women's were conservative and reluctant to resort to the caesarean, especially on young unmarried women who might want a family later.[91]

Prenatal diagnosis had now begun. The discovery that rubella in early pregnancy could produce blindness and/or deafness in the child posed grave ethical questions for parents and doctors. David Pitt's register of congenital malformations was the first study of their incidence in the general population, and his special study within that of the effects of maternal rubella won him the Katherine Bishop Harman prize in 1961.[92] W. M. Lemmon, of the Women's, found himself recommending terminations in cases of maternal rubella in pregnancy provided that the doctor protected himself with support from other obstetricians and a psychiatrist and that the operation was performed openly in the sight of the law.[93] By the mid 1950s amniocentesis, the examination of amniotic fluid at first to determine the severity of Rh-negative disease, widened the scope for pre-birth diagnosis and possible intervention.[94] Clinical and laboratory science, working in the interests of the child to be, now made claim for intervention in the natural process of reproduction as never before, but it also met with resistance from obstetricians who placed the interests of the mother before those of the baby. It remains a still unresolved contest between specialists in health care.

Mothers' Pain

The Lying-in Hospital was founded in the dawn of anaesthesia and Tracy had been to the forefront in the judicious use of chloroform in labour and for the treatment of eclampsia. In the labour ward at least, little had changed in ninety-five years: even the method of administration of chloroform on a cloth that was sniffed was essentially the same as it had been in the beginning. There were honorary anaesthetists, but most anaesthetics were given by general practitioners who came in, by residents and by midwives, and practice was cautious and conservative. But by the late 1940s the gynaecological surgeons needed better anaesthesia for the marathon Wertheim operations for uterine cancer which could take more than eight hours to perform. Then a woman died from inhalation of food, for which a nurse was blamed and the surgeons succeeded in persuading the hospital to find a director of anaesthesia who could bring the latest knowledge to the hospital.

A group of Australian doctors were staying in a house opposite the hospital in Bromley, in Kent in England, and happened to watch a young self-taught anaesthetist, Kevin McCaul, giving caudal and epidural anaesthetics. They suggested he come to Australia, he wrote off, and next thing he was being interviewed by Noel De Garis and it was arranged that he would come to Melbourne for two years. There was a world-wide shortage of anaesthetists and McCaul was finding his work load at Bromley too great. He arrived by ship in 1951 and was met on Station Pier by the medical superintendent, Dr William Refshauge. McCaul greeted him and Refshauge suddenly realised that the new director of anaesthesia at the Women's Hospital was Irish. Where had he qualified? Not at Trinity College, Dublin, which admitted only Protestants. Was he a Catholic? Yes. 'It's many years since we've had a Catholic at the Women's Hospital'. (Since 1918, in fact, apart from the odd resident like Frank Hayden who

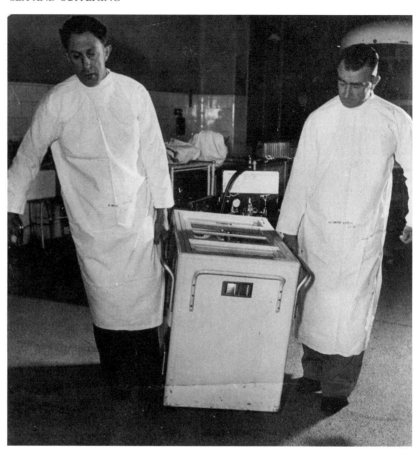

Premature baby hand ambulance, built in the hospital's workshop by the medical superintendent and the engineer *RWHA*

had felt frozen out of any further ambitions at the Women's.) Refshauge was worried about the tubal ligations and the therapeutic terminations the Women's had to perform; McCaul told him not to worry. The new director was shown proudly around the hospital. The operating theatre looked very old and had a strange metal contraption suspended over the operating table: 'What's that?' 'That's the old gas lighting', 'Oh, said McCaul without thinking twice, 'Fanny by gaslight'. The story flashed around stuffy Melbourne 'like wildfire and those gaslights came down in a few weeks'.[95]

McCaul's father had been a doctor in Ireland who had been ruined in the Depression and died prematurely, leaving a young family, and McCaul had seen a level of deprivation unknown in Australia:

> The poverty at that time was absolutely extraordinary. Very few working people would ever eat meat. Even in my young days the main food for any working man was porridge or potatoes mixed with cabbage and fatty bacon which was imported from America. And most women were anaemic. Tuberculosis was absolutely rampant. Several of my cousins — and we were well off — died of tuberculosis, particularly the females. The diet was deficient in Ireland. There were really no good iron preparations available. In fact at the Richmond Hospital in Dublin when I was a student, there was a form of anaemia called chlorosis — I've never met anyone here who's even seen it, but it was

quite common in Ireland. The hospital used to give a patient a pound of nails and they were told to soak that overnight and drink it in the morning. It blackened their teeth.

I despise the shift of wealth from the small. I just don't understand it. I don't understand greed as such. I suppose I'm reasonably greedy myself, but I've never wanted to be a business man — never. I never did medicine to make money. It was a calling, a profession — my grandfather, father, great uncle, a fairly long family tradition.

McCaul arrived to find the hospital had a new anaesthesia machine which no one could use; but what he found in the labour ward was even worse:

Every woman expected an anaesthetic — they came in screaming for it — and it almost became a religion that you had to have an anaesthetic to have a baby — even to the extent of holding the head back on the point of delivery so they could have an anaesthetic. A lot of patients came from Camp Pell — it was absolutely horrifying.

Private patients expected the doctor to do the delivery and would challenge the fee if he wasn't there, but that didn't matter so much in a public hospital. But when I arrived there I was told that my job was to train all the midwives going through the Women's to give twenty anaesthetics each to fit in with the nurses' registration. I decided that this wasn't on. I decided in the secrecy of my own mind that I wasn't training nurses to give anaesthetics — if a nurse had a fatality, she'd be blamed.

I had nobody to discuss this with, nobody knew anything about obstetric anaesthesia. First I went to C.I.G. [Commonwealth Industrial Gases] and said — would you pipe in nitrous oxide and oxygen to every labour ward in the Women's. And Harry Adams who was in charge of the medical section could see that if this was a success, it was going to help C.I.G. enormously. And he devised a rubber piping system — we had a bank of cylinders in a little shed adjacent to the labour ward and we piped every bed. And we modified an old dental anaesthetic machine which is still the basis for the nitrous oxide machine, so that it would give not less than 30 per cent oxygen and no more than 70 per cent nitrous oxide. And I had that installed within a year of coming here.

McCaul had made the Women's Hospital a world leader in obstetric anaesthesia, but the management of labour had to change also. There were certain senior midwives who had to go: technically they were excellent, emotionally they were disastrous for the reforms he had in mind, so he set examinations which a number failed and they were moved to other positions. Then,

I immediately started classes for women — we called them relaxation classes, and I persuaded a couple of enthusiastic young nurses to whom I'm forever grateful to come and help me. We had a basement room and we had all these women lying around like stranded whales and we

Camp Pell: emergency housing for poor families in the former US Army Camp in Royal Park

Dr Kevin McCaul and Sister Jessica Place teaching *RWHA*

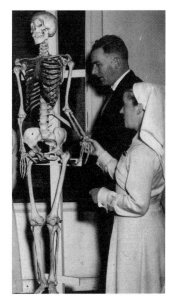

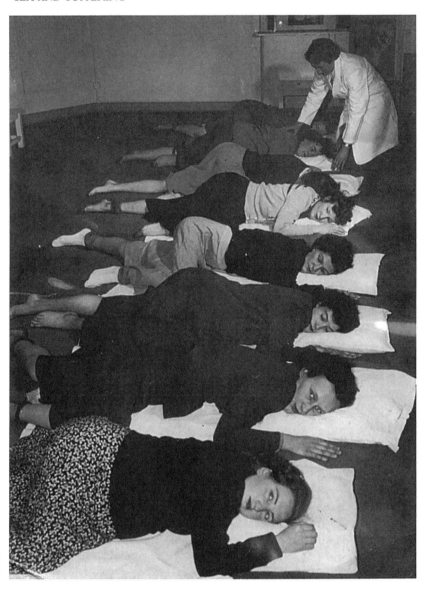

Relaxation clinic, 1948
RWHA

taught them how to breathe and how to relax and think of something
else. And how to inhale nitrous oxide. And of course it was essential
that nurses should follow this up, so I started doing regular nurses'
lectures. There was certainly a lot of enthusiasm.

I also involved the physiotherapists — they in fact tried to take over.
The problem was that they were very enthusiastic, but they really
didn't understand midwifery. And they didn't like working at night-
time or weekends — they weren't there when you really wanted them.
They had a goddess in England whose philosophy they followed to a
T. However that was all useful.

At the end of the year I suddenly got a rush request from the
matron to sign up the nurses' papers as being supervised for twenty
anaesthetics and I said 'nothing doing'. 'I've trained them in analgesia

and I've trained them for nitrous oxide and all the rest, but I will not sign them up to be trained in anaesthesia.' So I was called out to a meeting of some Cabinet group and they said, 'Why won't you sign?' 'Do you want me to sign a lie?' And that fixed the argument and I was asked what to do. And I said, you alter the regulations that nurses are not allowed to administer anaesthetics, but they are allowed to administer analgesia. That's all you have to do. And the regulation did come in.

By the end of 1952 it was accepted that you did not require an anaesthetic except when there was an indication for it. It was not a normal part of labour. We did all the training and it involved an enormous amount of work. I was a bachelor at the time, or I couldn't have done it.

McCaul had achieved a revolution by the end of his two-year contract, but barely had he arrived back in England before an urgent request came that he was wanted back in Melbourne. He returned permanently, pioneering spinal anaesthesia in Australia and contributing vastly to the knowledge and practice of resuscitation. Throughout his long career, he was never to have an anaesthetic death and was to remain a trenchant critic of poor practice in medicine. Like many of his generation, his practice was too busy to permit the time for publication that his work deserved.

By the end of the 1950s the experience of childbirth had dramatically

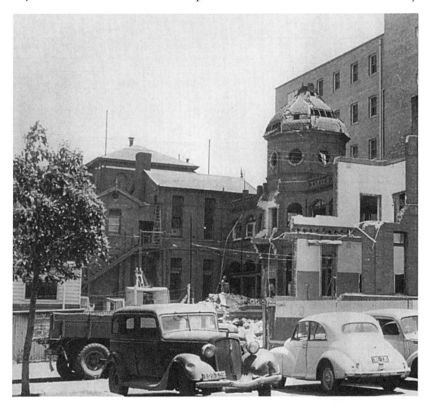

Demolition of Genevieve Ward Wing in 1956: Gertrude Kumm Wing to the right in Cardigan Street *RWHA*

changed for Australian women. Virtually all, except in the most remote places, gave birth in a hospital; and virtually all had received antenatal care. As a tertiary care hospital the Women's now had problematic cases booked and cared for antenatally rather than rushed in as emergency admissions: in 1930 1 in 4 had been an unbooked admission, in 1940 it was 1 in 5. By 1950 it was 1 in 12, and by 1960 1 in 15.[96] Antibiotics had apparently conquered all bacterial foes, lost blood could be replaced, and some of the more puzzling and elusive causes of foetal and maternal death or morbidity could be managed and reduced. In a short time, the world had travelled a long way from those 'old, colourful, rich warm, deadly days of clinical medicine at their worst and their best'.

VI

Human Relations
1945–1970

Managing Difference 12

'Those Migrant Women'

If the post-antibiotic world was a transformed one biologically, it was matched by a social revolution in cultural change which reshaped both the tone and composition of Australian society. European Australia was a new society created by conquest and immigration, but it had within a century and a half assimilated its different ethnicities from the British Isles, while remaining divided over religion and social class. The long Depression of the 1920s and 1930s had hardened prejudices against new immigrants, even Protestant, English-speaking ones. Few Australians, other than members of the armed forces, had travelled overseas. Languages other than English were rarely heard, and those immigrants who came before the 1950s learnt fast to speak Australian English and lose their accent. Australian Chinese hid in the shadows of society, as market gardeners, cafe owners, cooks and laundrymen. There were a handful of Italian restaurants in Melbourne, but the pre-war Italians, including those who were anti-Fascist, had been interned as enemy aliens; and as for Greeks, many people thought they were 'dagoes' also and could see no difference between them and Italians. Melbourne's small Jewish community was an old one, largely of English origin and Sephardic tradition, but during the inter-war period first immigrants from Palestine and later refugees from Europe, who had missed out on getting into the United States of America, found themselves instead at the bottom end of the world. In Carlton thrived a Yiddish-speaking community with a theatre group, library and political life, both Zionist and Bundist. Anti-Semitism, despite the horrific revelations of the Holocaust, still existed in Australian society, most conspicuously among the upper classes.

Those who came before the war encountered a society that was unsympathetic to cultural difference, and perhaps the most rigid expectations were those involving perceived strength of character. It was a puritanical society where emotional excess was feared. Most Australians were restrained about the display of feelings and physical affection, middle-class Australians especially so. And the medical and nursing staff were middle-class people, at the Women's almost entirely Protestant, with the doctors, and quite often the nurses, from private schools.

Part of being a mature person was to be able to endure pain in silence. A Methodist minister's daughter afflicted with osteomyelitis which left her with a discharging open wound for three years, remembers never being allowed to cry, even to 'shed a few quiet tears'. The family was never to raise their voices in anger, for they had to be the model Christian family for the community. In many happy and loving families, children were never cuddled or kissed: one dentist's family in Kew which transgressed were even advised by their family doctor, Dr Winifred Kennan, to desist lest they pass on too many germs.[1] Childbirth was sent to try women and they should do everything they could to control themselves. Screaming was only forgivable in extreme pain; it was not acceptable as a pure social custom. 'Dot' had a bad labour in 1939:

> In the labour ward there was only me and an Italian woman screaming and yelling, and I was trying to press a pillow into my face — I didn't want to make a fool of myself, I didn't want to make any trouble. And the nurses were lovely — they came and patted my face and said, 'hang on'. One of the nurses came in and slapped the other woman over the face — she wasn't in so advanced labour as me.[2]

'Jenny' had her first baby in the Women's at the age of nineteen in 1940:

> The labour ward was petrifying. There were a lot of migrants, just got out of Europe in time, who couldn't speak English and they'd be screaming out 'mamma mia'. The nurses or nurses aides would give these women a slap on the tail for screaming out 'mamma mia'. When you're only young yourself you're petrified — you lay there and held in your screams till you couldn't hold on any longer.[3]

The migrants brought disorder: noise, incomprehension, conflict. The pioneer sociologist, Jean Martin, noted that much of the hostility aroused by New Australians in Old Australians came from finding themselves unable to cope with language barriers and cultural differences. People who were accustomed to coping, like nurses and doctors, school teachers and social workers, were now at times out of their depth; and the migrant person before them unwittingly was eroding their professional persona.[4] Most migrants were young and about to start families, so that the maternity hospital was for many their first intimate encounter with a mainstream Australian institution. Hospitals along with schools were to find themselves charged with being the principal public agencies receiving and serving the new arrivals. And hospitals did so both as carers of the sick or parturient and as employers.

The hospital also was having its greatest crisis of accommodation since the 1880s. Between 1945 and 1955 its total annual admissions doubled from 8000 to 16000. In the nine months to March 1949 the Women's had the largest number of admissions of any public hospital in

Melbourne.[5] Everyone was busy having babies as soon as the war finished. Increasingly women expected to deliver in a hospital and home births all but disappeared. The new emphasis on compulsory antenatal care reinforced women's attachment to hospital childbirth, but at the very moment that women shifted their allegiances, the Women's Hospital for one became so overcrowded that it was unable to provide proper lying-in. By October 1946 the shortage of both midwifery beds and nurses forced the hospital to send women home after the fifth or sixth day. In 1949 the hospital set up a convalescent home at the old 'Villa Alba' in Kew, naming it in honour of Henry Pride; in 1951 a domiciliary nursing service was established where midwives visited lying-in mothers in their homes, making it possible to send women home after just two days in the postnatal wards. In 1952–53, the nine domiciliary sisters made 16 747 visits between them on 1446 patients, and were proud to report that 94 per cent of mothers visited were able to breast-feed.[6] In the hospital, rooming-in was extended to reduce the need for space and nursing staff in the nursery, and early ambulation of midwifery patients was tentatively suggested by the honorary medical staff.[7]

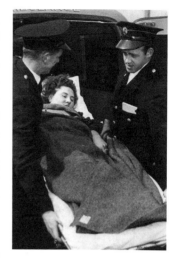

Going home on domiciliary care *RWHA*

In 1946 A. J. (Jim) Cunningham was appointed assistant secretary and manager, and he would administer the non-medical side of the hospital for the next three decades. Cunningham was devoted to the Women's and was a fine strategic thinker. He set about purchasing small properties around the hospital and in 1951 the hospital was fortunate to obtain the patronage of a commercial radio station, 3AW, for a 'Mother's Day' Appeal. It was very proud in 1954 to be given a Royal Charter. But as the demands on all hospitals grew, especially on maternity hospitals, a new scale of costs of public health and the fearsome (to many) example of the National Health Scheme in the United Kingdom strengthened the hand of those who wanted health care to lie in private hands. The Menzies government by 1952 sought to force public hospitals to become private: in the case of the Women's that it should charge midwifery patients eighteen shillings a day. The Labor state government counselled the Board to resist the Commonwealth's overtures and the hospital argued back that it could not afford to provide patients with the necessary high protein diet under such a financial regime; and reminded the government that since midwifery patients were uninsurable, such high fees would damage their health. But by October the Women's was 'going backwards' at the rate of £500 a month and tradesmen had not been paid for twelve weeks.[8] Nursing shortages continued as young women married at the highest rate in modern times, but fund-raising was giving the hospital more flexibility in forward planning and it was able to exert moral pressure on governments to keep it afloat in its vital national role of 'populate or perish'.

Bringing home the new family member *RWHA*

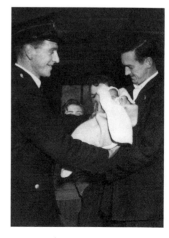

The rise in admissions went in steps. The first between 1945 and 1948 reflected the returning war servicemen and women starting their families, whereas the second from 1951 to 1954 was the coming of the migrants. Australia had grudgingly agreed to take 15 000 Jews fleeing Nazism in 1938, but only 6475 refugees had arrived by the time the war began. In 1945 Arthur Calwell had persuaded Cabinet that Australia should open its doors to Holocaust survivors, but most Australians wanted only immi-

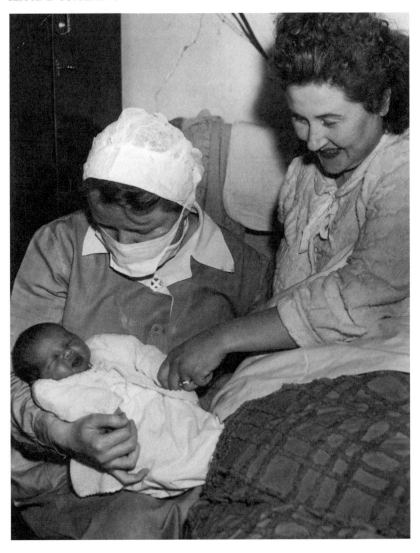

Domiciliary care *RWHA*

grants from Britain, preferably blue-eyed and blonde. When the expected
numbers of British immigrants did not apply to come, hostility reared
as Jewish refugees were alleged to be arriving in numbers. A fierce campaign was waged against Jewish immigration in 1946–47, including the
infamous letter to the *Argus* from H. B. S. Gullett, MHR for Henty and
future Coalition Whip in the lower house, which alleged that the Jews,
after securing 'a stranglehold on Germany after the last war during the
inflation period' had 'in a very large part brought upon themselves the
persecution which they subsequently suffered'. By 1947 the expected
numbers of British immigrants had not met the projected targets and
Calwell courageously negotiated with the International Refugee
Organisation to receive 4000 displaced persons for that year, and 12 000
in each succeeding year. It was the first step on the path to multiculturalism which would transform the nation.[9]

  'Luba' was fifteen when the Nazis invaded Poland, and with her father
and brother was among the very few Polish Jews to survive the labour

and concentration camps. Liberation did not bring freedom, however, and she had to spend another four years in Bergen–Belsen displaced persons camp, waiting with her new husband for a country that would accept them. They never expected to come to Australia, but once here, they were delighted:

> My husband found work right away. It was a good time and we were very happy to come. We were really feeling equal and free for the first time. I was exceptionally happy here — the people were so obliging. Once I went shopping and I had some coupons and £7 — it was a lot of money. I lost my purse, and what do you know, a lady brought it back. I was so thrilled. I spoke a little English and I told her 'I'm much obliged to you'. I was so happy I could express myself.[10]

But her limited English was not enough to enable her to negotiate her way through the rigidities of the Women's Hospital. Her first baby was born two months after she arrived in Australia. It was a long, painful labour of a big baby to a small mother:

> After I had my baby, they took me to the ward, very large. On the second or third day I called for a pan. These were the days when you had to stay in bed. The matron came and said 'No, you're not getting the pan. The nurse is bringing them around for all the patients. No you're not getting. If you insist, I will prove to you that you don't need the pan,' and she put the catheter through to show to me that I don't need to pass the water. But I did, and apparently that is when I got the infection. She was a nasty person, she was so rude to me. This I never forget.

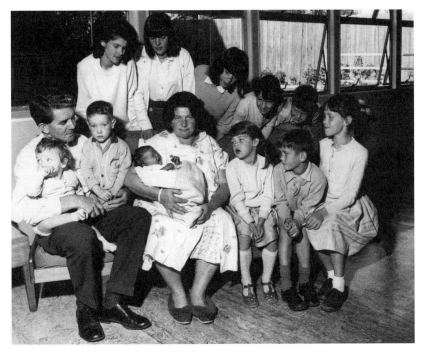

Dutch family with eleven children *RWHA*

Then they put me in an after-care. My husband came to visit me at the Women's and I wasn't there. I was waiting for him in the after-care, in Victoria Street. That was very unthoughtful to do to people that don't have relatives.

Then after I was sent home I got an infection and the doctor said I had to go back to hospital for treatment — penicillin, and I said 'I'm not going back to that hospital, for nothing in the world am I going back to that hospital — they treated me so badly. Then she got the penicillin and I got better but I was really in a very dangerous situation. I'll never forgive them for doing it to me. The doctors didn't care and neither did the matron. This is why I had such a grudge against them.

'Trudi' was Viennese, and had fled to Prague after her Jewish father was imprisoned. She escaped the camps but suffered extreme privation. Ten days after arriving in Australia she gave birth in the Women's Hospital:

I tell you, I was not happy there because I just arrived to Australia, my knowledge of English was pathetic. I did not know what to expect. There was no one to bring me chocolates and flowers, I was just lying in a passage there. It was a time that was really difficult, but it was a time that I knew would pass. Mind you, there were no real physical hardships.

At the antenatal clinic the doctors did teaching rounds with young students. The doctor was showing on me [demonstrating] and they were all pushing and prodding my belly. They were looking terribly concerned and I was really terrified. What was it all about? They must have told me but I didn't really understand.

I had to change my clothes and hang them behind a curtain. Somebody stole some of my things and some money. I was so upset, I cried and cried. In those days I cried all the time.

I had some contractions and went into hospital but the contractions stopped and the baby wasn't born for two days. They gave us things to do, we rolled cotton wool, we were folding things, we were not in bed, we walked around. There weren't enough beds, we were not in a proper ward yet.

After the baby was born [forceps delivery with anaesthetic] they would ask me a question and I didn't understand and I would say 'I beg your pardon', and they would just shout at me just as fast because they had never learned another language. So I would just say yes or no [to questions] and if I could see they weren't happy, I would change my answer to the opposite.

I had [postnatal depression] I thought something was terribly wrong. I didn't realise it was natural. I was unhappy it was a girl because I wanted a boy.

The food was awful, I wasn't used to it and I didn't like it. They couldn't cook. It was all mashy and wishy-washy. I remember the rice was boiled up to a blob; they overcooked things — I didn't know what it was. Bread was that horrible white bread that I don't like. There was no nice underdone meat. I was very frustrated about the food. I thought, 'They have the things, why can't they do something with it?' The lunches and dinners were boring. I didn't like the food there at all.

The place was clean but it was ugly. I don't remember a picture or anything. It was all utilitarian. I don't think there was anything there that was pretty. There was an impression of bleakness, of being lost and lonely and unhappy.

I thought the staff were dreadful but that wasn't their fault. They couldn't identify with anyone like me at all. They were not very patient because I did not speak the language. They didn't know I had just arrived.

In those days it was still something awesome and frightening for me to have a child. One knew of all the things that can go wrong, . . . mothers dying and so on. Maybe it was caused by me being on my own, and my husband was certainly no help.[11]

It was a story that would be repeated a thousand times. In midwifery in a public hospital, each admission was like an emergency admission. The labour ward staff knew nothing of the patient. No relationship had been established before, and the most important means of rapidly establishing a relationship was denied them by the language barrier. The labouring woman could not be counselled, questioned, instructed or soothed. It was crucial that the patient be kept calm, but the only means of calming distress was physical, and nurses were reluctant to touch patients. This was not just reticence or rules, it was also self-preservation because women out of control in labour bit and hit nurses' arms and hands, seized hold of any nearby body parts, including breasts. Labour ward could be stressful at any time, but with women screaming continuously at the top of their lungs, the noise could become unendurable both to staff and to other

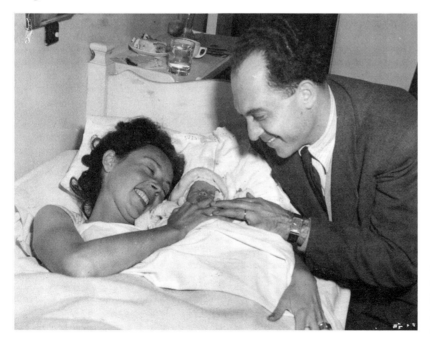

'New Australians All: 914 New Australians had babies in the Women's Hospital this year', 1954
RWHA

patients. And scream the migrants did, especially the Italians. They came in the second wave of immigration and between 1951 and 1954, and total annual admissions rose from 12 000 to 15 000 in just three years. Women were being delivered in beds in the corridors and then sent out after two days, either to Henry Pride or home with support from the domiciliary nurses. Some have no doubt they were sent home too soon. 'Don't take any notice of her screaming — she's just a migrant', remembers one mother who delivered there in 1954.[12]

Most of the Italians were proxy brides, who had scarcely, if at all, seen their future husbands before arriving in Australia. They emigrated without their families; many had little schooling because of the war. They were young, sexually ignorant, alone and terribly frightened. 'Gina' was just twenty-one years old, a proxy bride with her first baby:

> I had a very little experience at the hospital. I went for my check up regularly, once a month, then every fortnight, then every week. They help me very well. They save my life and my baby.
>
> In the labour ward, I had pain, they help with medicine. They done what they had to do, but they don't help me or any kindness. They treat me very strange. They treat me not a friendly. They done their proper job that they have to do, and of course it was the main thing but no one come to me and say 'I'm sorry for you', or some nice kind word. I remember one nurse who say 'Shut up you, you naughty girl', because of I don't care, I was screaming, I don't care. I was a scream because they expect me not to scream. I can't be quiet. I was screaming because I was lonely. I was scared. I did not know anything about labour because we were brought up strictly in a respectable family. We not allowed to talk about these things.[13]

'Marina' had no real complaints except the sadness her linguistic isolation brought:

> The food was good, I was happy but I wanted to come home straight away because of the language difficulty. It was a clean hospital. Everybody was very nice, the only thing was the language difficulty. The sadness was, a sister would go and talk to a patient and they would have a good laugh and I was sitting there like a stupid woman and there was nobody I could communicate with and that was the sadness.
>
> When I went the second time, there was this Italian woman screaming for her mother — she really had contractions. I had nothing (no contractions — I'd told them I was in labour in order to go in early). That made me laugh really. I had nobody to communicate [with], I sat in bed very quietly, reading. I was living in a boarding house then with many families, we had a bedroom, but I had nobody, because everybody went to work in the boarding house, so I thought I should go to the hospital to wait for the event.[14]

There were no professional interpreters, just domestic staff who might be called in during an emergency, or accompanying relatives or friends.

One unfortunate Italian woman came in to interpret for a friend — she was pregnant also, but certainly not in labour. No matter, she was also showered and was 'on the table before she was able to make herself understood that she was not in labour'.[15] Then in 1955 the hospital employed its first proper interpreter. She was a young proxy bride herself, from Egypt. Liliana Ferrara's father was Italian, her mother Greek and not only did she speak their languages, but she spoke Arabic, French and English. She had a diploma in Italian language and her new husband, whom she had met just once as his ship sailed through on its way to Australia, was Italian, but she has never been to Italy.

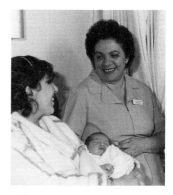

Liliana Ferrara with a patient *RWHA*

> I was discovering the Italians in Australia. I had spoken Italian with my family and studied it at school, I had my diploma of Italian, but when I saw them, they were different, strange — they spoke different dialects and had different customs — it was quite a discovery for me too.

Medical terminology and sexual knowledge was also a discovery for her; there was no school for medical interpreters as there would be later:

> I am from the old school. I was twenty-one, a young bride. And the first time I had this Italian patient who came to me saying that she had to see a doctor because she had a terrible pain in her stomach. And I said, 'What happened?' 'I don't know — I've got a ring inside me'. And I interpreted for the doctor. I thought the only way you got a ring in your stomach was that you swallowed it. I said, 'I think this patient has swallowed a ring', and the whole clinic was laughing at me. I was twenty-one with no experience.

She would go on to interpreting for men and women in the sexual counselling and infertility clinics, among the most difficult of all interpreting tasks. The migrant women would not discuss sexual problems and had little knowledge of their own bodies:

> It was a taboo subject, unless a woman was dying of discomfort:
> But now it's out in the open. We have sexual counselling clinics, although many of my migrants will not admit to having a problem. An interpreter can pick up many things if she's got a lot of experience. They might be coming many times to the clinic complaining of aches and pains, but in actual fact there is a hidden problem and I can pick it up.
> When you take a history you can tell if there are personal problems and I usually asked the doctor whether I can ask her is she has any personal problems. It helped the doctor if he was aware if she had a bad problem at home — the husband, the son, the daughter.
> And if the doctor asked a very intelligent question, I had to simplify it for the patient so she can understand. And out of a very simple answer I have to rephrase it in a more intelligent way for the doctor to understand.
> I not only interpreted the language, but the ways of thinking — the third language, I call it. You cannot use medical terminology that

the doctors use because they'll never understand. For instance, a hysterectomy: they see the uterus as very big, but in actual fact it is the size of my fist and you have to tell them that, because the way they think of the body is so distorted. They don't know that they've got two ovaries — they think they've got a lot of ovaries. So you have to put them at their ease and make sure that the patient understands because they will say 'yes' always.

You have to be warm before the patient — she has to trust you — you had a sixth sense. It's not like a court of law where it's all in the third person, word by word — hospitals is a different skill.

For Liliana, what had started out as a job became 'a mission', and it required both intellectual precision and emotional strength:

The girls in Italy were sheltered: they don't know about anything, they don't know what's going to happen when they get married. They were terrified.

And the others who'd already had a baby, they'd had their baby at home with a midwife and didn't have to go through all those examinations during their pregnancy.

So everything was terribly frightening for them. So I was there for the examination and I had to relax them and talk to them. I had to explain what was going to happen. I used to hold their hand, caress their head.

I sat through labour every day.

Often when she arrived in labour ward, sister would be too busy to tell her which patient needed an interpreter, so she would follow the 'Mumma mias':

In a strange country, no extended family, on their own: sometimes they call God, but they called their mothers: 'oh mumma mia, dio mia, oh Madonna mia, or Sant Antonio — a lot of St Antonio. Because you have all those saints in Italy that you call out if you are distressed. St Antonio is a saint for the mothers-to-be. With Anglo-Saxons St Gerard is sent for the expecting mothers. This would annoy the sister in labour ward: 'You must stop this "mumma mia'. No need for "mumma mia" and push'. But it comes naturally — when my time came I called for my mother too.

'Olivia' had already had three children in home births in Italy when she had the first of the seven she was to have in the Women's in Australia:

I was patient at the Women's with my first pregnancy that happened to me in Australia. I was always very pleased to be there, apart from the fact that it was a novelty to be in a hospital at all. It was a treat for me to go to the hospital. I met some very nice people there. There was a soft mattress, a beautiful clean linen, I feel a special patient. There were people to take care of me.

There was an enormous difference in having a baby in hospital after

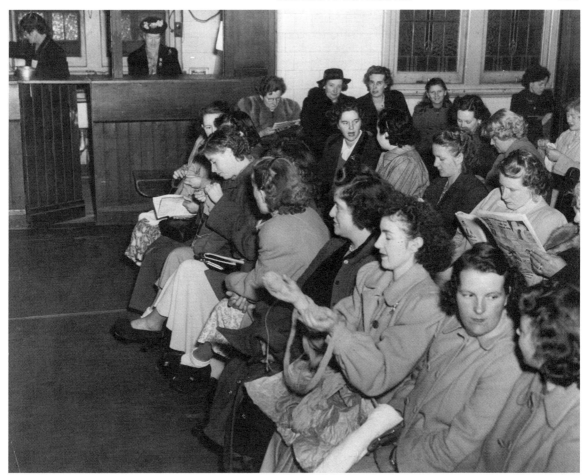

Some of the hospital's 60 000 outpatients for 1954 *RWHA*

having the others at home: at home you are surrounded by the people who love you, you feel not so scared. In hospital I had a terrible feeling that something will happen to me and I never see my husband and children again — isolated from your family. I was so terrified, I didn't know who is beside me. The labour was probably longer because I acted the way I did. They gave me an injection before the baby was born. They make me stupid. I was afraid of the mask, I thought it would put me to sleep, but it was just probably helping me. But subsequent deliveries were much better.

The doctor in charge of the Women's Hospital — he has a lot of time for me. I remember one day when I had to have an injection I was very very upset. I cry and I cry and I cry. And they say to me, 'What can we do for you? Why do you cry to have an injection?' I said they should ask the doctor to come. He came over and sat beside me and said that I had to have it, and I did. I have a beautiful memory of Henry Pride. It is like a motel for ladies. It was just a beautiful holiday, the park was just fantastic.

The food was very good. I liked the tray, [all set up with salt and pepper etc] the thing that surprised me mentally was the breakfast — I was used to just some bread or toast, but there was always something

— some meat, some kidney, some liver, some stewed fruit. I had never had a cooking breakfast. I liked just the consommé for morning tea and afternoon tea.

I am very grateful to the hospital. I had seven children in there and I never pay a bill. If I was rich I would give a donation.[16]

The Italians were far from ungrateful. They appreciated the medical care, the cleanliness of the hospital, the plentiful if unpalatable food. But those who had already given birth in Italy found the vaginal examinations, the shaving, the stirrups for delivery, the mask for anaesthesia, the loneliness amidst a crowd of busy professionals difficult to bear.

As interpreter, Liliana's role was different from the social worker's. She was a broker between cultures as well as individuals. Hers was a unique perspective that saw the needs and requirements of the hospital and society in conflict with the realities of the migrants' lives. The proxy brides came to Australia in a new suit of clothes, a trousseau and gold jewellery: 'it was part of their culture to give them gold'. The Australians saw new clothes and gold and concluded they were well off:

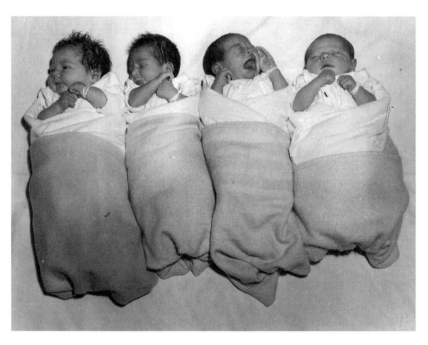

'Italy, Malta, Ceylon, Ireland' *RWHA*

Everybody was assessed. You had to go through a means test and that was very painful sometimes. It was enough for a husband to earn ten shillings over a week and that would have you 'above income'. And I was with the patient from the time she walked in the door. They'd walk in: scared, frightened, in this unknown world, this different language and I was everything for them — their mother, their sister. They had nobody — not a sister who spoke English, or children, like they do now.

So I had to be with them when they were assessed and they were very often crying because they were above income, yet they lived in a room and had their fares to pay back. But that was not taken into account.

I would say that 85 per cent were in debt — they had big debts. Money lenders from here and from Italy. They were under terrible conditions.

But the most intense culture clash took place in the postnatal wards, over food. The food at the Women's was now plentiful, even over-generous in the 1950s with extra butter on the mashed potatoes and a double serve of meat if you wanted, but to the Continental palate it was 'awful': 'the salad was without oil, the vegetables were overcooked' and everything was drenched with either white sauce or brown gravy, which was delivered to the wards by the jugful:

In Italy, especially in the villages, they fussed a lot over a woman who had just had a baby, because of the breast feeding. So they'd make them a good chicken soup and for breast-feeding they'd give them a glass of milk and a piece of bread. But at the Women's at 5.30 a tray came with two big sausages with sauce and they don't know what it was. The gravy was a terrible thing. They'd say to me, 'Please tell them not to put any gravy — they forever put gravy'. The Anglo-Saxons could not understand how you can eat this kind of meat without any gravy. Maybe they were prepared to try it — a bit of meat — but as soon as the nurses put this white sauce over it, they would leave everything.

They would not eat and their husband would come with a sandwich of provolone cheese, of salami. But the sister in charge would say, 'Naughty girl — she didn't have her dinner or her lunch and look at what she's eating'. And the mother-in-law, or mother or cousin would bring a thermos with a bit of chicken soup and she would enjoy that. And they would say, 'What's that? Little white worms?' The pasta — the very fine noodles.

I was a referee. I used to get very upset because I had to explain to the nursing staff the type of food and on the other side, I had to tell the poor patient that they don't know what you're eating and they think it's little worms.

Every day there was soup, even in the summer. And there were two white buckets — one was a dark mixture of soup and the other was a white one. So they came around with a ladle, 'White or dark?' 'No, no, no soup; no, no, no gravy'.

They would sit and eat a bit of chocolate that the visitors brought them and in those years you had to stay in hospital for many days.

'Stella' coped, and remembers the young Liliana:

I didn't like the food at first — shock — one piece of carrot, no oil, some potatoes, and the gravy! My husband brought food in, but I ate what I like of the hospital food. I always had a good appetite.

The doctors were good, very good. Nurses — 'not so noise'. I remember one dark skinned nurse, she was the best. They didn't teach us much about care for the baby. They helped me with the feeding but at Henry Pride you had to fend for yourself.

When I came to Australia I was very happy with the [warm] temperatures, but it was a real drag trying to learn the language. I had an interpreter, from Egypt — she was a very serious lady. I used to have plenty of visitors.[17]

The migrants' visitors also changed the hospital. 'Miriam' had herself come as a migrant from Palestine in 1929. In the 1960s she was a gynaecological patient in the Women's and was an acute social observer:

When I was woken up early for breakfast, you had a thick mug with very strong tea like railway tea which had been brewing for hours. Then there was a bowl that was porridge. There were Maltese women there, strangers in a strange country.

After that sister came along with your obligatory penicillin injection. Honestly, the needles were twelve inches long. Everyone was yelling. Sister lifted up the nightie of one of the women who was screaming and said, 'Look, I haven't even put it in yet.'

Evening came and through the double glass doors you could see everybody waiting. The nurses watched the big clock to the second. It was like a Myers sale. I thought — this is mad. When the doors were opened, the men, women and grandmothers — all the rellies burst in with pots, casseroles, covered with towels, all filled with food. There were delicious spaghettis, salami. I said to my husband, 'The smells are driving me mad, go get me a pie or something'. It was because they wouldn't eat the food.[18]

The migrants themselves found the Australians strange, even amusing. 'Despina' was diabetic and had long stays in the hospital:

Henry Pride was good. The matron was a bit like a sergeant, . . . Queue up every morning. She didn't want the nurses to slack. But she was good, she look after us good. I always managed my English, I never had to ask for an interpreter. I never had to take my husband with me.

Some of the mothers were funny — one screamed all night about her husband what he had done to her — she was in pain. Another hummed all the time.[19]

And 'Trudi', just ten days in Australia before giving birth, was struck by a beautiful young Australian woman in the bed opposite:

She smiled at me, then she took her teeth out and washed them. I got such a shock. I found out that a lot of these young women had false teeth. We were not used to that. I think it was a sort of 'investment' for the girl — they got rid of their teeth and didn't have to worry about them again.

In 1954 and 1955 new suburban hospitals opened in Footscray and Williamstown, and with the new hospital at Box Hill from 1957, the growth of admissions at the Women's had eased. But the migrants continued to come, and from a wider range of national groups than before. A German interpreter had to be employed, but Liliana was equipped to look after the Greeks until she left herself in 1964 to have her own family. Intending migrants were strictly screened medically before being allowed to enter Australia, especially for tuberculosis and syphilis, but the desperate bought clear X-rays on the black market so that there was some tuberculosis among the immigrant population, as well as a significant degree of infertility caused by pelvic tuberculosis and past venereal infec-

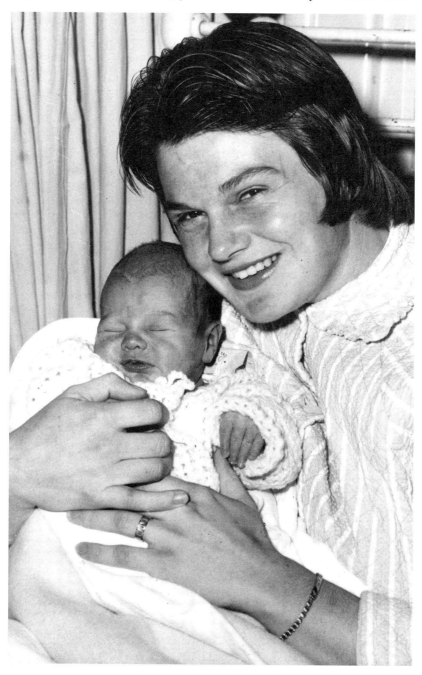

Mother and baby
RWHA

tions. These new Australians of the 1950s and early 1960s were fit, on the whole, and they were to enjoy better than average physical health compared to the old Australian population.[20] But many had not escaped the privations of war and it was the Greeks, with the long civil war following World War II, who displayed the most damage from past malnutrition. Sub-clinical rickets resulting in small pelves reappeared at the hospital after an interval of a century since the Irish and Scottish Highland famine victims of its founding years.[21] 'Toula' from Rhodes was a child when the war began. The Italians and the Germans took everything: meat they had only once every two or three weeks, they collected wild vegetables and leaves, made a little cheese, lived on olives and bread. She did not stop growing until she was twenty; reached menarche at seventeen, whereas her Australian-born daughters did so at ten and eleven. By 1963 when she was in the Women's, she coped well, with the interpreter's support, and ate everything: 'I still today have a lot of courage'. She reads her Bible daily and keeps fit with Greek dancing.[22]

The Mediterranean migrants did have one special health problem: thalassaemia, a genetic mutation which had conferred on the carriers (the heterozygotes) some protection against malaria, but which exposed the homozygotes to fatal anaemia. The first case of the disease in Australia was reported from Brisbane in 1961.[23] By 1974 the Royal Women's had established a Thalassaemia Clinic, where in 1976 Dr Rex Betheras was the first in Australia to conduct prenatal diagnosis for homozygous thalassaemia by fetoscopy and foetal blood sampling.

The cultural education of both sides of the migrant divide was mediated by people such as Liliana Ferrara and the scores of immigrants who found work in the hospitals of Australia. Here, even more than in factories, multiculturalism was born as Greek, Italian, Dutch, Yugoslav, Polish, English, Scottish and many others worked together. The domestic staff

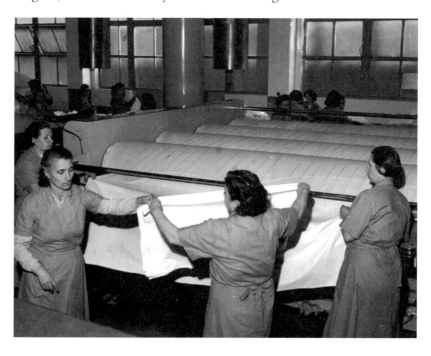

Migrant workers in the laundry *RWHA*

of the hospital became predominantly immigrant and these men and women formed cross-cultural friendship groups which eased their integration into mainstream Australian society. In doing things for patients and working with medical and nursing staff, they were able to display their competence and true capacity. They became colleagues and friends, and thus it was in workplaces first of all that prejudice began to break down. Old Australians might tease and say terrible things about Greeks, for instance, but say of their neighbour who was also Greek, 'Oh but she's lovely'. Multiculturalism was born of ordinary kindness — kindness offered on both sides. The migrant workers in the hospital enjoyed great companionship and support in their workmates from all nations; they shared problems and achievements, and found much fun and independence. The canteen was daily filled with teams of domestics, laughing and arguing, fractured Aussie English uniting them. And as 'those migrant women' became less threatening, the old Australians began to move towards meeting them part of the way.

'A' Mothers

The Women's Hospital continued to shoulder the largest burden of delivering unmarried women. If between 1860 and 1895 it had delivered more than 20 per cent of Victoria's ex-nuptial births, by 1967 it was 40 per cent, and most Melbourne maternity homes for the unmarried sent their inmates there.[24] But as the problems of the biological world were yielding to the advances of rational science, so too could social problems be solved by rational practices. The unfortunate Magdalene could be purged of her mistake and permitted to begin a new life; while her baby could fill an empty cradle in a loving, stable but childless home.

Until the Act of 1929 adoption had been irregular and haphazard. The children were at risk from poor supervision of prospective adopting families, but also adoption carried a stigma. The eugenics craze had aroused fears of inherited criminality or alcoholism or syphilis and people feared families 'with tuberculosis in them'. As Shurlee Swain and Renate Howe have shown, for adoption to become respectable there had to be a discursive shift from hereditarianism to environmentalism, where moral viciousness and physical degeneracy could be blamed on 'slum living' and poverty, and corrected by physical rescue, love, Christian training, good food, clean air and wholesome exercise.[25] The illegitimate child, as long as it was free of disability, could be a *tabula rasa* for its new family. The unfortunate biological mother, if she was the victim of deception or even her own immaturity, could 'put it all behind her' and face her future as if nothing had ever happened.

The 1929 Victorian Act made it possible for a hospital to be an adoption agency in its own right, and in 1941 the Board of the Women's Hospital formally gave its Social Work Department the responsibility of arranging the adoption of babies born within the hospital: it grew from 21 in that first year to 351 during 1968, having accelerated in growth during the 1960s.[26] Isobel Strahan and Connie Hunt carried the full work load from 1942 to the mid 1960s, a time in which social work changed in its focus.

Adoption was to become almost the dominant work of the department and the staff developed a high level of expertise in the placing of babies with adopting families. But post-war prosperity also transformed their work:

> One mother whose first baby was born in this hospital in October 1937 had her twelfth baby here in October 1956. We have watched the varying fortunes of the family. In 1937 her husband was on sustenance, receiving 22/- a week. By 1948 we find him working as a cleaner with a wage of £6/13/- per week. By 1954 his earnings have risen to £12/13/- per week. In 1956 his weekly wage has risen to £13/6/- per week and the family has graduated from living with her mother to a Housing Commission home.

A more complex story came from another big family:

> We met the mother first in 1936 when she came to have her third baby — the first two having been born in 1930 and 1933 respectively. Her husband had been out of work for three years. He received 22/- per week for sustenance and paid 8/- for rent. By the time they had four children, the sustenance was £2/10/6 per week and their rent 15/-. He joined the Army in 1940 and with six children the mother received the allotment of £11/4/- per fortnight. Soon after this they moved into a Housing Commission home (which they still occupy) at a weekly rental of 19/-. By 1950 when the tenth child was born, her husband's weekly wage had risen to £8, but the two eldest were earning. Today the eldest is attending university, the second is comfortably settled in a home of his own and both his children have been born in this hospital. The eldest daughter is married too and owns her own home. Their mother still keeps in touch with us. Her difficulties are manifold, but now she works — looks ten years younger and enjoys the love and respect of all her children. Her husband deteriorated with the struggle, but she rose above it.[27]

While material aid and financial counselling remained important, funded by the department's own Babaneek Auxiliary, by the end of the 1950s Isobel Strahan could report that counselling for emotional and social problems was becoming more important and that 'alcoholism, and illegitimate and unwanted pregnancies' had become their most frequent concerns.[28]

That illegitimate or unwanted babies should be found better homes, and that everyone — the child, the mother and the adopting family — would be better off was an unshakeable conviction. Everyone agreed that a single mother was unable to provide both financially and socially and that she owed it to her child to give it a better chance in life. Don Lawson, by 1960 senior obstetric consultant at the Women's, argued, as the R. H. Fetherston Memorial Lecturer, that the obstetrician had a duty to 'urge' the unmarried to relinquish their babies, to break the cycles of poverty and parental dysfunction, and that adoption was a case where the rule 'when in doubt, do' should prevail. Shot-gun marriages too often ended in disaster and a single mother was doomed to poverty and marginality.

Science now endorsed this: 'a good environment will make a better job of bad genes than a bad environment will make of good genes'. As for the biological mother, often she was matured by 'the experience' and he had seen 'many happily-adjusted married women who have had a child out of wedlock'.[29]

The Women's led the field in this new rational management of ex-nuptial birthing, and its trainees took the practices to other hospitals both public and private. Unmarried and pregnant, you were by definition a social work case. The social work theory, argue Swain and Howe, focused on the pregnant girl's 'mental anguish' rather than on her social or economic problems, and the first question she was asked was whether she was going to keep the baby. Inevitably, 'consenting to adoption was an instant way of regaining the social approval which most single mothers had lost immediately their pregnancy became obvious'.[30] The decision to adopt most often was driven by the single girl's own family, but it was left to the professionals to take responsibility. Most of this interaction with clients was kindly, but in the midst of kindness and concern it was harder to refuse the moral imperative to relinquish the child. Isobel Strahan was a deeply kind woman, widely respected and admired. Liliana Ferrara, as interpreter, worked under her supervision:

> She was a wonderful, wonderful person — very understanding. I had a lot of Italian and Greek patients who were single mothers and I used to go everywhere with her. I went to St Joseph's in Broadmeadows for the single girls, and there was another St Joseph's house for the single girls opposite the hospital in Grattan Street. A lot of girls from the country stayed there.

Some mothers did resist and keep their babies, and then the social work

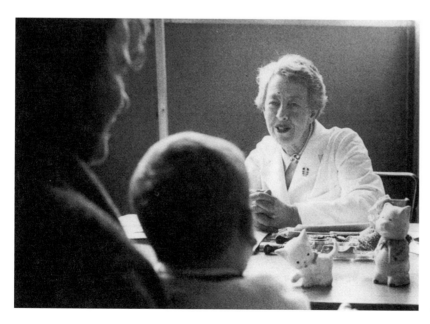

Isobel Strahan
Mark Strizic, RWHA

department and the domiciliary nursing service would support them:

> Those who kept their babies were given some help, but they didn't even have clothes. They'd give them an old singlet and maybe a better one and two nappies. There was no money, no clothes, they had nobody knitting and crocheting for them. They didn't have a toothbrush or toothpaste. I had to go with the social worker and give them a bit of money — they had nothing, not a nightie, it was terrible. And they had to hide from the relatives, most of them. We had to usher them through a different door — painful times.

The plight of migrant single mothers was made all the more acute by their isolation and the harsh moral standards of their communities. Liliana again:

> I had a couple of cases where I suspect it was incest, but the girls were so frightened.
>
> But mainly it was Greek girls because they would come in shiploads, not married by proxy like the Italians, and you'd find a lot of young Greek boys waiting for them . . . 'Oh we've got a room' . . . and promise to marry them. Some were promised from Greece, but once they'd seen each other they would not like them and would take advantage of them.
>
> If I close my eyes now, I can see them. But you have to be very careful, because if I'd meet them in the street and they'd look at me, looking very worried, and I'd turn my face and pretend not to know them. But once I was really shocked because I had this Greek lady coming with her husband and I looked at her and said, 'How are you?' — you know your patients quite well, especially the single mothers because you're dealing so much with them. And she turned her head and said, 'I'm here to have my first baby' and I knew very well that she had given her earlier baby up for adoption. And I said to her in the cubicle, 'Did you have to come to this hospital — you shocked me'. And she said, 'My husband doesn't know'.
>
> Most of them were having their babies adopted, and that was very traumatic. They'd either want to have their baby and run away or they did it in a very painful way. They'd beg me, 'Can I see my baby?' 'No, you're not allowed to see it if you leave it for adoption'. That was terrible. I became a different person — I became an interpreter with so much experience of human nature, of suffering, of pain. Oh, I grew up very quickly.

The Women's Hospital method relied on denial. If a single mother had decided on adoption, then she would get over losing her baby more quickly if the baby did not exist. The foetus became a large lump that had to be removed: if it never became a baby she saw, touched, held, caressed, fed with her own breasts, then perhaps she would recover more quickly. Allowing her foetus to become her baby, even for just a few minutes, would only make it harder for her to put the experience and her moral lapse behind her. While many nurses and doctors may have

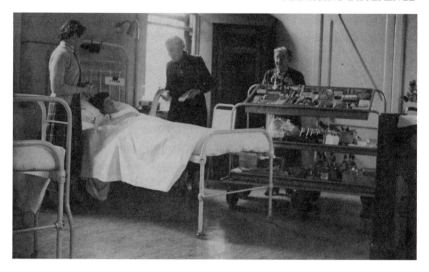

Patient trolley service, 1957 *RWHA*

had private misgivings, that was the way it should be done. Most staff sincerely believed that it was for the best for all concerned. Moreover, many of the single mothers were adolescents, scarcely out of childhood. They knew nothing of childbirth, they felt unable to resist the kindly advice of all these professional people who 'wanted only the best for the baby' yet they were going to lose something — perhaps the most important thing — they had created. Their extreme youth, and sometimes their poverty and personal neglect increased their chances of obstetric complications, but perhaps even more, Val Lissenden as a midwife can see with hindsight, their mental state delayed labour: 'When it was over, they'd have to give the baby up — whereas all the time it was inside her, it was safe'.[31] These teenage single mothers were therefore conspicuous for their long labours. Not all these lingering labours were painful, but some were and Cathy Hallam has vivid memories of 'little first-time teenage mothers in a lot of pain and out of control — so frightened'.[32] Heroin or morphine were used still in the 1970s for these girls, and labours of thirty-six to forty hours were common, but in the 1950s many staff took pride in very long labours.[33] Some of the senior obstetric staff, to make matters worse, refused to perform a caesarean section on an unmarried woman unless her life was in danger. They did not want to leave a scar on the uterus for fear that it might rupture in a subsequent pregnancy; and since the unfortunate might one day rehabilitate herself into a respectable married woman, she should be able to start her legitimate family as though she were virginal. They argued that 'once a caesar, always a caesar' and that the uterus could only tolerate two such sections, ignoring the possibility of lower segment caesarean sections, which while more difficult, could be repeated. Others disagreed, but that was hospital policy. Dr Kevin McCaul:

> Even the good obstetricians took a delight in saying, 'I had a woman
> in labour for three days and the baby's all right'. But you knew bloody
> well the baby wasn't all right. It would have been much better if it
> had been delivered on Monday. The mathematics of this were
> extraordinarily simple — but no, they took sheer delight in saying

'we didn't interfere'. The people suffering from that were the poor women. And I had to intervene in many cases. I used to live opposite where there's now a car park, and I would wander over at night time to the hospital, and I'd hear someone screaming and occasionally I'd intervene. One unit had an order against me that I was not to see their patients, because they knew perfectly well, that if I saw them, I'd intervene.

This remains one of the most painful issues in the hospital's history. Those who defend the obstetricians and midwives argue that they were doing what they thought was best; those who criticise see cruelty and wilful ignorance. McCaul first heard about the lower segment caesarean just after the war at a special lecture at the Royal Society of Medicine in London. As Australia's largest specialist women's hospital, the Women's should have been a national leader in practising and teaching the new techniques by the early 1950s. Instead McCaul found himself fighting an obstetric hierarchy that was deeply conservative and obsessed with the mechanics of labour. His later struggle to introduce spinal anaesthesia for caesarean sections so that women could be conscious for the arrival of their baby, was 'a grubby, dreadful battle: they ignored things and I've never understood why they did it'. He found strong support from the gynaecologists and widely throughout the hospital community, but the older, senior obstetricians were not being encouraged into research by the hospital with its penny-pinching ways, and they remained uninterested in pharmacology.

While the hospital took pains not to make single mothers suffer by giving them cheap wedding rings and removing their 'lumps' so that they could go back into the world unscarred, there was also an unconscious, and at times conscious, punitiveness, especially towards the unrepentant. One progressive obstetrician later observed that 'there was an attitude that you made her sweat it out a bit more if she was unmarried, and that she could not be respectable if she got married and had a caesarean scar'.[34] And some midwives and doctors took the chance as the mother reached transition, psychologically the most vulnerable time in labour, to administer 'the lecture': relinquishing mothers now testify to being examined with deliberate roughness and to cutting and cruel remarks at times of deep personal crisis.[35] The baby was rushed away as soon as it was delivered, towels placed over faces or heads turned away so that the new mother could not see and say goodbye.

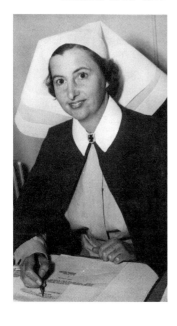

Miss Betty Lawson, matron 1955–1977

They became 'A' mothers, mothers whose babies were up for adoption, and the babies went into full-time nursery care. Roman Catholic girls were said to be numerous, because they would not have abortions. They had decided to keep their babies alive in utero, but had to relinquish them once out in the world. They were kept together, usually on the old balconies, because it was thought that they would have more in common, and, unlike the other postnatal patients, they did not have their babies with them. Betty Lawson realised as matron:

There was a phenomenon we didn't realise for a long time. We got into the habit of putting the single girls out on a balcony because we

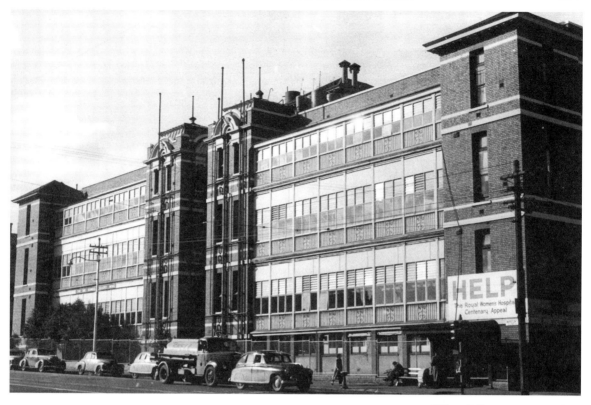

Gillott Wing (1927) and Druids' Wing (1912) on the corner of Swanston and Grattan streets in 1956 *RWHA*

thought it was nice for them, but it came to be assumed by them that they were out there for punishment. That wasn't the intention at all — it was to protect them from closer contact with ward babies.

In the postnatal wards, nurses did their best, but were often too immature themselves to help these girls with their grief. Cathy Hallam:

> We had a number of very young teenage girls and we did feel for them, although I remember first coming into an antenatal ward with perhaps half-a-dozen unmarried mothers and there was a definite moral stigma. A couple were there for their second and we'd think, 'Oh these poor women cannot be helped — this is really it. How could they possibly be stupid enough to come in for their second'.
>
> I don't suppose we tried to dissuade them from keeping their babies, but we certainly didn't encourage them. The idea was that it wouldn't have helped a baby to be lumped with a teenage mother. And these poor souls wouldn't even see their babies — they might go through a hideous labour, then their babies would be taken away.
>
> I can remember a few who were distressed postnatally and a few very ambivalent. I must admit I can remember a few having a cuddle a few days later and trying to decide. And the torment of those poor girls. We were just totally inadequate to cope with that — at least, I was, I shouldn't speak for others — but I can't remember getting much in the way of assistance in our training.
>
> I'll always be somewhat ashamed of that part of mid. — it was

handled very badly. And again, once you've had children yourself, you realise that attachment.

However efficient and skilful the hospital was in dealing with the body, many staff, both nursing and medical, had no aptitude in dealing with feelings. These were superb professionals, who worked long hours, who were brave and highly disciplined, and were therefore often constitutionally incapable of empathising with the emotions of people different from themselves. George Robinson, who came as a resident anaesthetist under Kevin McCaul, was appalled, as were many medical students and young doctors, by the insensitivity of the institution: 'I think that if you were faced with a situation where there's nothing you can do about something — people in long wearying labours — you just close up shop and say "that's life"'. But also, underlying this insensitivity, was a conviction that public patients were a slightly different species of human being, whose feelings were somehow not like one's own. A Melbourne gynaecologist told a medical congress at the Women's in 1948 or 1950 that from their observation of public patients, they knew that such people were very different from themselves. 'This must not be misconstrued as an attempt to place us in a snobbish society group', he continued, 'but we are college men, university graduates and are supposed to be intelligent and intellectual'. And it was from their own class that 'most of the superior minds develop'. His immediate concern was the higher incidence of endometriosis in wives of such men, who delayed childbearing and thereby risked infertility, allowing the 'inferior' classes to outbreed them.[36] Few would subscribe to such eugenicist fears, but many underneath assumed that the poor and uneducated did not feel things as deeply or with the same intensity as the refined and educated. Just as Aboriginal parents would not feel the loss of children stolen from them by well-meaning persons, these young relinquishing mothers would 'get over it' quickly, were rough and therefore could be treated roughly, would grieve for their lost babies a while, but have plenty more later and forget all about it.

After many years in the labour ward at the Women's, Sheila Haynes finished her nursing career on a mixed ward in a country hospital:

> It was quiet and there was time to talk and I found that women over seventy, who might have been coming in for gynaecological problems, would say, 'You're a midwife?' 'Yes.' 'Well I lost my baby years ago' and it was the first time that they'd plucked up courage to talk about it, because you had the time to sit there. And those women have suffered all their lives — they've never forgotten it. It's a real myth to say that it's over and done with.
>
> It's never over and it's never done with and it ruins their lives. It ruins their family lives — their ability to rear their families. They admit it themselves when you get them sitting down — that they could have been better mothers. They were always looking for the child that went — the child that was given up.[37]

Nurses 13

No wonder some of us are peculiar.

You never had any social life. To start with, you weren't allowed to be married and you couldn't do this and you couldn't do that. Besides you never met anybody — only a doctor, which you wouldn't give the time of day to. Then there were the broken shifts, so what did you do? You ate, you slept and you worked and that went on for at least twenty years of your career.[38]

We were treated like ladies. When you had a white uniform on and you became a charge sister, it was a real boost to your career. You had your separate dining room and you used to go to the Sitting Room for morning tea. And you moved to the sixth floor of the nurses' home and there was a dining room where you could entertain.

We used to get silver service in the Sisters' Dining Room. Your meal was brought to you. You had table cloths on the table. You had a serviette ring with your name on it. We were the last of the ladies.[39]

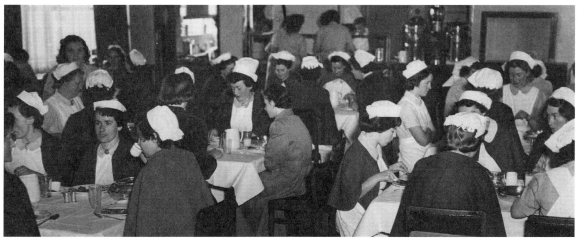

Nurses dining room, c. 1950 *RWHA*

If male doctors and administrators ruled, the hospital none the less was a woman's world. Men passed through as doctors, visitors, cleaners and tradesmen, but for as long as nursing remained a feminised profession, it was a universe run by women for women. Most of the human interaction day in and day out was between women. Charge sisters had ground rules set for them, but the wards were their places. Nurses sustained the culture of the hospital. And their world was held together by stories, jokes, customs, eccentricities, petty tyrannies, exhilarations, griefs and fears. Until the 1980s they would call each other by their surnames and privately more often by a nickname than a given name. They worked together under great stress and their enemies were in common. They saw more of each other than any other human beings in their lives. They drew deep comfort from a very real sisterhood, a connectiveness akin to that of soldiers in war. Their relationship with doctors was always ambiguous: few doctors still in the 1950s treated them as colleagues, too many took advantage of the young and attractive (although some fell in love and married them). But where the Women's Hospital was unusual, even the labour ward was the domain of the midwives rather than the obstetricians.

The Labour Ward

Beryl Shannon, after five years as a staff nurse around the hospital, went into Labour Ward 30 in 1947 and remained a charge midwife until she retired in 1972. The hospital was her entire world. She lived in the Nurses' Home throughout: 'It was a great relief to get to my room and just rest for a while if it had been a busy day'; and the only time she left the premises was on her days off. It was an entirely absorbing universe — 'there was so much to think about and do' — and she never lost her wonder at childbirth:

Marble slab in Labour Ward 30 *RWHA*

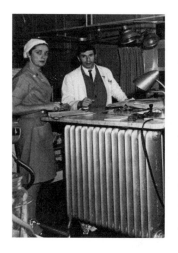

> It was always a joyous time and the mothers loved to see their babies. Quite often I liked to put the baby up to the breast and the baby was wanting to suck anyway and the mother was quite pleased to be able to do that. And that made the uterus contract which helped a bit.
>
> And the Italian babies with all their hair — they were so pretty when they were born.

And busy they were in the 1950s. The hospital delivered around seven thousand babies a year and provided one of the most dramatic stages for the first act of Australia's biggest experiment with mass migration and multiculturalism since the gold rush of a century before.

The setting was still 'Dickensian' to most observers. Labour Ward 30, with its great barn-like roof, was more reminiscent of a church than a modern hospital. In 1950 it had nineteen beds in the complex and Shannon remembers it minutely. There was one very large room with seven beds for patients in 'good labour' and in a corner was the baby area with six cots, a premature cot and a bath, a bench with baby scales and a ruler for measuring the baby's length. On the other side of the baby corner was the scrub-up area with a long metal bench on which

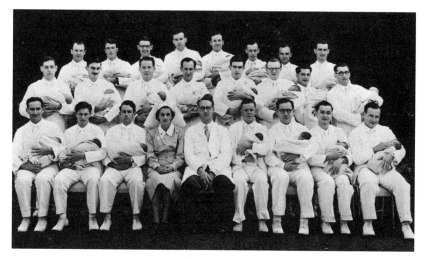

Sister Beryl Shannon and Professor (Sir) Lance Townsend, with student group in 1953 *RWHA*

were large drums for sterile gowns, gloves, face masks and lotions, nail brushes, tins of sterile powder and a copper scrub-up basin. Finally another small area had an anaesthetic trolley and oxygen cylinders.

In the centre of the ward stood a glass case for instruments, cat gut, needles and syringes, and on each side of that were two large marble slabs. The first marble slab was where the charge sister stood to do the clerical work such as completing the patient's charts after delivering a baby. Each birth was written in ink into a large leather-bound book with every detail of the type of delivery. At the change of each shift, the on-coming staff gathered there to receive the report of the staff going off duty. Sisters rarely sat and only a high stool was provided. The other slab held bowls of zephiran swabs, foetal and maternal stethoscopes, an ether machine and blood pressure machine and rubber face-masks.

First-time mothers were put into a small two-bed room, known as 'the Cottage', to insulate them from the noise of the 'old hands' and another small room called 'Top Special' was for prolonged or difficult labours. There was a day room where the trained staff had their morning and afternoon tea. There was the linen room and finally at the end of the corridor was the bathroom and admitting area. At the other side of the ward was the 'eclamps room' where patients with pre-eclampsia or eclampsia were kept sedated with paraldehyde administered rectally, or morphine if they were very early in labour. The room was darkened and quiet, with a padded spoon tied on each locker and oxygen ready. The patient was never left unattended, the nurse having to sit very still and watch every sign. There was a bell to ring if a patient began to fit and there were sides to the bed to draw up if necessary. Any patient with much protein in her urine was placed in the special ward for observation. The complex was completed by the sterilising room, the pan room and another ward of eight beds called the Labour Ward Annexe which accommodated patients in early labour. Finally on the balcony were three beds for use in the busiest times and 'there resided a torso and dummy and old Neville Barnes forceps for medical students to practise their forceps deliveries'.

It was a place both for delivering babies and teaching and the labour ward sister did the book work for both, as well as making up the rosters and duties of trained staff and pupil midwives. Pupil midwives did their lectures while off duty. This clerical work was done when the ward was quiet, or more often when the sister herself was off duty. Each week the sister-in-charge was responsible for the order books like the big store book for equipment such as syringes, rubber gloves, razor blades, suture needles, hanks of string, crepe bandages, catheters, glass connections for the mucus catheters, stationery and cotton wool. The food store book recorded tea, sugar and biscuits for both patients' and staff's morning and afternoon tea. Once a week all the empty bottles from the Dispensary were collected and placed in a large basket to be refilled, and brought back by the porter. Dangerous drugs were ordered in a separate book and the Dispensary rang the ward so that a nurse could collect them. Every Sunday the walls were washed by the nursing staff and the curtains between each bed changed. Once a year they were notified of the linen count and the labour ward linen room had everything counted in tens, with a piece of paper between for easy counting. The beds had to be made exactly the same way for easy identification of the linen and pillows. Another inventory was of the stainless steel and instruments which were counted every six months. At the end of each financial year, the charge sister added up the total number of deliveries as well as the number of breeches, forceps, premature babies, caesarean sections, maternal and foetal deaths. The medical superintendent also did this job in his office, and if the totals did not match, there had to be a recount. The rewards were intangible rather than monetary. In 1950 the pay for senior staff was £8 5s a week; five shillings a fortnight was taken out for uniforms and veils and they worked from five to thirteen hours overtime a fortnight. Time off was at a premium, however, as nursing shortages continued after the war. As a result, trained staff usually received only one day off in one week and two days off in the next. The overall staffing was of thirteen to fourteen charge sisters and staff nurses with twenty-one pupil midwives, with seven on each day shift, fewer at night because there was no cleaning done. There were always three trained staff on a shift. Mostly it was enough, but sometimes, such as one memorable Christmas Day, as Sheila Haynes remembers:

> We came on in the morning and the night charge sister had tears rolling down her cheeks — 'We've had the most dreadful night'. They'd had eight or nine deliveries and it didn't stop, it continued. And it went on for three shifts and it was a record — twenty-seven babies born on a Christmas Day.

The seven pupil midwives were allocated various tasks in rotation. The 'short straw' was the sterilising room and pan room. There was no Central Sterilising Department and so the sterilising work on the ward was almost continuous. The autoclave (known as 'the bomb') took an hour and the nurse on duty never stopped, washing, sterilising, drying and packing. She autoclaved the normal delivery trays with drapes, Spencer Wells forceps, towel clips and a mucus catheter. Neville Barnes forceps were wrapped in cotton wool covered by gauze stitched around the edge. This covering was made by the nursing staff. There were bowls of dry swabs, also rolled by the nurses in their spare time, and the sheets of cotton wool were fluffed up over the steam of the steriliser to make them go further. Large drums held small stainless steel bowls and kidney dishes for autoclaving. Rubber gloves also went into the large drums, but not until they had been washed, dried and tested for holes and repaired with small pieces of rubber cut out of discarded gloves, then powdered and put into special calico two-sided packets. (This job was carried out on a bed in the freezing balcony ward.) Everything possible was recycled. The syringes were autoclaved in paper bags with the size marked on the outside of the bag. And everything went into the bomb, even the 'Ungvita' ointment used for sore nipples in the postnatal ward was cleaned out of the nipple bowls, put in 'the bomb', melted down and made ready for the next patient.

Everyone was busy. Because the domestic staff were not allowed in the labour ward, pupils swept the floor with tea leaves three times a day to collect the dust that harboured the bacteria they now knew to be so dangerous to parturient women. The newest pupil found herself making tea for the whole ward; the 'eclamps' nurse had only to sit still and watch and hope her bladder would last the distance because no one had time to take over while she went to the toilet. The most restful job was as the baby nurse. A cot was always warmed and kept ready to receive a baby. After about a quarter to half an hour after the birth, the baby was weighed and measured. This procedure was checked by Sister and the particulars were written on the baby label which was placed on the singlet (including the name of each nurse who had weighed, checked and cleaned the baby); the tape which was already on the baby's wrist was stitched on after the

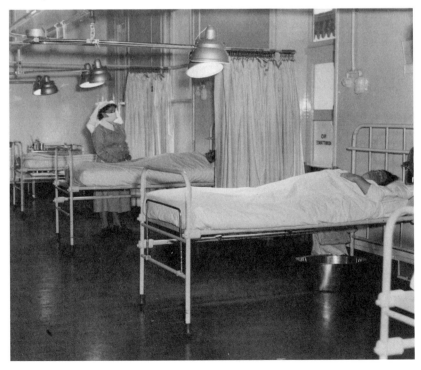

Labour Ward 30, west side
RWHA

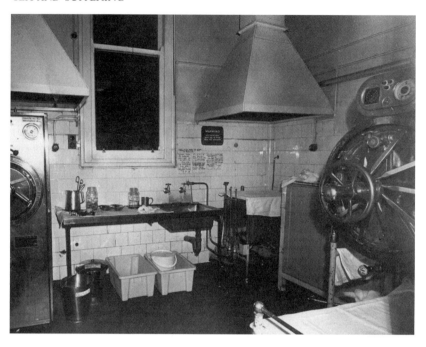

Labour Ward 30, sterilising room *RWHA*

baby was cleansed. In the early days the babies were washed with soap and water in the baby bath; later, after the golden staphylococcus outbreak, they were cleaned with hexachlorophane cream and not bathed. The baby was then transferred in its cot to the postnatal ward, but, before leaving, Sister again checked the sex and the particulars on the baby's label, double-checking the information already recorded in the big leather-bound book on the marble slab in the centre of the ward and initialling the baby label.

One pupil was allocated to the bathroom where patients were admitted. Women had no privacy from each other in the bleak bathroom with its red concrete floor. The woman was grabbed as she came in — not knowing what was going to happen to her. She was showered, shaved and given an enema. The shower and shave were compulsory, no matter how far a woman was advanced in labour: 'some in poor circumstances had nits in their hair and in the early years there were quite a few ones who really needed a shower'. With ferocious efficiency, women were shaved even while they had contractions. They were put into the stiff hospital night-dresses (often conspicuously patched), dressing gowns and slippers and their own clothes sent home. The history was taken and the chart shown to the charge sister who informed the doctor that the patient was being admitted. If it was an uncomplicated case, he gave permission for the sister to admit her. The patient was admitted, a medical student or pupil midwife made a pelvic examination, and the book in the admitting area was filled in with her name and address. The patient then had her enema: in the 1950s soap and water were given with an enema tube and funnel. The solution had been made up by the staff using Velvet soap and water boiled up in an enamel jug placed in a steriliser. Later a more sophisti-cated pack was introduced, which was already sterile and ready for use. In busy times it could be peremptory. But nature also could be peremp-tory, and many a new Australian entered the world in the shower or into

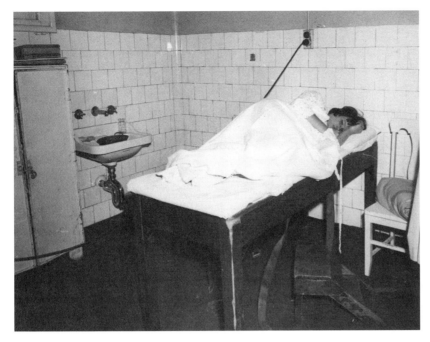

Labour Ward 30 bathroom in 1969, where patients were also examined, hence 'pelvic in the bathroom' *RWHA*

a bed pan. 'Jean' gave birth to six of her ten children at the Women's:

> I came in a taxi. The taxi driver kept saying, 'Don't have this baby in my cab.' I just made it. They were angry at me because you weren't supposed to go to hospital in labour on your own, but I didn't have anybody to bring. I was shaved — that was the worst. I can only remember having an enema once. I was always so quick. When I arrived you'd go into the one room and you could hear all the other ladies screaming, but after he was born, I used to think, 'What were they screaming about?' I went home to Moorabbin on the train and bus with the first and second.
>
> I'd still go back to the Women's if I had to.[40]

Most had a longer wait, however. They began in the Labour Ward Annexe, where a pupil midwife watched and timed their contractions. Shannon would encourage them to walk about, even take another shower which often helped. The progress of labour was assessed by rectal examination and palpation of the abdomen. Sometimes, if a woman needed to be brought into labour, the nurses would prepare her a vile mixture of orange juice and castor oil, fizzed up with bicarbonate of soda and put her into a hot bath. The mess, if she suddenly came into labour, was dreadful. Once strong labour was in progress, she moved to the delivery room, with only curtains between each patient. The screens were drawn only to give pans or for delivery, so the women could call out to the staff and to each other. Shannon liked it that way: the patients 'seemed more relaxed when they could see the nursing staff and the sisters' and the Charge midwife was attuned to each mother. Marlene Kavanagh ('Kav') remembers Sister Parsons: 'she'd be at the marble slab writing up and she'd say 'Set up over there'. Nothing would seem to be different, but this woman had just made an 'hmmg' or a 'hmph' or a something, and 999 times out of a thousand she was right'. If many women were horrified at sharing their childbed with five or six others in the same plight, there were some who were delighted. 'Grace' had a baby there in 1951 after three in private hospitals:

> I loved the feeling of not being alone having my babies. There was a feeling that we were all equal — there were some mothers who were unmarried and in those days there was a stigma, and they were all called Mrs. So and So, and I think were provided with wedding rings. You liked it that nobody was looked askance at.
>
> Also, I didn't mind going to the antenatal check ups. Of course sometimes the doctors treated you as if you didn't have a brain... 'Oh! you're reading a book!'[41]

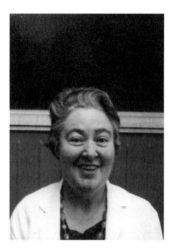

Miss Dott, chief of Pharmacy *RWHA*

Few women were prepared for labour pain with other than fear, ignorance and old wives' tales. Anaesthesia was offered for the delivery using the ether machine but, during labour, pain relief was helped by the nitrous oxide piped in beside each delivery bed. Stronger analgesia was offered only to those who became distressed. Heroin was the drug of choice at the Women's, its euphoric qualities doing wonders for new mothers' morale, but it was confined to primiparas lest women become too fond of it, and morphine and later pethidine were preferred for the multiparas. Chloral hydrate, a hypnotic, was also used extensively in the 1940s and 1950s. Opiates were never given less than four hours before delivery in case the baby was slow to breathe. When heroin was withdrawn from the market the dispenser, Miss Dott, had bought in advance huge supplies and the Women's was able to continue giving heroin in labour for many years: 'we found the patients did very well and were relaxed'. Initially heroin came in tablet form which had to be dissolved in a spoon of water boiled over a flame.

The pupil midwives had two tasks — the delivery itself or working at the 'head end' trying to keep the mother calm and helping with anaesthesia, and, after delivery and the third stage, giving the ergometrine injection. There were trolleys to attend to at the end of the bed, differently equipped for normal and abnormal deliveries. On the top shelf would be small sterile canisters with swabs, string for tying the baby's cord, cord dressings and a tray with a lid containing sterile mucus catheters and Spencer forceps, clamps and scissors. The bottom shelf held large billies with sterile towels and sterile 'mother pads', draw sheets and leggings. The leggings amazed Dr Kevin McCaul when he arrived fresh from the United Kingdom in 1951:

> An extraordinary garment I've never seen before or since. It was a type of pyjama made of linen, heavy, with a hole in the centre, and if you put a woman up, that was the only exposure — you weren't allowed to look at the legs. I remember the horror one day when a woman came up to theatre refusing to have this thing on. It was reported to the Board of Management and there were all sorts of discussions and meetings.

The progress of labour was often not the calm, ordered routine described in the textbooks. Patients lost control, became violent, and the screaming of the screamers became unbearable for the tired and stressed. Lorraine Danson was once pulled under the shower by a distraught migrant woman and was saturated.[42] Idealistic visions of natural child-birth stood no chance against the hysteria unleashed by many patients. Helen Ferguson:

> It was very, very loud and it was very hard to explain to these people that you were just trying to help them, because it was all so foreign to them. And a lot of us suffered minor injuries from the kicking, scratching and the punching and so forth — because they were fighting against something they didn't understand.[43]

'Peg', coming in to have her second baby in 1954, remembers the noise of the labour ward above all: 'The labour ward was a huge room filled with all these screaming migrant ladies giving birth to their babies. There were doctors and nurses running everywhere. The hospital was absolutely overflowing with migrants. They had to make up beds anywhere they could to make everybody comfortable'.[44] Liliana Ferrara remembers Shannon as particularly understanding with the migrants and later she delivered three of Liliana's own babies: 'she was very delicate':

> Before I had my baby I used to say to patients, 'There's no need to scream like that — you push now, you don't push now'. You have to encourage them to push and not to push.
>
> And when my time came I thought — Oh, ho — I'd better keep my mouth closed. And Sister Shannon said to the doctors, 'Mrs Ferrara's a bit inhibited because she's worked here'. 'If you feel like screaming, you just go ahead and do it', she said to me. And I did.

Shannon remembers the careful routine of a normal delivery: the patients were delivered in the left lateral position. If it was a delivery for a medical student, he had to remember to bring another student to hold up the leg. If a pupil midwife was given the delivery, then another nurse had to hold the leg up. Then stirrups were introduced to do this job. If a delivery for a medical student occurred at night-time, there was a bell outside the Labour ward door activating a bell under the student's pillow. Each trainee midwife and medical student had twenty normal deliveries and as well as three forceps, a breech, a caesarean section and for the medical students an artificial rupture of the membranes. There was an intake of thirty medical students every three months. Each trainee mid-wife and medical student had to do three pelvic and three rectal examin-ations. For the first three deliveries a sister had to scrub up and assist and instruct. For the pupil midwives Shannon liked to page a tutor sister for one of the pupil's first three deliveries. The remainder of the twenty deliveries were supervised by a sister.

Cathy Hallam was a pupil midwife at the Women's in the early 1970s. She had followed her mother's footsteps — general nursing at the Alfred, midwifery at the Women's. She was apprehensive — how would she 'cope with the embarrassment of looking at bottoms all day', but also how would she cope with actually delivering babies?

> I did enjoy it at the end, but I can remember being very overcome the first time. It was such a messy experience. It's funny — I was overcome about this little baby, but at the same time slightly revolted by all the mess and what the baby looked like because I'd never seen one born before. But I do remember a time when I did become very emotional, and that was when I was assisting with a father there, and that was very unusual. He'd specially asked, this father, and the ward sister didn't want him and there was a lot of discussion about whether he should or should not be there. Eventually he was allowed and it was a beautiful delivery to watch because the mother and father supported each other fairly well (probably not as well as now because the instruction wasn't all there, but he was very encouraging). And at the time the baby was born there were tears and laughing, and I had so many tears in my eyes I couldn't even put the injection in — I couldn't find this jolly vein — because if you didn't get the ergometrine injection in quickly you were roasted.

Like many students, both midwifery and medical, she was impressed with the skill of the trained midwives:

> The trained midwives used to do episiotomies and they were very good at it — sometimes the resident doctors were not so good, because the midwives did many, many more. But they would try their darnedest to get the baby out without any episiotomy at all. They really tried very hard, and if they had to resort to one they'd feel bad; if there was a tear, particularly a large tear — that was something to be ashamed of. And delivering babies, that was the foremost thing in my mind. I can still remember the pressure on that thumb, trying to keep the chin flexed — trying to keep control. You'd feel for the chin — you'd have your right hand on the head, trying to slow it down. You'd have the other hand on the perineum, trying to feel the chin as it

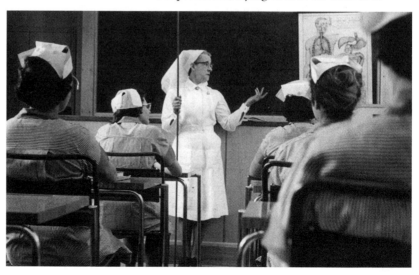

Tutor Sister Jessica Place
Mark Strizic RWHA

came up and assisting the perineum to expand. You'd push the chin — gosh it must have hurt, but the poor mother probably couldn't feel anything at that stage. You'd push it in so you'd keep the crown coming first up. The amount of pressure on that thumb caused a lot of aching, although I guess the more experienced you were, the less inclined you were to traumatise your thumb.

The pupil midwives had to conduct their normal deliveries without a doctor being present:

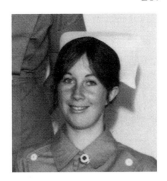

Sister Catherine Hallam, pupil midwife, September State Group, 1971 *RWHA*

And the first three were done with hands over the midwife's so you weren't doing anything much except feeling what to do. Then we did all the deliveries ourselves but with the midwife looking on and very much in control — our faces were just inches away. In the twenty deliveries there had to be three to five complicated ones where a doctor was present — breeches and forceps. The breeches were very frightening and they were more commonplace then — it was more acceptable to do a breech vaginally than to do a caesar. You knew there was a hazard involved and you were just a bit anxious about the baby because you'd heard all the stories about babies getting stuck. We helped too with versions — mostly they were successful and a lot depended if it was a specialist doing it or a resident. The mother had to be very, very relaxed, so that was our role.

I thought the forceps themselves were revolting. We used to usher them in quickly so the mother wouldn't see — for good reason, they do look awful. I saw a high forceps done and I think it was because they tried very hard not to do caesars. It's quite the reverse now. Again it wasn't out of preference, but I often wondered if some of the residents would quite like the experience. You'd get this feeling — like in all teaching hospitals — oh, here's a chance, let's go for it. Epidurals were not very common in the early 1970s, but they did try and do epidurals, and what we called pudendal blocks — for forceps. I could never bear watching those — a huge injection and a huge needle because they had to be very long. I remember when I had Ellen, I was wheeled into a delivery room with all the instruments laid out and I often thought if I was a mother with no experience of that, it must be a dreadful sight, so I hope they're still being careful in what they show.

The third stage of the delivery had its own stresses: the ergometrine injection had to be timed properly — given too soon, the uterus might begin to contract down before the placenta was fully detached; given too late, the mother might bleed:

I didn't enjoy doing grande multips because you knew they had a really lax uterus, particularly if they were already starting to bleed quite heavily. So sometimes panic would set in. And if the poor junior nurse was having trouble with the ergot, there'd be lots of abuse thrown around. It could be very tense in a delivery room.

And that is what she finds so different now: 'it's not nearly as tense now with what they call natural childbirth'.

Before there were certain expectations of the delivery. You were supposed to do things in certain times — everything was very rigid. First stage was a certain length; second stage was a certain length; you had to get your procedures done in a certain time and in a certain order. You had to maintain sterility at all times, and I honestly don't think that they are as strict as that any more. Staph. has always been there, but we were always very concerned about it because Staph. on babies is always taken seriously.

Babies were whisked away — they weren't' allowed to stay on the mother. We thought the babies would chill, so we'd wrap them up tightly. And if they came back, it was only for a short time. It was all very controlled. The poor mother had very little 'say'. It was rigid because it was a large institution and conservative as well. In fact it wasn't very different from the Alfred, so I didn't question it. But it was the only place I had to wear a veil — they went out soon afterwards, and they were almost dangerous. They were not the old soft type that draped over your shoulders; they were very stiff and starched solid and they went straight out the back at right angles, so if you turned your head quickly, you could poke somebody in the eye. They were lethal. We wore caps for delivery, which again wasn't very reassuring for the mother.

Cathy's memories are of the new labour wards in operation by the 1970s. Labour Ward 30 in the 1950s could be hectic beyond belief. Kav's worst day was a Saturday morning in July:

It was just myself, one other trained staff and five pupil midwives. If it hadn't been for the medical students who were on labour ward duty, we would never have coped. We had eighteen admissions, sixteen deliveries and fourteen of those were forceps. In the meantime we got a transfer from Prince Henry's — an eclamptic who had the afibrinogenaemia, so was about to die.

afibrinogenaemia: complete absence of the coagulation factor fibrinogen in the blood (*OMD*)

Oh God, I've never had a day like it. I started work at 7 o'clock in the morning and got off at 9 o'clock at night and I still left the afternoon charge sister with about four charts to do. And there were a couple of medical students, and if it hadn't been for them . . .

The woman in eclamps was found in a street in South Melbourne unconscious and was taken to Prince Henry's where they found she was pregnant but couldn't find what else was wrong with her, so they sent her up in an ambulance to us. On the way in the ambulance she started pouring blood — she just about died. She'd been to an abortionist. She was about twenty-four weeks pregnant and she must have fitted at the abortionists and they just threw her out. Amazingly she lived — had no recollection of what happened to her. But then we had this big hassle because the family said she had $700 on her when she went out — to buy a lounge suite or something. And when she came from Prince Henry's, all she had was a hospital gown.

And those who trained in the 1950s, saw more death. Kav again:

The first time a patient died on me was when I was a student, on

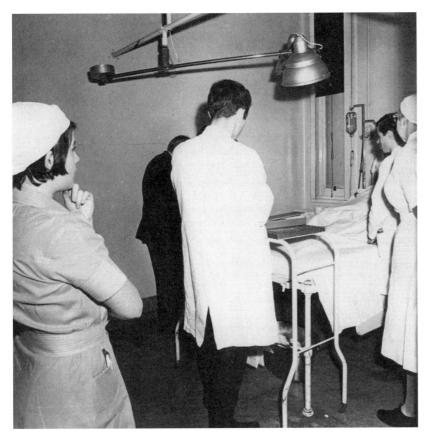

Labour Ward 30
consultation *RWHA*

night duty. It was a woman from the country, a diabetic who'd been told never to have children—she had polycystic kidneys and her diabetes was very brittle. And she desperately wanted a baby so went to a GP who didn't know her and who said, 'You're a strong healthy girl, of course you can have a baby'. And she died and I remember being absolutely shattered. Two student midwives on—we didn't expect that. We'd come to do mid because patients didn't die. The babies might die, but the mothers didn't. That was our perception of it. These were young healthy women. The husband was staying at Peter Poynton's pub. It was 2 a.m. and the local priest in Carlton arranged with the country priest to get the parents down. The priest came and we almost confessed to him—we just weren't coping, it was so unexpected.

But the worst I saw was a young girl of nineteen sent down from William Angliss, and she bled to death. The poor husband—he was about twenty-two and this baby was three hours old. He couldn't take it in. He really couldn't understand what the doctor was trying to tell him. It was just terrible.

When things went wrong, the Women's Hospital could swing into disciplined action. Cathy Hallam again:

If a mother had to go up to theatre for a caesar—it was not unusual but it was not like it is today—it was almost with a sense as though someone had failed. Something had gone wrong—what a shame.

Or in the case of an emergency like a prolapsed cord — and that's where the Women's worked *very* well. As soon as it occurred, all the right procedures would happen: the mother would be put in the right position and they'd be up in theatre in minutes. It was very, very efficient.

And it all depended on control, control of every activity in every corner of the labour ward, a control which was very hard to relinquish even in the face of the new natural childbirth. 'Vera' was by profession a social worker who had done her placements as a student at the Women's. Her husband was a medical student and he had been permitted to attend her first confinement at the Queen Victoria Hospital, where she had delivered without analgesia. It was 1953 and her obstetrician was J. W. ('Hoppy') Johnstone, acting professor:

> Before my second confinement I had regularly attended exercise classes and I was all prepared for natural childbirth.
> 'Hoppy' was away when I went into labour and I had a registrar and my husband was with me. When I went into the second stage, they

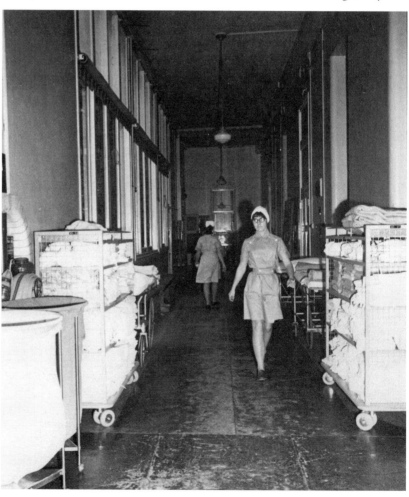

**Corridor outside Labour
Ward 30** *RWHA*

asked my husband to leave. He had been present at the Queen Vic
confinement. On top of that they urged me to have nitrous oxide and
I sort of refused and set the whole hospital off balance.

They called the director of nursing and she started arguing with
me. You know how vulnerable you are. I clearly remember having one
whiff to please her. Here I was, being told to have some help and my
husband shoved out — I was really angry.[45]

If doctors took the ultimate professional responsibility, the senior nursing
staff none the less exercised considerable power, especially in the labour
ward. Midwifery was paradoxical. Midwives were trained to deliver babies
on their own, provided the delivery was normal. As Shannon remembers:
'Any professor coming to Melbourne was surprised at the amount of
responsibility we took in the labour ward. It was very different from
America. The doctors relied on us because they couldn't be in the ward
very often'. Often the midwives knew more than the young doctors,
and often were more manually adept. They learnt to manage doctors,
recalls Kav: 'You learnt to say 'Doctor — do you want to do this *now?*
instead of 'You'd better do so-an-so'. And there were times when it ran-
kled as raw young medicos ordered them about as mere underlings. But
other medical students, residents and honoraries respected the skill and
dedication of the midwives, while the nursing staff 'felt safe' because expert
help was always near at hand. Few forgot Labour Ward 30.

After-care

The patients mostly remember the after-care, however. Births were too
rushed and anaesthesia removed memory, therefore the days after are the
real 'hospital experience' and here nurses overwhelmingly dominated the
patient's world. And for all the tragedies and the social problems that passed
through its doors, the Women's was found by most to be a very happy
hospital. Cathy Hallam was pleasantly surprised:

I'd had some foreboding about it because people said it was very strict
and it was extremely busy and the ward sisters weren't very nice. But I
felt it had a lovely atmosphere and I thoroughly enjoyed it. The whole
hospital had a lighter feel to it — it was a happy form of nursing.
And those bits of tension I had are really to be expected for an
inexperienced nurse trying to deal with things which she's not
sure about.

The atmosphere of the hospital softened considerably from the 1940s to
the 1970s, as a new generation of nurses and doctors rose to positions
of authority. And despite the financial difficulties of the 1950s as the hospital staggered under the baby boom, food was no longer an acceptable
area for financial stringency. Everyone was very conscious that many of
their patients needed rest and feeding up. There was sugared Aktavite with
every meal and in the 1950s ward sisters often served out double T-bone
steaks to patients, and again so much of the tension and misunderstanding

between the hospital and its migrant patients arose from the hospital's determination that British styles of eating be imposed because they were nutritionally superior to home Italian food. Patients *had* to eat up, it was good for them, *and* they had to stay in bed.

The ordinary wards were therefore a social stage for great dramas of class and cultural conflict. 'Monica' had eight babies in the Women's between 1942 and 1959: 'The wards were a bit frowzy and noisy, but they improved as time went on. I never grizzled about the food and I thought it was a wonderful place because every time I was there I had another baby'.[46] Many whose expectations of a public hospital were modest found no hardship and instead enjoyed the warmth and occasional earthiness, as did 'Sheila' who had four confinements there at the height of the baby boom:

> I found the service was excellent. They were always cheerful. There were returned nurses there and they were always good for a laugh. There must have been a miscarriage one day and one of the Army nurses came in and said, 'I never knew so many women fall over logs of wood'. I was treated with respect. I couldn't fault it.[47]

'Gwenda' had longer to observe. She was a social worker who had herself worked with clients at the hospital.

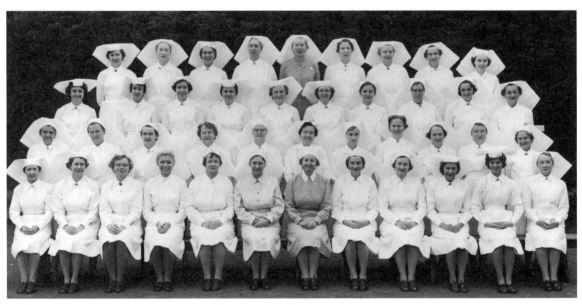

The Royal Women's Hospital, Matron and Charge Sisters photographed for *A Century of Nurse Training, 1862–1962* Back row: Sisters D. Williams, P. Taylor, G. Barnard, M. Parsons, C. McPherson, L. Durrant, A. Forbes, P. Geyer, T. Matson. Third row: Sisters D. Hanrahan, C. Oswald, L. Fowler, M. Mabbitt, M. Cole, C. Reichert, M. Corkill, F. Weppner, E. Brereton, B. Shannon Second row: Sisters E. Lewis, E. Henderson, V. Campbell, C. Murnane, M. Morgan, L. Dredge, E. Lambert, J. Filsell, S. Findlay, M. Gleisner, V. Page Front: Sisters P. Lloyd, G. McAlister, E. Block, S. Orzel, W. Mulqueen, J. Crameri, Matron B. C. Lawson, Sisters E. Begg, H. Ferguson, M. Patching, J. Barton, J. Place *RWHA*

In 1950 I took a very young retarded teenager, thirteen or fourteen years, from Travancore to the hospital. She had been taken advantage of by a man and became pregnant. The staff at the Women's were very kind to her. It was very well handled. She had her baby there. She saw it once and then they whipped it away. She said, 'Other people have a husband and a mother to visit but I have no one. They all get to see their baby but I don't.' But she said that she gave her a nice name — 'Sylvia.'

The other women had flowers and were showered with presents. I brought her flowers but it was nothing like the others. But my impression was that the girl was a little bit of a V.I.P. in there. People thought, 'What a shame, this poor little girl, let's be nice to her and plan for the future.' The nurses and doctors were very sympathetic and understanding.

'Gwenda' became pregnant with twins while her husband was a medical student and at seven months she had to be admitted to the antenatal ward:

There was a really nice nurse there. She said, 'You won't be lonely will you, with your two babies?' I think she was Dutch. The ward looked out on to a big tree. I just used to lie and relax and look at it. I had been doing a really traumatic job with neglected children and it was so nice to relax. I stayed in bed a month. The food was probably not too bad — it's a complete blank. I was due to be induced as my blood pressure was up and it was for the babies' sake and my sake. I couldn't put my shoes on or my ring on. It was the optimal time for delivery, then three hours before the induction I went into labour spontaneously.

I was taken to the labour ward and had an epidural. They had those awful stirrups, and they shaved me and I had an enema. I was in labour from 5.00 am to 11.00 am when the first one was born — he was a breech. The doctor said, 'You've done your duty.' I was shocked — a little girl would have been just as welcome. The twins were born vaginally. I had forceps for the second one, half an hour later. He was a bit bruised, and one of the sisters said, 'He's going blue.' I didn't see him for three days. When I finally had mustered up my courage to ask why, they said, 'He had a rough passage and so had you'. The other was up in intensive care, I saw him the next day — they took me up in a wheel chair. Right after they were born they brought in a beautiful tray of food and orange juice and milk. I drank a little, then I was sick. Everything went everywhere. When I woke up I was in a single room with a nurse sitting there in a pool of light with a padded spoon. Perhaps I'd had a fit. They took my blood pressure quite a bit.

I didn't have either baby with me which was hard, especially as I was having difficulties expressing milk. I was expressing till 10.00 o'clock every night. I had no idea how much was needed. I asked a nurse was it enough? and she laughed very unkindly and said, 'Oh goodness gracious me, that's not nearly enough.' It was a terrible ward, one of those Florence Nightingale wards, with those horrible nighties. They were hard as a board and patched. The ward was terribly

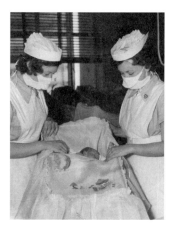

Christmas 1952, Premature Nursery. Hand-printed muslin cot covers were used at Christmas for many years. Note the masks which were worn constantly in the nursery. *RWHA*

noisy and the clatter and clang of trolleys — radio on full-blast at times with terrible commercials. Once we had 'Your Choice' program and I was allowed to make a choice. I chose 'One enchanted evening' — it was really popular at the time. The food was inferior to that in the other ward. It wasn't very palatable and the crockery wasn't much, but the nurses were nice to all the patients.

The babies came eleven months after we were married. They were born bang in the middle of 'Ian's' exams. He was doing the gynaecology and obstetrics exam on the day they were born and he was asked the complications of twins. We thought it was very funny and so did the examiners — they knew what was going on.

There was a single mother outside on the verandah. She was crying a lot. She seemed pretty well educated. A nice young doctor or student said to her, 'Your baby looks a lot like you.' She didn't have any visitors. And there was a young girl from Camp Pell. She was cheery, bouncy and optimistic and loud. A very nice attentive young man of about seventeen came to visit, obviously the father. She had a lot of pain, and yelled. Straight away after that they hurried to give her the baby — that cheered her up. She looked about sixteen. The visiting hours were a bit rigid — just husbands and mothers. It was a bit short. It was a pity that they weren't more flexible — but I wouldn't have wanted great hordes coming in. A lot were migrants — there was a Dutch lady next to me.

Possibly I got a slightly privileged treatment because I was Dr Churches' patient, and 'Ian' was doing a medical course. 'Ian' was at a celebratory party because of the twins and came just after visiting hours closed but they let him in, just for a minute.

I stayed for ages at the Queen Elizabeth. We had no place to live, not even a cot for the two babies. Eventually they woke up to the fact that I had been here so long and I then went to my mum's.[48]

'Anne' was another eclamptic, rushed from a private hospital for a caesarean section in 1948. For her the culture shock was more profound:

In those days no one would have gone there by choice — it was too rugged. The food was pretty 'off'. It was so nondescript, it was just awful, there was no taste in it or anything — mostly stews and stuff; you ate it because you had to eat something.

Once you were what they thought was OK you were tossed out on the verandah and that was it. It was bleak, it was cold. It was early in September, you could hear the wind blowing. I hardly slept out there — people were travelling past. I was cold: they said, 'You've got enough blankets', but there was no heating on the verandah.

Nobody could have looked after me better while I was as ill as what I was. The younger nurses were lovely and attentive. The old girl (the 'fishwife') was hard. She brought me my baby for his first feed, and here was I, thirty-three years old, I'd never fed a baby, and I'd got this great gash here, and she said, 'Here, feed your baby'. I had no idea — she wasn't helpful. I ended up crying . She said, 'You modern females don't know how to have babies.' A young nurse came and helped me.

She got a pillow underneath and said, 'Don't pay any attention to her'.

I'd been brought in from St George's and dumped down, and it was visiting hours and all these people were filing past me with dusty shoes. My husband complained. He told the doctor, 'My wife is dangerously ill and she can't have people staring at her.'

After the anaesthetic wore off they said to me, 'You've got a beautiful boy'. I was in that special ward after I was delivered. There was a great big ward with about twelve women in it. I felt how awful, to be in a ward like that — they would have found it more rugged than I did.

I felt there were not enough people to do what had to be done. It was an old fashioned and rundown type of place compared to St George's. It was as clean as they could possibly keep it. It had these old fashioned enamel beds with lumps of enamel knocked off them. The bathrooms were arctic — half the time the water was only luke-warm. There were no curtains on the alcoves — there was no privacy, you turned your back on people when you were drying yourself and put on your dressing gown as quickly as you could. The hospital was so clattery and noisy and it never seemed quite clean.

I know if I hadn't gone to the Women's I wouldn't be here now — I know that in my heart. I suppose they ran it as well as they could on what they had. I felt sorry for people who had to go there.[49]

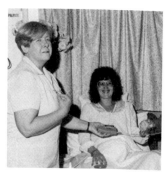

Sister Helen Johnstone with a patient *RWHA*

Helen Johnstone was one of the young nurses who stayed. Her father was a distinguished obstetrician who was acting professor of obstetrics between the death of Marshall Allan and the appointment of Lance Townsend. He was famous for his manual skill as an accoucheur and Helen had known the hospital from childhood, when he slipped in after hours to see patients. After doing her general nursing at the Royal Melbourne Hospital and the Associated Hospitals' School of Nursing, she commenced midwifery at the Women's:

I think I was expected to be better than I was and I thought I'd killed the kid in my first delivery — even though it was a sick baby and it didn't breathe, but I thought it was my fault and I'd wrung its neck. So I didn't want to go back to labour ward.

But I did like the mothers and babies afterwards — postnatal. And I liked it because they weren't sick. I liked a bit of drama now and then, but I didn't like critically ill people who were dying. In Labour ward they were transient — they had their baby and left, whereas in postnatal, we got to know them. We knew them as family.

By the time she retired, she estimated that she had cared for around 30 000 babies. Her ward became a home away from home. At Christmas time, especially while in the old hospital, the ward sisters competed to have the best decorated wards, paying for most of it out of their own pockets. Helen would visit the Queen Victoria Market in the early morning to buy flowers and in her first years used her imagination: 'painted I.V. bottles and bought flowers, but after a while that became an impossibility and so you bought decorations'. Light-fingered visitors went off with a lot

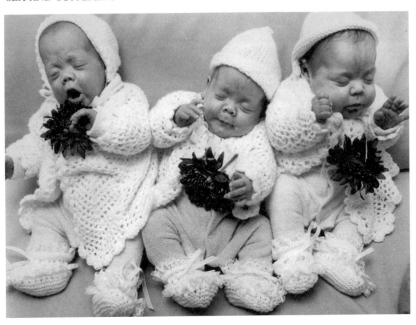

Decorated babies *RWHA*

of it ('everything that wasn't screwed down, you lost' says Kav), but Christmas was special with the wards packed for carol singing led by visiting choirs. 'Betty' had two Christmases there: 'it was lovely — the nurses decorated the wards, sang carols and I received a hamper from the Smith family as my husband was unemployed. It contained baby clothes and food'.[50]

Helen liked to keep the mothers busy with 'hospital cottage indus-try'. She had to do much of the sterilising for the rest of the hospital and had her postnatal patients, sitting up in their hair-curlers and smoking cigarettes, making cotton wool balls and maternity pads. Doctors often encouraged women to smoke in bed to 'settle their nerves', and they puffed away while breast-feeding, reading *True Confessions* magazines, curlers in, moccasins at the ready. Liliana Ferrara, fresh from Egypt, had not expected poverty in Australia: 'I was shocked and astonished — I was very inquisitive, everything was very new to me'. Some patients were unkempt, occasionally intoxicated: 'I asked Isobel Strahan once and she said that it started with childhood — that they never had a chance'. The staff felt for them, so many looked worn and old beyond their years. Helen Ferguson:

> When we first went to do midwifery we all couldn't understand the mothers who didn't want to see their babies after they were born: 'I don't want to see it, take it away'.

Kav had an even more disillusioning introduction to maternal feelings:

> When I started Mid I was put out on the balcony with the 'A' mothers — those whose babies were to be adopted — so I'd never actually seen a mother and a baby together.
> One week I asked if I could be moved inside and I can remember

someone brought up a woman from Labour ward and I looked at her
card and it didn't have an 'A' on and she'd had seven other babies. And
I said, 'Oh Mrs So and so, I've seen your baby in the nursery — he's
lovely.

She said: 'The little bastard — I'm having him adopted.'

It absolutely shattered my world.

Many young student midwives were shocked by the poverty still
evident in the late 1950s. Margaret Mabbitt:

They hadn't been exposed to the depth of the problems you saw here,
even in a general hospital where you saw another sort of poverty.

And the things that men did to women. It's still going on, but you
don't see it as much in here. You got a lot of battered women — a
woman with a broken beer bottle shoved up her vagina, black eyes,
broken ribs. It was not unusual for women to come in with things
inserted in them.

And so often you'd hear the women say — I've got to go home
today because it's pay day and if I'm not there when he comes home,
he'll drink it all and we won't have anything to eat for the week.

There were forty-year-olds with no teeth, varicose veins, hair
cropped short, socks — and they looked like their children's
grandmothers. And yet they always put on a front when they came
into hospital. If they had no nighties, they'd borrow from their
neighbours, even though we supplied everything. Their hair went into
curlers almost as soon as they hit the place and the only time they
came out was at visiting hours in the evening, and then they went
straight back in again. The majority of them smoked — there was no
restriction and they could smoke whenever they wanted.

I've no memory of any coarse language, except when they were in
labour and the barriers dropped. But in the wards they were putting
on side — they felt that when they came into hospital they had to
'behave themselves'.

But among themselves a lot of friendships grew up — and they all
got to know each other because they were in for so long. They
swapped problems and they supported each other — exchanging life
stories, telling each other how to deal with things. Especially the older
women with the younger one having her first baby — that was very
evident.

You got many who were very thin, and a lot who were very flabby
rather than overweight. Not a very nutritious diet and they didn't
particularly like what they were given in here — a lot of them had
lived on fish and chips for years.[51]

Day two, postnatal ward, with Sister Tai *RWHA*

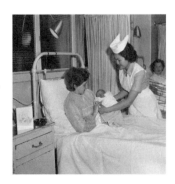

Breast-feeding often became a battleground, because there were staff
who were fanatical and unsympathetic to those who were just too harried
to bother or who had to return to work. They knew that some with five
or six children would have the oldest feeding the baby with a bottle, so
they would breast-feed in hospital and change to the bottle as soon as
they got home. 'Oh, it's all right love', said one woman to Kav, it's so

much easier if I breast-feed in hospital — that old bitch won't get at me, but I'll bottle feed when I get home'. Another told Mary Logan that she breast-fed in hospital because it was 'easier for you girls'. While the hospital was committed strongly to breast-feeding, practice often fell short. Liliana observed in the 1950s that the staff were often too busy to persevere with a patient having difficulties, and as it was migrant women usually who were planning to return to work, leaving the baby with grandparents. When she returned to interpreting at the hospital in the 1970s, it seemed like 90 per cent were breast-feeding and 'ninety-five per cent of my Lebanese girls would not even think of the bottle':

> The Lebanese are family orientated — because of the culture and religion, the wife is not allowed to go out and is there to produce children. Therefore she has to stay home, look after her children, breast-feed them and cook for the whole family.

Breast-feeding also failed because science misunderstood it. Demand feeding seemed incompatible with discipline and routine. While small and frail babies were fed three-hourly, larger babies were fed four-hourly on the dot, and when inexperienced but law-abiding mothers went home and tried to keep the hospital's — and the Infant Welfare Centre's — timetables, they ended up with either guilt, hysteria or insufficiency. The physiology of milk production and suckling were not taken as seriously as child training and home management. With the best will in the world, ward sisters and trainee midwives got it wrong too often. Cathy Hallam:

Dr Truby King: New Zealand expert on infant feeding and rearing who advocated feeding babies only on a strict schedule

> In the 1970s it was all fairly rigid, though not as rigid as it had been in the Truby King days. There were four-hourly schedules — no demand stuff at all. And for the smaller babies that would be three-hourly. I was still learning and there must have been a lot of things I missed out of ignorance. And they were always encouraging us to take note of things like mother's bonding with the baby. But I'm not sure I was very good at that.
>
> We seemed to grab the baby with one hand — I've seen it done still — grab the baby behind the neck, grab the mother's boob and go *crunch* — in one hard action. And if they didn't instantly click then I used to think — oh what do I do? I was not very good at helping and a lot of those women depended on our skill and we didn't necessarily have a lot. I guess that's a disadvantage of a teaching hospital. You have to depend on the fact that if a nurse has a lot of difficulty that they'll go and ask.

One of the shocks of midwifery nursing for most students was that the patients were well, remembers Kav:

> All our lives nursing we had been doing things for people because people were sick. When you got to midwifery, these were well women who were having a baby and you had to teach them, but you didn't have to look after them in the sense that you had to look after patients in a general hospital. They didn't *need* you and the biggest thing you

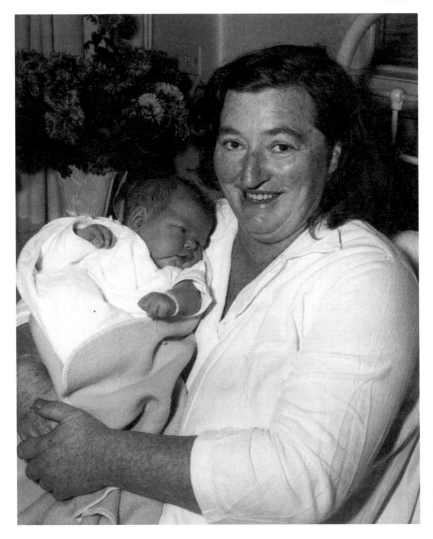

**Proud mother with her
fifteenth baby, May 1962**
RWHA

had to learn was to stop doing things. It was much quicker for us to change the baby's napkin or feed it, burp it or put it back in its cot than it was to watch the mother breast-feed it and change the napkin. We had to stop taking over and that was very hard to learn.

'Mavis', however, did need special attention because she was blind:

I was hospitalised several times before the baby was due because of blood pressure. A doctor asked me during one stay, 'Have you thought about how you're going to manage this baby?' I was extremely indignant as I am almost totally independent (though blind) and have been all my life. It never occurred to me that I wouldn't manage.

They were going to induce the baby in ten days but I went into labour early. I came into hospital and I remember going to the lounge and it all started to happen. You weren't told what was going to happen. It was all a bit of a shock and surprise. It was frightening, very frightening. Antenatal classes had not quite started yet.

My first baby had a breathing problem and I didn't see him for three days. I was crying and the sister said, 'What's wrong with you?' 'I haven't seen my baby'. They quickly brought the baby to me but after a few seconds they whipped him away. They didn't explain anything, they didn't tell you anything — he could have been dead.

My strong memories would be the helpfulness to me in the handling of my baby. When I got him back with me I said, 'Would you teach me everything about the care of the baby right from the word go'. Of course you had to be in bed but you learned to feed them, change them, bathe them.

The nursing staff were very good. I'm full of praise. They were just starting rooming in with the baby and I found that extremely good.

I was having trouble breast-feeding — he kept falling asleep. A New Zealand nurse walked out of the ward saying, 'That blind woman is hopeless': that gave me a lot of confidence. It was her technique that was hopeless. There were bath demonstrations but I had to listen to what was said around me — no one offered extra explanations.

We had to make our own beds, dress the baby, but we didn't have to get dressed, we could lie down any time. We had to keep the baby beside us all night, but one nurse, when another woman and I were having our third, said, 'You know what to do. I know I'm breaking the rules but I'm taking your babies out.' She gave us a sleeping pill and we had a good sleep.[52]

Antenatal care underwent great change, and again it was a generational transformation. Dr James Smibert was convinced that early ambulation would be better for women, especially in improving the drainage of the lochia as well as their general circulation. The age-old fear of prolapse was retreating. He worked his reforms through hand-picked charge sisters. Helen Johnstone was one:

Patients had to stay in bed two days and we'd give them wash-downs twice a day. But when I was in charge of Ward 18, Dr Smibert came to me and said that he didn't think there needed to be any more bedpans for normal midwifery and that the ladies could get straight up out of bed. So I said, 'Yes Dr Smibert'. I didn't know the hospital politics and I didn't say anything — I just got the ladies up. And when Sister —— came around on Friday lunchtime to supervise the meals serving out, as she frequently did, she did a round and I'd have to say the names: 'Mrs so-n-so, day two, she must be in the bathroom'. Well Sister hit the roof. 'These women will be fainting on you Johnstone. We'll be sued!' 'But Dr Smibert told me to.' 'You don't do anything the doctors tell you! You see me first.'

And that was the beginning of early ambulation. It made a big difference — it reduced the number of smears and cultures we had to do and resulted in fewer postnatal infections.

But nurses had many frustrations with doctors. Those who worked many years on postnatal wards became very aware of postnatal depression, yet many doctors did not recognise it. Margaret Mabbitt can remember fighting women to get paraldehyde into them. As for Helen Johnstone:

> I've had a telephone cord swung around my body — I've been twisted round and round until the phone came out of the socket — by a lady who had postnatal depression. One of the problems was getting the medical staff to see there was a problem — they wouldn't believe the nursing staff, yet we were with the patients twenty-four hours a day. The doctor would walk in for five minutes and they'd be all sweetness and smiles — no problem. So getting someone to see these women would take several days and by that time they were in a very distressed state.

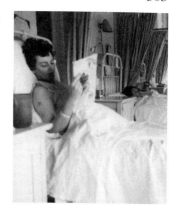

Postnatal ward *RWHA*

Many staff, including nurses, were not good at handling grief and loss in a maternity hospital, which was meant to be all about new life. Stillborn and desperately sick babies were whisked out of sight in the hope they would be soon out of mind. 'Flora"s third baby was stillborn after a birth accident:

> I went into hospital in the evening and I was swabbed. I felt I was on fire. The woman doctor was called away and never examined my stomach. She didn't see that it was breech. In my innocence I believed that my records would have been transferred from the outpatients clinic. I was put in a ten bed ward, there was one girl on duty. All the blankets were wet. I had to put on my dressing gown to keep warm. I knew something was wrong but I don't say much as a rule.
> Near daylight I couldn't lie on my back, I had to lie on my side. I called to the nurse, she got the doctor. I feel I always want to curse this bloke. While he was examining me, he said, 'It's a breech'. They didn't know in the ward that it was although it had been known for two months, because I hadn't been examined when I was brought in. I had no anaesthetic, they cut me to get the baby out. They brought the baby out and I wouldn't look. I closed my eyes. Another doctor came back and said, 'We've done all we could, but he hasn't survived'. I touched his hand and said, 'You've done what you could.' I felt I had to comfort him.
> The sister who telephoned my husband couldn't find him at work and I knew he was going home to grieve in an empty house and I burst into tears. The sister who had tried to phone ran right down the ward and held me tight. Then the social worker came round and asked me what I wanted to do with the baby — did I want a funeral. I said no — he wasn't my baby, he was a little person who had come and gone. We didn't even name him. It took me eighteen years to get over it. The cord strangled him. If they had tried to turn him the night before the labour really started . . . but he was small, only five pounds. Something else was wrong.[53]

Fear of infection, especially in the special care nursery, aggravated the problems. Women whose babies went into intensive care could suffer dreadfully, unable to visit and touch, often not being told anything much or anything at all about what was going on. Some panicked and assumed their baby had died and no one would tell them. The experience of a trainee like Cathy Hallam reveals the special qualities of those who dedicated themselves to intensive care:

> We had to do our stint in intensive care and that was very scary — we had some very sick babies with what we considered was a lot of monitoring, but by today's standards wouldn't have been. There would be two nurses — one to do obs and one to feed.
>
> I spent most of the time being frightened. And sometimes the little prems in the ordinary isolettes would stop breathing — you might be the only one in the room and you'd see one of them lying very still and going a bit blue, so you'd hit the isolette and the little thing would go WHOOF — jump up in the air, almost leap out of the bed and then back down again and start breathing. They were darling babies but I was just too anxious to enjoy it completely.

Most nurses had 'narrow squeaks' looking after babies and the stories become part of nurses' lore. Cathy again:

> I can remember having to look after a room with about eighteen babies and I would say that sixteen of the eighteen were crying or wanting to be fed and I was the only one there and it was a nightmare — a real nightmare. It was taboo to feed more than one; you had to feed them in your arms; you weren't to feed them in the cot — you'd be practically sent to Matron if you were caught doing something like that. And if the poor little thing vomited, you had to start again.
>
> In the prem ward, where you had eight babies, some of the babies were gavaged — fed by a tiny tube down the nose. You had to make sure you had the tube in the right place, because you'd been taught

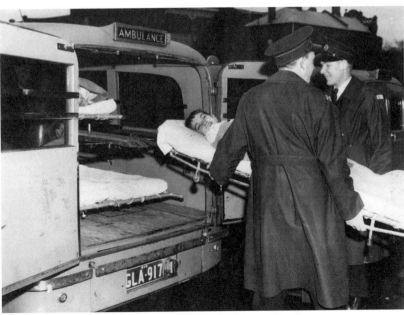

Off to Henry Pride, packed in 'like Adam's Cakes' *RWHA*

how to check and you'd think Oh hell, the baby might get a lung full of milk, what am I going to do?

It was a constant chain of feeding and changing. The poor little things had no other attention given to them really. And you'd just finished putting 30 mls down one and it would go BLURGGH and you'd have to start again.

The post-war baby boom had forced the hospital to develop both domiciliary care and its after-care annexe, Henry Pride. Trainee midwives went out with the domiciliary nurses and for Cathy Hallam it was a wonderful experience: 'they were lovely nurses, very good at what they did and I admired them a lot, not really thinking that I'd end up doing a very similar thing'. Still in the 1960s, Marg Mabbitt remembers the 'Dom' nurses taking baby clothes and blankets to destitute mothers and finding babies sleeping in drawers.

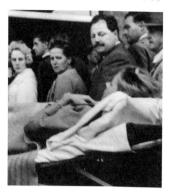

Coming in by ambulance as an emergency admission: photograph taken to publicise the lack of privacy for patients in the old building *RWHA*

Henry Pride was another world unto itself. Kav:

On night duty you worked from 8 p.m. to 6.30 a.m. and two nights a week we had lectures from 6.30 to 8. So going out to Henry Pride was like going out into the country — it was a great relief: thirteen weeks of night duty was over and you were out in the country in this beautiful garden. It was spring and all the blossoms were out.

Sometimes patients' journeys to Henry Pride were less idyllic:

In the ambulance to Henry Pride, I was on the top deck (there were four women to an ambulance). It was hot, I was waiting and waiting to be moved, it was in February, I was just about expiring, babies yelling with heat and exhaustion. We finally got to the Henry Pride and I was given a bed. There were sixteen in a ward at Henry Pride and they were partitioned into four bed sections. You ate your meals at a dining table in another room. [54]

Another patient felt she was like a rack of cakes in an Adams' delivery truck in the ambulance. But the whole atmosphere at Henry Pride was more relaxed and patients enjoyed the chance to recuperate and get to know their babies while under care. For 'Gina' it was healing after a terrifying labour: she remembers the garden, the kindness of the nurses, the baby care she learnt.[55]

'Emerge' and 'Gynae'

If the labour ward and the antenatal and postnatal wards were mostly places of new life and the triumph over illness and disability, 'emerge' or the emergency department and 'gynae' or the 'gynaecological side' saw more of the tragedies both of nature and society. Here the hospital was closer to a general hospital, yet here also the suffering that sex brought women was more starkly seen. The 1950s saw the growth of major surgery: Dr Graeme Godfrey's Wertheim operations for uterine cancer could take all day, with patients going to theatre at 8 a.m. and not returning for twelve hours. But despite antibiotics and better birth control, the pathological consequences of induced abortion continued to dominate the non-midwifery side of the Women's. Septic abortions did not start to fall significantly until 1971, after the clarifiction of the psychological and medical grounds for legal termination of pregnancy by Mr Justice Menhennit in 1969. By 1972 the clinical report could state that 'septic abortion is a rare cause for admission', and cases of Welch infection were down to four for the year. While Welch infections were averaging around twenty a year in the 1950s and 1960s, the septic ward had treated thirty-seven cases in 1961, but with no deaths; the last such death was to be in 1970.[56]

There was still the shock of what women in their desperation did to themselves: syringing the womb with Rinso, Persil, Dettol, copper sulphate solution, even flammable liquids; and one who died had a notice attached to her bed that she was 'flammable'. They douched themselves with hoses at high pressure. They inserted sticks, twigs, knitting needles, umbrella ribs into their cervixes. 'Emerge' was Kav's domain for twenty-five years:

> I can remember a fifteen-year-old girl coming in who aborted herself with an umbrella rib and she'd given herself 'Welch' — at the age of fifteen and she had to have a hysterectomy. And then her kidneys gave out. She didn't die luckily — she went across to the Royal Melbourne and was put on dialysis. She was one of the first. And it was only because of 'Bung' Hill that she survived: he'd picked it up quickly — no one would have wanted to do a hysterectomy on a fifteen-year-old, but that was her only chance to live.

Another shot herself:

> This woman had had a baby eleven months before and found she was pregnant again. She was twenty-four or twenty-six weeks, so it was too late to have an abortion. She got her husband's shot gun and shot herself in the abdomen.
>
> And I can always remember Margaret Mackie saying: 'This woman I cannot believe'. She took her to theatre and she had not damaged anything. If she had had an X-ray and a graph on the X-ray, she couldn't have done a better job. She'd shot herself through the abdomen, missed all the main arteries, ureters, the works; went through the uterus, straight through the baby's head and out through the other side. And Margaret Mackie said, 'I opened her up and all I had to do was to take the baby out and sew up the holes.'

Most of the induced abortions did not end up septic or physically traumatic, however. They required a straightforward curette, but since the Women's Hospital was the only hospital where women could walk off the street for treatment for an incomplete or threatened 'AB', the work load of the hospital was horrific. There were three theatre lists a day for D & Cs of incomplete ABs. Kav again:

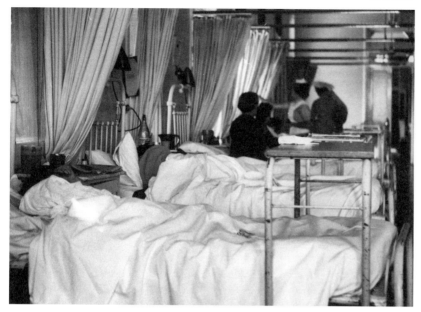

Gynaecology ward in Druids' Wing, 1960 *RWHA*

There used to be a receiving gynae resident, a receiving obstetric resident and a receiving AB resident. Every day you had a resident who did nothing but ABs. And this poor fellow once — one of his mates had told him 'For God's sake get there at the crack of dawn because you can have anything up to thirty a day. And so he arrived at the dot of 8 o'clock: 'Where are they all?' And I think we had only eight in for the whole day which was most unusual. And he thought 'This is a breeze — only eight'. And the next day they had twenty-seven incomplete ABs come. Those were the sort of numbers you had. Whereas in the last years I worked there, after the Menhennit Ruling, you'd be lucky if you'd get eight a day.

The women would walk in with their stories of falls and furniture moving. Some even brought foetuses purchased from an enterprising lady who sold them — 'Where she got them, God alone knows' — 'I passed this'.

Liliana Ferrara was also constantly on call for 'Emerge':

I had a lot of migrant women begging me to ask the doctor to terminate a pregnancy. That was heartbreaking too — because they had four children. And the idea was for her to go to work in a factory to be able to help her husband put a deposit on a house or pay off their fare. Terrible — so much debt! And all of a sudden she was expecting and she'd kneel down and beg the doctor. Nothing doing. Absolutely no.

So what happened? Because of that I was forever at Emergency Department with miscarriages. They'd never admit they'd interfered or it was interfered with God knows where — back-yard abortions. They all denied it — they push the table, they lift a mattress, they had a fall, but in fact they were abortions. I've seen women with those infections — and a couple that died too.

I was forever at Emergency — maybe two or three times a day I was called. And I've seen so many little foetuses — you've no idea — that I was able to tell eventually how far pregnant she was. They called it 'Johnny' — 'Johnny' was coming — she was bleeding with clots, and then the foetus would come out. They'd say, 'Oh yes, eight weeks, ten weeks.

The doctors used to say 'Mrs Ferrara, would you please ask her — she must tell us — did she do anything or go anywhere? There's infection — it smells infected'. They were so scared — it was done word of mouth where to go.

I remember one Greek patient who admitted that she'd terminated a pregnancy. She'd get a branch from a tree — a very fine branch — and irritate the cervix. She had about ten or twelve and she was lucky. 'Oh my God, how could you do that?' 'Oh, very easily.'

The women driven to such dangerous and dreadful acts came from all walks of life. While those who ended up septic and sick were more likely to have been unmarried and being both terrified and ignorant, had left it too long before seeking a curette, the majority of admissions for incomplete abortions which the hospital suspected were induced were still married women. A study conducted by the hospital's Social Work Department in 1956 found financial and family planning reasons dominating the motives for terminating a pregnancy. In fact research was suggesting that single women increasingly were going through with a pregnancy.[57] Of the 196 studied, only thirty-one women admitted interference, and of those only six had sought assistance: two from a doctor, two from a nurse and two from abortionists of 'unspecified qualifications'. The cost in 1956 had varied from £11 to £30, making it beyond the means of many. The other twenty-five had induced the miscarriage themselves: twenty still by syringing, plus there were, either singly or in combination, six attempts with abortifacients, three with an intra-uterine catheter, two with curettage, two with heavy exercise and only one with the traditional slippery elm bark. The thirty-one's reasons, including those who gave more than one, were:

financial difficulties	15
number of children in family (i.e. financial difficulties also)	14
fear of social stigma	14
insecurity because separated, being a de facto or single	7
marital disharmony (including drink)	6
pregnancy too soon after last child	4
pregnancy too soon after marriage	4
housing difficulties	3
fear of pregnancy	3
deserted since pregnancy occurred	2
eugenic reasons — fear of genetic abnormality	2
husband's ill health	2
husband's hostility to children	1
patient's erotic entanglement	1
pregnancy too late in life	1

The almoner was impressed by the seriousness of their plight and their responses:

> To all of these women . . . the difficulties had appeared overwhelming and few of them appeared unrealistic. None had light heartedly contemplated interference. Whenever it had been embarked upon for the first time this act had resulted from panic or from despair; the second abortion would be less anxiously planned if no complications had arisen after the first.[58]

Above all 'these women, with few exceptions, were not moved by selfish reasons, but by concern for their present and future children'. If their own health were a primary concern, that too would affect their families; and the single were acutely aware of the repercussions of the pregnancy on their families. Few also felt a sense of loss or genuine guilt: for all the distress and fear of procuring a termination, their overwhelming sentiment was relief.[59]

Of the one hundred former patients interviewed for this history, eleven admitted to having had a termination: six were Australian-born and three of those sought terminations because of life-threatening complications of pregnancy: eclampsia and hyperemesis. The remaining five were all immigrants, two being Holocaust victims and displaced persons, fearful of not being allowed into Australia if they had children. Others were caught in the emotional and financial dislocations of flight from Europe and finding their feet in a new society. Two others of the eleven had become pregnant to their fiancés and just two were unlucky from affairs. One Australian had three young children and her husband on sustenance in the Depression. Their experiences ranged from the safe and expensive Collins Street specialist abortion in private rooms, to being syringed by a relative or catheterised illegally. One woman had a nervous breakdown afterwards, having found herself septic and bleeding in the Queen Victoria Hospital. Many had degrading and brutal experiences.

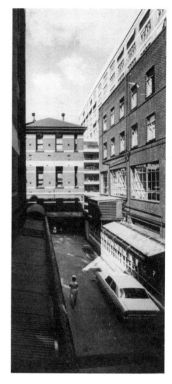

Courtyard *RWHA*

If there were so many conceiving babies they could not afford to bear, there were also some who were not able to conceive the babies they wanted. The 1950s were a decade awash with babies and the infertile suffered acutely. Phantom pregnancies were not uncommon and they would come into the labour ward screaming '"It's coming, it's coming" and be all blown up'. One old prostitute, who preyed on innocent young men, had it down to a fine art, remembers Sheila Haynes: 'She'd tell them in the morning that they'd got her pregnant and if he didn't pay up, she'd go down to the Women's and tell them. She'd get herself all blown up, holding breath, and the doctor knew her of old and would try to get her to take a breath: "General anaesthetic nurse" — and she upped and walked out'. It seemed to the nurses that migrant couples suffered especially when they were unable to have children: 'sterility for the migrants was a terrible thing', recalls Liliana. Many husbands would not countenance adopting 'someone else's bastard'. For the men, it was often the only time they received some respect; for the women pregnancy was the only time that their husbands made no sexual demands. Later in her career, Sheila began to understand that there were men who were always 'at their wives', giving them a respite only in pregnancy:

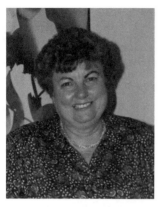

Marlene Kavanagh
RWHA

In the '70s in the Greek community, we still have some women we admitted over night when there was nothing wrong with them. But they knew that if they put on a big scene and came on, we would at least keep them for the night — to find out. It was psychology. But in the 1950s there was no psychology — it was fact or it was fiction. And those poor infertile women — there was no help for them. But to have this moment of glory — I've been to the maternity hospital. At least the neighbours might think 'She is' or 'she was'.

And while many proxy marriages became love matches, others were emotional and sexual disasters. Kav:

Do you remember 'Sophie', the Greek proxy bride who literally from the day she was pregnant, vomited and spent the entire pregnancy in ward 14. And the moment they'd say — she hasn't vomited for three days, the girls would catch her vomiting again. She said later that she hated her husband — proxy bride to a fellow she didn't even know, and the moment the boat hit the shore, she hated his guts, and this was her way out.

But it was perhaps 'Emerge' where life in the raw was more visible. It could be dangerous. Kav was assaulted by a Spanish woman who had refused to have an interpreter:

A nice doctor, a woman, began to examine her and she went berserk — tried to strangle the doctor with her stethoscope. I got the doctor out and asked, 'What have we done, why are you so upset?' and with that she took her umbrella to me and bashed me and spat at me. She lifted the bedrails off and broke them. Broke the Agar plates we had in there. One of the doctors rang security only to get the message that all the security had gone to lunch. She then went out and to this day we don't know why she did it.

I was very badly bruised and I got quite upset because no one had ever done that before in all the time I'd worked in the department. We'd had people who were a bit strange, but they'd never attacked any of the staff.

The nurses grieved with those who lost their babies, especially those they had nursed for weeks antenatally, but they coped with much of the dramatic and bizarre with black humour. Kav again:

It has to be black humour or else you wouldn't survive. I think of the laughs we used to get out of poor 'Penelope' who used to come out of Royal Park mental hospital and she was right off her tree. 'Penelope' had no perception of personal space — she'd nose to nose you. She'd drive us mad. She'd come in and say, 'I want a hysterectomy'.

'Penelope. You know we don't do hysterectomies on Mondays — they're only done on Fridays'.

'Oh all right then — can I have a baby?'

But that's how you had to cope with them.

VII

Transformations
1970–1996

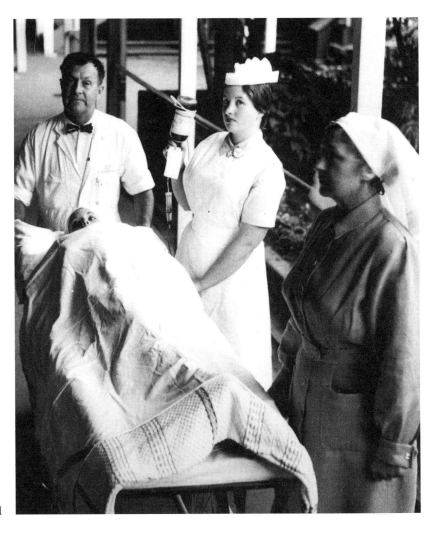

Hospital scene *RWHA*

Values *14*

In 1958 Percy Rogers came to the Women's as a medical student:

> I recall going on a ward round with a consultant and there was a full
> entourage of the lord, his faithful retainer, his third in command and a
> rag taggle of students with bum freezers on. And we were standing
> around the bed of a woman whose baby had died. It had died and the
> cervix had clamped around the neck — it was a prem breech birth.
> And the method of extracting this was to put weights on the end of
> the baby's legs, hang them over the end of the bed, then adjust the
> weights and let the cervix dilate up slowly. He described this in
> graphic detail standing around the bed — the poor woman sobbing her
> heart out. And us standing there unable to express sympathy with the
> patient and I felt it was a brutal thing to do.
>
> This was my first introduction to obstetrics and I felt it was
> absolutely appalling, so I was determined when I entered practice to
> endeavour to do something about this.[1]

For all its efficiency and achievements, the Women's Hospital was still
erratic in its psychic treatment of patients. There were kindly staff and
moments of genuine compassion, but there were also unacceptable lapses
of empathy and sensitivity, sins of omission more often than of commission by busy professionals simply not aware that a patient was embarrassed by a lack of privacy, or hurt by an off-hand remark, or grieving,
or simply lonely and frightened. These were failures of moral imagination, deficiencies of fellow feeling which had their origin in the class
and gender divisions which persisted in the prosperous 1960s and 1970s.
If the Queen Victoria Hospital had its own peculiarities, it was none the
less softer in its treatment of patients, more respectful of them as women
than its rival up the road.

Other medical students and pupil midwives were more fortunate than
Percy Rogers in their first experience of labour ward, and many were

captivated by the processes of birth. For medical students their time at the Women's was their first hands-on experience, the first chance to become involved with a patient and to follow one of the great moments of human existence. Some fell in love with obstetrics for life, but many did feel uneasy about the military efficiency of the place, the assumption of Anglo-Saxon ascendancy, the class distinctions and the deep conservatism of the hospital's hierarchies.

By the early 1960s it was an immense institution to run effectively. It had over 11 000 midwifery admissions annually and delivered around 7000 babies. Well over a thousand babies were admitted to the premature or sick babies' wards each year. More than a third of the patients were born overseas, with those from non-English-speaking countries outnumbering the British. It was still the leading obstetric and gynaecological teaching hospital in Victoria, and under the leadership of Professor Lance Townsend from 1951 until 1977, its research and teaching grew in stature and extent. Townsend was a gifted teacher and he was determined that the Women's hold a place among the leading specialist teaching hospitals of the world. He also placed it at the centre of obstetrics and gynaecology for the region, personally monitoring standards of practice, advising doctors in private practice or peripheral or rural hospitals.[2] Over time, he had taught so many Victorian doctors that his personal relationships enabled him to form a network of informally integrated care throughout the state. A cytology unit had begun in 1958 after Hans Bettinger returned from an overseas study tour, and in 1960 an endocrine unit was established with the appointment of an endocrinologist through the professorial unit. Joining forces with the fertility and sterility clinic which had started in 1945, this was the beginning of the reproductive biology research which would capture the limelight in the 1980s. By 1966 the professorial unit was able to report significant success in the induction of ovulation.[3] In 1963 the new professorial unit was opened. To support the growing research culture in the hospital, a medical librarian was appointed in 1960 and the Marshall Allan Library opened the following year. A long-serving generation was reaching retirement age and Townsend recruited young Australian talent and overseas expertise. He was a shrewd judge of academic potential and protected new staff from the domination of senior staff now set in their ways. The research culture blossomed and it became an exciting place to work. The second half of the 1960s saw the first successes with the anti-D immune globulin in rhesus-immunised women; the coming of the laparoscope and endoscope in the late 1960s which would revolutionise abdominal surgery and knowledge of internal structures and conditions; ultrasound; and in 1970, the computerisation of medical records, facilitating epidemiological research as well as improving efficiency.

The Women's remained deeply conservative socially, however. The big teaching hospitals were all dominated by cliques of senior staff who came from restricted circles of Melbourne society. The same small group of boys' private schools had educated most of the doctors. Many were sons of doctors, some sons of former honoraries at the same hospital. Unselfconsciously, the old boys cherished those bonds and caused far more offence than they ever realised when they inquired of each new resident,

medical student, even pupil midwife: 'And where did you go to school?'
Nowhere was this more entrenched than at the Women's, where the honoraries formed, as the Annual Report boasted in 1962, a 'strong social
and traditional bond such as exists in no other hospital in Australia'.[4]
Much was due to 'the personality' of Dr Arthur Hill, the social secretary,
and Dr Colin Macdonald, the hospital historian. The Tracy Maund dinners
were famous and the honorary staff had their own cellar. Their world
was far from that of their patients. Politically most were anti-Labor, one
exception being Don Lawson who openly campaigned against nuclear
weapons.[5] The older members accepted no professional authority over
them other than that of their peers and their college: a patient might
legitimately make a request, but never a demand or a condition. Their
medical authority was absolute and their dedication to healing and pre-
serving life could, *in extremis,* exempt them from respect for a patient's
self-hood and autonomy. They were people accustomed to giving orders
and having them obeyed; they were also people capable of undertaking
awesome responsibilities, of tackling problems that most ordinary mor-
tals shrink from, of taking very hard decisions. They lived on a chronic
shortage of sleep and they lived with the fear that one slip, one lapse of
attention, one moment of carelessness could cost a life. Their wives and
children saw little of them; they were for the most part people obsessed
with medicine.

They took very seriously the obligations and duties of an honorary
appointment. They prided themselves on being on call for their public

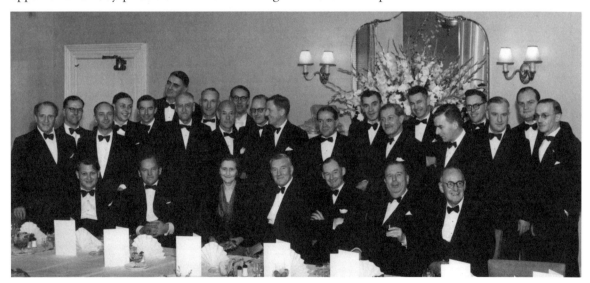

Honorary medical staff dinner
Back from left: Drs Hans Bettinger, Alwyn Long, Barry Kneale,
Tom Madison, Eric Mackay, John Laver, Colin Macdonald, Vernon
Hollyhock, A. M. ('Bung') Hill, Professor Lance Townsend, Gordon
Ley, Don Lawson, Bruce Anderson, Noel De Garis, Bill Rawlings,
Kelvin Churches, Kevin McCaul, Frank Forster, Ronald Rome,
Paul Jeffrey, James Smibert
Front: J. W. Johnstone, Harold Hattam, Kate Campbell, George
Simpson, John Colebatch, George Bearham, Bill Lemmon *RWHA*

patients, and many women who were seriously ill were surprised that the specialist came to see them at 3 in the morning. They came only when needed, and in fact, to the gratification of the nursing staff, remembers Margaret Peters, the honoraries rarely interfered, the resident medical staff were too busy, so the midwives and nurses had the wards and the patients to themselves.[6] If the honorary staff enjoyed privileges and prestige on account of their position, it was a justifiable reward for their honorary service to the hospital. And the patients should be grateful for the favour done them. Not all senior doctors were at ease in the culture, nor were all younger practitioners welcome to join, so new blood with different ideas found it difficult to enter the magic circle. At least one such young practitioner, who was to have one of the most profound effects on the hospital's practice from the mid-1970s, found it very difficult to obtain his initial appointment.

The nursing structure also was inevitably conservative. This vast hospital was run by a small core of staff nurses, most of whom stayed for decades and who had the unusual distinction of enjoying an internal promotional structure. But their role was supervisory and educational: the midwifery section actually operated on the labour of students — a workforce that arrived in four staggered cohorts a year. Margaret Peters remembers it as 'students everywhere', because the hospital had the biggest midwifery school in the country. One night she did 'eighteen double scrubs', that is eighteen times she had to scrub up and take a learner through a delivery. Margaret Mabbitt remembers doing so many in a shift that she could be interrupted in her spiel to a student to attend to another problem, and then with prompting, pick up from the exact word where she left off. And still they had to be ready to deal with extreme emergencies: women in 'high-risk, diabolical situations, who required a lot of care in difficult surroundings'. Engraved on Margaret Peters' memory is the woman who was brought in by ambulance from the hills:

> We knew she was coming and we knew she was APH, probably placenta praevia. And we put her on to the bed and had a look at her. She didn't look that good. We pulled back the blankets and she'd actually delivered the placenta and the baby after it. I've never seen anything like it — and she lived!

Fewer and fewer women died in childbirth — in 1961–62, none at all for the first time since 1858, but when women did die, the staff were devastated and still grieve for women who died thirty years ago. Pulmonary and amniotic fluid embolisms were now the leading cause of death, and so seemingly unjust in their happening suddenly and without warning.[7] The technical skill of the midwifery staff was outstanding, but the physical and administrative structure of this great, old hospital made a more relaxed and sensitive approach to normal childbirth very difficult. The hospital was softening, none the less, with restrictions on adult visitors to obstetrical patients lifted in 1958, and those on children in 1963. By 1964 the administration had awakened to the value of multilingual pamphlets for the visiting public, and so they were in German, French, Italian, Polish, Hungarian and Greek.

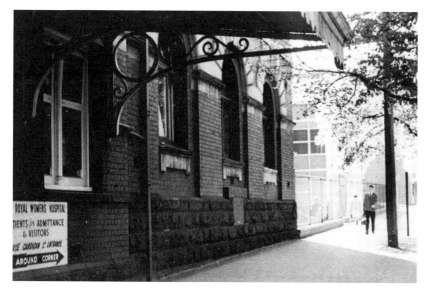

Grattan Street entrance, children's play centre behind wire *RWHA*

The student workforce was kept in control with strict uniform and conduct rules, a regimen which seemed to forget that they were already registered nurses, many with experience in intensive care or casualty. Netta McArthur, coming to the hospital in 1979, was astounded: 'the students were treated as though they were beginning student nurses': they could not check drugs even though under the law they were qualified; they were reinstructed in basics like taking blood pressure.

> The whole atmosphere of the place was like the military — they all had these tied-up brown shoes with five holes in them — good, sensible shoes on their feet. Half of them were still in veils, and wearing nurses' uniforms and caps working in management.
>
> It was controlling — the unit managers, or charge nurses as they were called, were afraid to make decisions to change any procedures. They had to ask permission of the School of Nursing or senior nurses in administration. It was outdated — the controls over the rosters, the patient care. The whole atmosphere of the place was less than friendly. And they all called themselves by their surnames.
>
> The doctors in their own way were the same, although they never saw themselves that way.[8]

The senior nursing administration had a fierce dedication to women, especially poor, disadvantaged women, and an equally strong loyalty to the nursing profession. But the matron's contract placed her under the authority of the medical superintendent and she did not have a place on the Board of Management. Every effort at reform was inevitably a power struggle, so the strategies for coping with large numbers of patients and student staff remained military rather than civilian. There was genuine interest in change and in patient welfare, but there was no process for change, and during the 1960s the building of a new hospital took precedence over any strategy for the future.

Preparation had begun in the 1950s and the master building plan was completed by 1960. Building commenced in 1964, part occupation took place in 1968 and the completed complex was officially opened as the 3AW Community Block in 1972. In a time of rapid social change in private life and public values, the hospital that faced the future brand new in the 1970s conceptually was a product of the 1950s. By the time it was opened it was already old-fashioned. No one envisaged the end of the midwifery school, therefore it would continue to be staffed by students who required constant surveillance. Accordingly, although the new hospital recognised that women's strongest desire was for privacy in labour, viewing windows were placed between the single labour wards, walls were merely partitions and everything was within lines of sight of the charge sister if the curtains in the four-bed wards were drawn aside. With babies rooming-in, it was very noisy. And for efficiency in the labour ward the woman's perineum faced the door, so that if she was delivering as you opened the door, that is what you saw at once. As they admit now, the staff were so used to naked perineums that they simply ceased to realise that the patients minded. Nursing was still all about control — control of staff and control of patients. The staffing and management of the new hospital was done very well, however, because the matron, Betty Lawson, had engaged the services of a senior nursing educator, Jean Headberry, to review all nursing tasks and find a more rational division of labour. The Women's was finally given permission to abandon broken shifts — and have three shifts a day rather than two. There was now a central sterilisation unit so that ward staff no longer spent time auto-claving everything. Gone were the multi-bed labour wards: now with single wards perhaps husbands could be with their wives in labour. Betty Lawson also fought for the public wards to have new furniture: in every way the new hospital was to be new and morale rose accordingly.

More progressive doctors saw the move to the new hospital as an opportunity to reshape the nursing style of midwifery. A memo to the Honorary Staff argued that while the statistics suggested that technical standards were high, there remained 'a large, and in this hospital, unex-plored area in which great improvement can be anticipated and that is in the emotional support of the labouring mother'. It went on:

> The architecture of the old hospital is such that there is no close relation-ship between the staffs in the labour ward and the antenatal/postnatal complexes. Those of us who were alive at the time will recollect the marked improvement in the medical supervision of the patients when the medical unit system was introduced in 1951. However, there has been no comparable change in the nursing organisation and it is to the nurse who is continually in attendance in the labour ward that the labouring mother looks for emotional support. It is obvious that standards in this respect fall far short of those desirable. Efforts to continue techniques learnt in the relaxation classes have failed because of nursing staff resistance and lack of co-operation with the physiotherapists who have retired dismayed from the labour ward. This situation probably stems from the innate con-servatism of the labour ward staff and the fact that sisters remain too long in labour ward and, although becoming technically proficient, develop impersonal attitudes and become cortically deaf to the woman distressed in labour.[9]

The medical staff had a mixed agenda, however. Not only did they want a modern facility, with five floors of the new tower block each comprising a miniature maternity hospital complete unto itself serving each week-day clinic, but they wanted to bring private practice to the public institutions. They wanted their gravest private cases to have access to the expertise and equipment of the teaching hospital. But they also saw parsimoniousness and insensitivity as the legacy of 'workhouse' medicine, of the paupers' infirmary. They wanted to elevate the tone of the public hospital by including private patients and they wanted to be able to recruit future private patients from the public patients they attended without fee. The structure of Australian society was changing. The desperate poverty of the past had retreated and the time had come for public hospitals to serve a wider cross-section of the community, including those whose taxes sustained public health care. There were simply not enough private maternity beds available for the increasing numbers of women who did not qualify financially for a public bed.[10] Above all, the costs of health care now exceeded the fund-raising capacities of the old self-supporting hospitals: the distinction between public and private had blurred. In 1961 the Hospital and Charities Commission permitted the Women's to introduce 'intermediate beds' where a patient could be delivered by her own doctor, and all at once, doctors became more of a presence in the labour ward and births had to be delayed while the doctor was sent for. Midwives felt threatened, but still were in command of public patients. By 1964 the medical staff were still dissatisfied, especially by the fact that the Women's was now the only public hospital which did not have special wards for intermediate and private patients. The Hospital won the approval, but not the full financial support of the Hospitals and Charities Commission, for the building of a three-floor private hospital on top of the planned nine-floor main block.[11]

The doctors had clear ideas of what their private hospital should be like: that is, in every way different from the public hospital. It should have a special name, something historical and refined. The food, the furniture, the décor, the cutlery, the crockery and the linen, all had to be

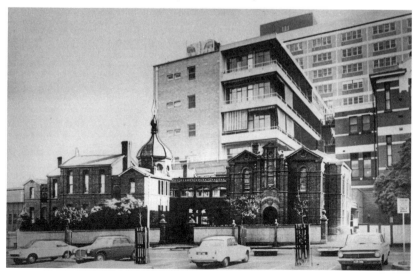

The new 3AW Community Service Block (1965–1969), with the old Genevieve Ward Wing (1888) superimposed. The Professorial Unit (1961) is to the left, the Gertrude Kumm Wing (1941) in the middle and the Edward Wilson Wing (1917) on the right. *RWHA*

distinctive and superior. The matron had to be different and new: she needed 'a pleasant personality' and 'business acumen'. Student midwives were to keep their distance, only registered midwives could attend the patients and each ward was to have three charge sisters on duty. Doctors expected to be called for all patient care. Private patients were to have priority in theatre bookings and husbands were to be admitted to labour wards 'when considered desirable'. On the top floor, luxury suites were built with adjoining bedrooms so that husbands or relatives could stay while a wealthy private patient had a delicate operation.[12] Frances Perry House opened on 2 November 1979, commemorating the Bishop's pious wife who had dreamed of a lying-in establishment for the married but homeless. When they planned it, there was no government restriction on what private patients could be charged, so that luxury could be profitable. This way the Royal Women's Hospital could serve all women, and be elevated from a charity hospital to a renowned hospital. As Australia advanced, the public sector would probably shrink. More intermediate patients would occupy once public beds and those public beds should be of a higher quality; private medicine would have lodged itself firmly in the public system, and the stigma of poverty and immorality erased from the public image of their institution.

The growth of private medicine on the premises began to affect the practices of the whole hospital. Intermediate and private patients were more likely to have caesarean sections, but then many had chosen a specialist obstetrician precisely because complications were expected. But between 1958 and 1976 the incidence of forceps doubled and the rate of caesarean section among public patients trebled, and in both the turning point came in the early 1970s with the opening of the new hospital and of Frances Perry House. But the most significant driving force was a change of attitude towards the desirability of prolonged labours. In his 1970 Clinical Report, Professor Townsend deplored the fact that 251 patients were in labour over 36 hours and 560 over 20 hours and committed the hospital to reducing the incidence. Of 1974 he reported: 'It is disturbing to note that 8.3 per cent of public patients had a prolonged labour . . . [while in] intermediate and private patients it varies between 3.4 per cent and 5.7 per cent'. The standards of private care had begun to raise the expectations of public care: labours of more than 24 hours could now 'rarely be justified under modern conditions'.[13]

But the hospital was no longer mistress of her own fate: no more a world unto itself. It found itself acted upon by forces from outside: political directive, governmental regulation and social change. The government and society were increasingly having a say in the practices and performance of the institution. As public hospitals, especially the old ones with deep historical roots, became steadily more dependent on both state and federal funding, they relinquished with each reform another piece of their autonomy. Coalition governments, both state and federal, had also endeavoured to force public patients to contribute more towards their medical care, but nothing seemed more threatening than the spectre of 'nationalisation' of medicine. The Labor Party had a new, educated, middle-class leader in Gough Whitlam, and national reform to health care took a prominent place in the revived Labor platform by 1969. The Australian

Medical Association feared that the proposed National Health Service would reduce medical practitioners to being 'quasi-public servants' and stimulate an overuse of clinical time, hospital beds and pharmaceuticals by both doctors and patients who no longer understood and appreciated the costs involved.[14] The new Royal Women's Hospital could not have been built without government assistance and this new relationship must lead to the modernisation of staffing. The Royal Children's Hospital had led the way with the abolition of the honorary system and the appointment of salaried senior staff; the Royal Women's was now the last of the great public hospitals to be contemplating this drastic break with a long and distinguished past. In almost every sphere, it was proving to be the public hospital most resistant to the forces of reform.

It had a close rival always in the Queen Victoria Hospital, but the Queen Vic also had its rigidities. Gytha Betheras had come down from Brisbane where women were not being appointed in obstetrics, to a residency at the Queen Vic. There the honorary staff networked: a decision would be made about the method of delivery of a second twin, and every doctor in the hospital would adhere to that practice until the policy changed. When Gytha moved to the Women's in 1957 with its five individual clinics with two doctors each, she discovered there were ten different ways of delivering a second twin. She found the male anarchy refreshing and more stimulating, however much she admired the Queen Vic women.[15] But since 1965 the Queen Vic had become part of the new Monash University Medical School, a modern medical course with a focus on social medicine and, under the leadership of Professor Carl Wood, it took the initiative in new thinking about childbirth practices, hospital care and women's reproductive health.

Even so, it was responding after the event to the profound changes in sexual behaviour and self-realisation which marked the beginnings of the second wave of feminism. The media and the pundits were quick to historicise it as 'the sexual revolution' — a sudden sexual freedom made possible by the new oral contraceptive 'pill'.[16] Field trials had begun in 1956 and the pill reached Australia in 1960. The first major clinical trials in Australia began to be published in 1962, with the Crown Street Women's Hospital in Sydney and private practitioners leading the way. Significantly the Crown Street report commented that it was 'never our intention to start a general contraceptive clinic', because Australian women's hospitals simply did not see themselves as having such a role in the community.[17] The results of the first trials were impressive: the contraceptive effectiveness was outstanding, the side-effects tolerable to most women, and the method aesthetically very pleasing.[18] Contraceptive advice was only given at the Women's when another pregnancy posed a medical risk to the woman's health, so that the 'pill' was mostly used for the regulation of dysfunctional bleeding. The pill was not eligible for pharmaceutical benefits and it was available only on prescription. Women had to ask their private doctors for it and few doctors felt comfortable about prescribing it for those unmarried women who had the nerve to ask. It cost them in 1965 five shillings a month. Its ease, its biological subtlety, its effectiveness provoked immediate anxiety in those opposed to all birth control. As the thalidomide tragedy unfolded during 1961–62, people

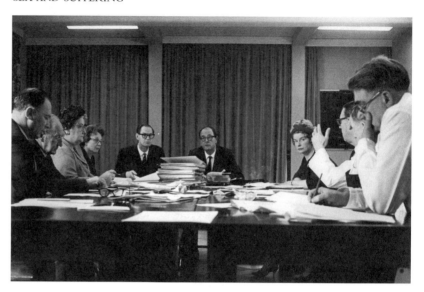

Finance Committee:
A. J. Cunningham,
manager, fifth from left
and Dr John Laver,
medical superintendent,
far right.
Mark Strizic, RWHA

became more fearful of the effects of drugs on the biology of reproduction: one Sydney pathologist warned that 'a certain popular contraceptive pill at present in use could possibly have more serious effects than
nuclear fallout on the health of unborn Australians'.[19] It became a debate
between Catholics and Protestants, in the *Medical Journal of Australia*, with
remarkable attention to theology and to the growing awareness of world
over-population. Almost none of this 'pill' discourse from doctors of the
1960s was about women and their rights to control over their reproductive lives.[20]

There was a new element in the contraceptive discourse after 1966:
the deleterious effects on unwanted children of parental stress, psychological incapacity and above all poverty. The work of Dr Dora Bialestock
and Drs Bob and John Birrell on neglected children and the 'battered
baby syndrome' distressed both the medical and wider communities.[21]
Their work was to become repeated referent points in public debate about
contraception, abortion, and adoption of illegitimate or neglected children. In 1968 Carl Wood delivered a remarkable lecture at the annual
general meeting of the Queen Vic: and when published the following
year, it was the first time in the history of Australia's medical literature
that a university professor of obstetrics and gynaecology could openly
affirm that making babies is a good thing, but so also was making love
and that 'we may and should make love, if no baby was intended'. All
babies should be planned and wanted. And the most ethical way to ensure
that was to prevent conception; however, there were situations where
'abortion is acceptable'. Some methods of contraception were morally
preferable and that was because they were aesthetically more acceptable,
not because they were 'artificial' or might 'interfere with a normal biological process'; for 'all medicine is an interference with natural biological
processes, using or outwitting them in either case for the sake of humanly
chosen ends'. Finally, such matters were matters for the private conscience,
and no one has the right to 'deprive their neighbours of their freedom
and responsibility to follow their conscience'. Central to his case was the

social and personal damage wrought by social problems which had their origin in our sexuality.[22]

Notwithstanding the impediments both moral and material placed in their way, Australian women soon became the greatest per capita users of oral contraceptives in the world. But it was not simply because of their relative affluence and their educational levels, it was also because birth control had remained difficult and unreliable. Contraceptives of all sorts were still hard to get in many parts of the country and were still expensive. Many rural pharmacists were reluctant to sell them, or sold them at the back door as though they were illegal, even though contraceptives had never been banned in Australia. If there was a sexual revolution in the 1960s, there had also been one in the 1950s when the parents of the baby boomers, through reading, decided that they wanted a modern, fulfilled marriage and not one of 'doing without' like their parents had done to control the size of their families. There were more conceptions in the 1950s partly because married couples were having more sex. Abortion remained an unspoken reality of Australian life, except that in the 1950s and early 1960s more middle-class married women were finding themselves forced to terminate a fifth or sixth pregnancy because they thought four children was a good family size and what they could afford. There were also too many young single girls who arrived in a dreadful state in emergency departments and still, in the 1960s, they died. The last woman to die of a *Clostridium welchii* post-abortal infection at the Women's died in 1970.[23] There were doctors who specialised in abortion and some were forced to pay protection money to police as the later Beach Inquiry revealed; but there were many other leading gynaecologists who performed non-therapeutic D & C's privately. One such practitioner estimated that 60 per cent of his private middle-class patients had had a pregnancy terminated.

For Catholic women, exhausted after seven, eight or nine pregnancies in almost as many years, a prescription of the pill for 'irregular bleeding' brought both intense relief and guilt. In the years before the Pope issued 'Humanae Vitae', many such women felt the church was sufficiently ambiguous in its messages for them to risk it; those who continued on the pill after it was proscribed resigned themselves to missing communion for years. Many Catholic marriages fell short of the ideal of Christian love: as one admitted, after failing with the rhythm method, they had to resort to 'twin beds'.[24] The one hundred former patients interviewed revealed that they had controlled their fertility in many ways: abstinence, withdrawal, prolonged breast-feeding, the rhythm and Billings methods, syringing, cocoa butter and quinine pessaries, diaphragms, sea sponges, condoms, the pill, sterilisation and abortion. Three non-Catholic working-class women who had known great poverty were all opposed to birth control and had never used it. Another three simply wanted many children and never bothered. One Catholic had argued with her priest and then took her own initiative; another, so fearful of repeated miscarriage after six of them that her marriage suffered, resorted to sterilisation amidst great guilt: 'My religion tells me no, but my heart tells me yes'. Italian and Greek husbands relied on coitus interruptus: 'The pill came too late for us. We didn't enjoy much the sex. Always I tell my husband, 'Be careful, be careful, be careful'.[25]

Those wanting to try the pill, took to it at once, only for many to find the side-effects of these early high-dose pills unacceptable. But for some it was a complete transformation:

> At age thirty-nine I began to use the pill. I was one of the first to use it — about 1960. My doctor rang each day to see how I was, blood pressure, smear tests etc. They were looking for side-effects. But it was wonderful. I felt so fit. I had no premenstrual tension. I took the pill all the time until my husband died. I think it was the most marvellous thing that has ever been invented. I thought I could enjoy sex so much more.[26]

For Gytha Betheras, as a gynaecologist who has specialised in family planning and sexual counselling, the pill marked the true beginning of women's biological emancipation: 'It was the answer to a woman's prayer. I don't think we'd have had the freedom to go to work, even to be feminists if it were not for what contraception, especially hormonal oral contraception has done'. The Hospital was quick to blame the pill in 1965 for the first significant fall in confinements in decades, although it also acknowledged the roles of rising affluence and private insurance.[27] However, the pill took longer to reach the poor and the inexperienced. In a landmark study for Australia in 1969 Carl Wood led a multi-disciplinary survey of two hundred mothers delivered at the Queen Victoria Hospital and discovered an alarming degree of both ignorance and neglect of contraception in premarital sex: fully one third knew nothing of birth control on starting to have coitus, and of all methods used, 77 per cent were dependent on the male. They also found pre-marital intercourse to be more common with women with a high libido.[28] (To quote one of the 'One hundred former patients' — one who became pregnant before marriage in the time before motor cars and motel rooms: 'You'd go off in the bush. Take a blanket. Where there's a will there's a way'.[29]) An even more ambitious study published two years later also revealed working-class women delivering in public hospitals to be poorly informed about birth control. Sixty-four per cent used some form of contraception, the most common method now being the pill (60 per cent), followed by withdrawal (37 per cent — this was the method chosen by 58 per cent of immigrants but only 25 per cent of Australians). Despite the fact that 23 per cent of the Australians and 47 per cent of the immigrants were Roman Catholics (36 per cent of the whole sample), merely 10 per cent used no birth control entirely for religious reasons. The overwhelming reason for using contraception was economic (64 per cent) and the dominant reason for not using it was a desire for a larger family (45 per cent).[30] These women appeared to be still in the old pattern of having their desired family in a hurry, and turning to birth control only when the family was completed. But the difficulty in obtaining professional advice continued.

The new interest in the social aspects of health and medical practice had also penetrated the Royal Women's Hospital and more such research was being undertaken. But the Board of Management also began to influence the interests of the hospital. As hospital management became more complex and medicine more scientific, the lay women on the Board were distanced from the work of the hospital. Their principal means of contact with the world of the patients was vicariously through the Social Work department. This was not always appropriate and at times intrusive, but it was work the Board thought it understood. It helped, however, with one of the hospital's greatest successes in the foster care scheme. Between 1955 and 1964 the proportion of the hospital's deliveries of single women had doubled, reaching 15 per cent. By 1968 it was 19 per cent, and the hospital could not place all the babies available for adoption, especially after the new Adoption Act reduced the number of adoption agencies. The babies could not be kept in the nurseries for weeks or even months — the costs were prohibitive and carers were now more aware of the emotional damage done to babies who were never cuddled or talked to. Valerie Douglas of the Social Work department organised a network of women who took babies into their home on a voluntary basis to care for them until they could be adopted, and among the keenest foster mothers was Mrs Joy Snedden, a member of the Board and the wife of a young government minister.[31]

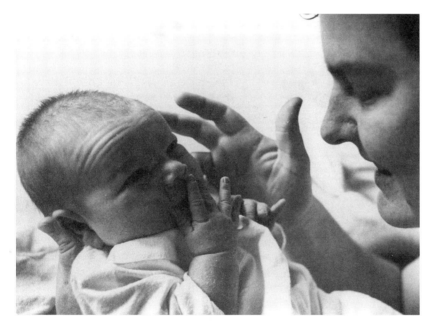

Mother and baby
Mark Strizic, RWHA

The Board also attracted women with a real concern for their fellow woman, and Dame Mabel Coles was a patron of the Family Planning Association. Thus pressure from Board members combined with the march of social change in the outside world, and the growing call for more public provision, persuaded the executive medical staff to overcome their traditional self-image as providers only of tertiary care while 'lesser doctors' attended to the everyday issues of health, sickness and living.[32] In November 1969 they resolved that the Royal Women's Hospital provide a Family Planning Clinic, and the medical superintendent, Gad Trevaks, asked Gytha Betheras whether she would lead it. It opened in May 1971 staffed by a group of women doctors who became known as

'Gytha's girls', and they were soon very busy: booking 120 on a Thursday and seeing eighty of them. The effects were immediate and dramatic: in a period where the Victorian birth rate dropped just 1.9 per cent, the Royal Women's birth rate dropped 18 per cent, while over eighteen months, that of the Queen Vic's post-natal patients who attended their family planning clinic, the birth rate dropped 40 per cent.[33]

The growing sexual freedom was more noticeable — and alarming to some — because it was visible in the middle class. But it was again only part of wider changes, ripples reaching Australia from the United Kingdom and the United States, which were strengthened by the expansion of higher education for both young men and women. Commonwealth scholarships and teaching studentships had been bringing working-class and lower middle-class young people in large numbers into the universities for the first time in Australian history. The suburban middle class were beginning to travel overseas and vast numbers of young people spent working holidays abroad. Young people could afford to leave home before they married; the standard of living continued to rise. There came a feeling of expansion, of adventure, except that for young men there was the prospect of conscription for the war in Vietnam. Political consciousness between the triumphant visit of American President Johnson in 1966 and the anti-Vietnam moratoriums of 1970 was quite transformed, and alongside that change of allegiance among the middle-class young and some of their parents were transformations in sexual behaviour, personal identity and religious adherence. American west coast cultural experiments began to affect young Australians quite as much as the Hollywood romance had since the 1930s, and integral to the whole baggage of self-realisation, natural living, spiritual and sensual freedom, creativity and holism — the full reaction against advanced industrial urban society — was a critique of the medicalisation of childbirth.

Again the movement to reform the human birth experience for both mother and baby had a longer history than merely from the 1960s. Numerous philosophers, reformers and zealots had railed against the unnaturalness of pain and suffering in what surely was the supremely natural event of human life. From Mary De Garis' theories of painless childbirth published in 1930, to Grantly Dick-Read just before the war, doctors had argued that pain was caused by fear and tension. Percy Rogers was impressed by a book by three doctors from the Soviet Union on pyschoprophylaxis. A French obstetrician, Lamaze, watched Russian women give birth with the method and burst into tears. He brought it back to France and began practising it in a metal workers' clinic. It was controversial, but in 1956 it was blessed by the Pope at an international congress of obstetricians and gynaecologists in Rome, and it spread widely through the Catholic world: 'One up for the Cold War' says Percy. A remarkable physiotherapist, Mrs Frame, began to train Melbourne physiotherapists and in 1962 Percy Rogers started his own classes. The purpose of the classes was to give the birthing process back to the couple: the husband was there as a partner in the labour ward; with panting and controlled breathing there was no need for routine analgesics although they were always given if required; there was no shaving and no enema. His practice was in Coburg and his working-class patients were unaccustomed to asking for things, but once aware of what he was offering, they were quite as keen as the middle-class women, now more educated and confident than ever before, who had begun to expect more of their obstetricians. There were many sceptics, especially among the obstetricians, but there was a growing recognition that women's feelings in labour mattered, and that a traumatic birth experience followed by insensitive postnatal care predisposed women to continuing depression and distress.[34]

Women were changing. Within the left around the developed world, the second wave of feminism was to unleash forces which were to change an institution like the Royal Women's Hospital more dramatically than any others in its past. It was to do this by empowering female staff, nurses above all, with a critique of practices and structures which transformed both themselves and their perceptions of their patients. Female nurses were forced into new loyalties — to their fellow nurses and to their patients as women. They felt themselves charged with a new responsibility of advocacy on behalf of fellow women. Feminism clarified the petty and gross indignities of nursing's traditional subservience to a predominantly male medical profession, and it obliged nurses to identify with their patients rather than with the authority of the hospital. Even some of the most conservative felt drawn into new ideas and feelings and the hospital was dragged to the forefront of some of the most troubled moral controversies of the times.

The turmoil over abortion in Victoria was aggravated in 1968 by the decision of the Victorian Homicide Squad to eliminate illegal abortion: six doctors were prosecuted and in 1969 eighteen prosecutions were launched, but at one of the trials Mr Justice Menhennit 'made a precise statement of the law regarding abortion' in Victoria which reassured doctors 'that termination of pregnancy performed in good faith in the interests of the mother's health is not unlawful'.[35] Within the Royal Women's Hospital there was immediate anxiety. What was 'the degree of "necessity" ' in making decisions to terminate? The Medical Staff asked the Board to seek a legal opinion.[36] By February 1970 the hospital was feeling the community pressure for it to become a major provider of therapeutic abortions on psychiatric grounds. The Board was concerned that any reform of the Victorian Abortion Law would force the Women's 'to undertake the major burden of the work' and the prospect was horrifying:

> Reports from ex-residents of this hospital working in the UK show that 30 per cent of the gynaecological beds are filled with termination of pregnancy cases. By far the greater proportion of these cases fall into the psychiatric category. There is insufficient psychiatric time to assess the patients thoroughly and it is easier to accede to the request after a short interview than for the psychiatrist to endure the prolonged and vituperative interview that refusal engenders. Refusal also leads to the patient 'shopping around' to other hospitals (they already do so in Melbourne) with further psychiatric time being spent going over the same ground in other hospitals. In the UK in some centres 'abortion on demand' is emerging and the formation of private abortion clinics. The entire situation, according to reports, is creating problems in resident medical staff and

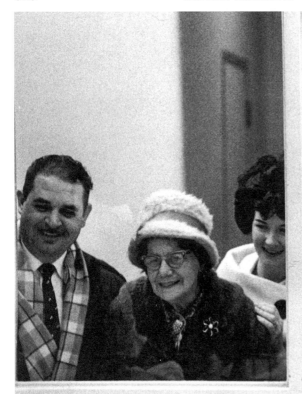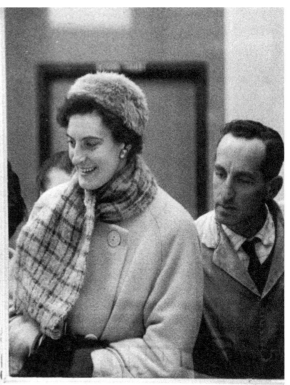

Looking at babies, 1960s
Mark Strizic, RWHA

nursing circles. To most doctors and nurses the operation of termination of pregnancy is distasteful even when the indications are convincing. The resident medical officers and nurses carry out the operation but have no part in making the decision. When the indications, to their mind, are tenuous, dissatisfaction in the staff becomes evident. This aspect seems to be overlooked by the 'abortion reformers' who seem to assume that there is an army of technical experts ready and willing to undertake the increased number of these operations that reform of the law will bring.[37]

Just as the Royal Women's Hospital was reinventing itself as a classless community hospital, the stigmas of its past threatened to return. Honorary medical staff who quietly terminated pregnancies for their private patients, were reluctant to perform them openly on public patients: the interpretation of the law might change overnight, but people could not. Already by mid 1972, the hospital's consultant psychiatric staff was overtaxed and there was urgent need for more outpatient accommodation.[38] Within the medical profession the debate was shifting slowly. Dr Rod Bretherton, son of Dr Albert Bretherton, was given space in the *MJA* in October 1969 to argue the case for abortion law reform and in July the following year a survey of ninety-two general practitioners in New South Wales revealed the majority to support abortion when the pregnancy threatened the woman's physical or mental health, and a sizeable number to support abortion on request.[39] In a decade attitudes to sexuality and gender had undergone a revolution in society outside; the 1970s were to see many of those transformations institutionalised.

Practices

15

If the 1960s saw values change, the 1970s saw institutions change, transformations made possible initially by the election of a federal Labor government in 1972. It unleashed a quarter of a century of pent-up frustration and reformist zeal: health, education and urban reform were at the top of the agenda, and health, with the Commonwealth's powers extending further into its various systems than they could in education, was the most vulnerable to drastic intervention.

The patients were also forcing the pace of change, deserting the public system for the private so that by early 1973 two labour wards had been closed.[40] Then in May 1973 the Royal Women's Hospital, at the behest of the Health Commission, finally began paying consultants by session, but the formal end of the honorary system did not come until the introduction of the federal Labor government's national health scheme, Medibank, in August 1975. The Royal Women's did not embrace change without reservations and regrets: 'The highest tribute must be paid to the hundreds of skilled medical practitioners who gave honorary service over the past 119 years. It is hoped that the remunerated service will provide that selfless devotion always common to its dedicated forebears'.[41] Medibank changed everything. The hospital received more money, but now could not take out an overdraft and had to operate within its means. There was a very real fear that this new dependence on Commonwealth funding with its inevitable bureaucratic control might in the long term hold the hospital back and prevent new ventures, or that it would even be unable to maintain existing services in times of national economic stringency.[42] They were prophetic words.

Such profound change came at the same time as rising inflation, fuelled by the international oil crisis and an explosion in wages and salaries. Expectations of professional services also changed: staff numbers, especially of medical and para-medical staff grew. Reform required more planners and administrators, and yet the hospital was constrained in raising revenue by the Medibank cap placed on fees for private beds. Luxury private medicine was not permitted so the Mabel Coles suite on the twelfth floor was virtually redundant within a few years of opening for business. In the decade 1967 to 1977, total costs in running the hospital were to multiply five-fold. The sacking of the Whitlam Labor government and the return of the coalition only brought more disruption as Medibank was sanitised into Medicare, marking the beginning of a period of constant uncertainty in medical and hospital administration in Australia. Margaret Mabbitt says she has lost count of the number of times cash registers were installed in Outpatients only to be removed again with yet another 'reform'. What did not change was the steady rise in salary costs, driven most of all by the expansion of medical work itself — the development of new sub-specialities and of new social concerns, as well as new technologies and therapies.

But as costs rose, midwifery patient numbers continued to fall, and not all of it was due to rising affluence or the pill. The radical critique of the medicalisation of childbirth had caused a backlash on the public maternity hospital system. Two organisations, the Association for Painless Childbirth and the Childbirth Education Association, had been keeping dossiers on Victorian obstetricians: on who could be trusted to respect a woman's wishes and who could not. In reaction, women turned to home birth, to the horror of the professionals, and a couple of avoidable tragedies received wide publicity. The Royal Women's decided to invite general practitioners with large obstetric practices to deliver in its wards in the hope of bringing more women into the hospital and providing a place for those who sought an alternative. Percy Rogers was delighted to make the transition from delivering in private hospitals, and he found the Women's happy and friendly, with people always ready to talk about obstetrics in the cafeteria. He appreciated also the strong culture of research, where the staff felt secure enough to commence long-term projects and were sustained by the interest and support of their colleagues. It was a very good hospital, whatever its oddities:

> The convenience of everything at the Women's was just absurd — it was great. But when I came into labour ward, sister said
> — Oh, you're the new doctor. What's your fad?
> — What do you mean?
> — Well, you put your fads down, you know, what you like your women to have on admission.
> — Nothing.
> — No — what analgesics? A cocktail?
> — No, I don't want anything.
> — But you'll have to give them something.
> — No. If you feel that they need analgesics, I want to be rung.
> — What, any time of the night?
> — Any time of the night or day. Ring me and I'll come down and assess her, because there has to be something wrong if she's not coping. They've all been trained.
> And no shaving.
> — What about infections?
> — There's a study done in India which shows that there were more

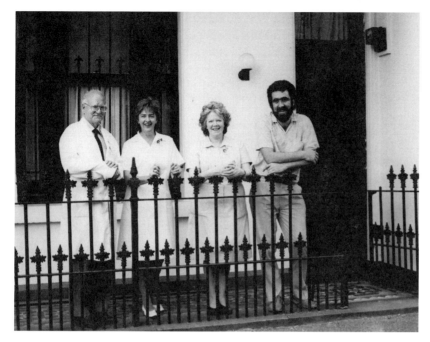

Dr Percy Rogers (far left) as head of the staff clinic in Cardigan Street, with Glenys Thurgood, Kate Collins and Stephen Swanborough *RWHA*

infections in the shaved women than in the non-.

— Enema?

— No, they've all emptied their bowels.

The edict went out — no shaving. I suffered in the ward rounds because the old consultants thought that it was a disgraceful habit not to shave.

Then came admitting the husbands into the ward which had not been done and I was insistent. But it was easier in the Women's than in the peripheral hospitals, they seemed to be more in tune.

His 'fads' were respected and kept — that was an advantage of rigidity in a hospital. Although as the doctors moved into the labour wards either with private patients or as members of the expanding salaried staff, the midwives felt their control over normal birth was slipping away. It was more than time that midwives took part in the reform of childbirth and reclaimed their place in the birthing process.

Margaret Peters was to be at the centre of the reforms of midwifery:

The early days of the Women's Movement weren't read correctly by the midwives until the mid-1970s onwards. I don't think the doctors read the Women's Movement, but they did read the stuff of evidence-based practice and they used that to increase staffing and to get more dominance. They've always been very dominant here, but they really took firm control.

Matron Betty Lawson and the younger charge nurses responded to the growing debate in the media about childbirth reform and home births, especially the work coming from the West Coast of America, even though much of it was not relevant to Australian practice. Betty Lawson supported Margaret Peters in her application for a three-month study tour in the United States to look at the midwifery movement that was newly emerging from the women's movement.[43] But Margaret had also had a personal experience which had shaken the nursing administration. It was Christmas Day 1974, and the charge sisters had an arrangement where they covered and relieved for each other. Margaret was relieving so that a charge nurse could have her Christmas Dinner:

> I was on a ward which only had three people, so I was having an easy time of it. But they had brought in that morning, off the Dom. Service, a Turkish woman whose baby was on the ninth floor in the Intensive Care Neo-natal ward, and she was said to be psychotic. They'd sedated her and she looked to be OK, so everyone went off and I was left alone. But she wasn't OK, and she was quite distressed and she attacked me and she really bashed me to bits. And after they'd rescued me from being stomped and put me back together again and carted her off to one of the mental hospitals, we all decided she was just psychotic.
>
> But then the psychiatrist told me that we were the ones who were mad because this woman was as sane as we were — the problem was she didn't speak English. Her husband had been informed fully about what was happening to the baby on the understanding that he would tell her. She thought we'd pinched her baby from her. She'd not been shown her baby, and she quite naturally was extremely distressed.
>
> I think she was a very courageous woman — she took it out on someone she saw as obstructing her from her baby, and that was fair enough.
>
> So out of that came the thought that what I should do is look at what happened with childbirth in Turkey and Greece since we were getting such a lot of women from those countries.

In the USA she looked at everything: alternative midwifery inside hospitals and outside. She met a new sort of midwife, who studied to Masters level, and who undertook 'a whole range of things that wouldn't be considered midwifery in this country — gynae care, family planning, and conducting births in their own right and separating out high risk from low, as to whose territory it was. And they were listening to what women were saying'. She also saw orthodox births: 'where you still had a woman strapped down on a delivery bed, attended by a whole plethora of people from the obstetrician, a nurse who'd done some OBGYN and then the paediatricians took control over the baby — things that were in some ways foreign to me and quite horrific'. On the West Coast, the talk was all of Suzanne Arms' new book *Immaculate Deception*; on the East Coast she visited the Maternity Centers Association's alternative birth centres, and met briefly one of their founders, Ruth Lubic. In Turkey she saw a tertiary referral hospital with no linen on the delivery beds — 'high rates of complications, high mortality' — and she became aware of the gender issues for Turkish women; in Greece it was no better: private hospitals that banned family support where 'long hard labours were had by all' and the public wards were worse. But before this she went to

Lausanne for her first meeting of the International Confederation of Midwives, where 'the most telling experience was in a small workshop and we had some midwives from the West Coast of Africa — and their wants were clean running water and a basin to collect it in and some clean swabs — all things we took for granted'. She also went to the United Kingdom where legislation decreed that every woman must be attended in childbirth by a midwife: 'Men have been taken through the courts for attending a woman in childbirth there, even though it's their own child and own wife'. She returned 'hyped up on the needs of women in less affluent societies', and it was the beginning of a close involvement of the hospital through her activism in the international midwives' movement. And it made her determined to work to establish midwifery as a profession separate from nursing and from medical domination, and for a national organisation of midwives.

Within the hospital nursing staff change would not be easy, but there were allies among the British midwives who emigrated in the 1960s and Matron Lawson herself who supported Margaret Peters in speaking out. Betty Lawson was due to retire in 1977 and, to celebrate her long and distinguished career, a seminar 'The Hand that Rocks the Cradle' was organised with Ruth Lubic, Director General of the Maternity Center Association of New York, as the keynote speaker. She inspired her audience with a new concept of the role of the midwife:

> If you expect me to perform as a 'junior obstetrician', you ask me to misapply my skills. Let me teach care for mothers and families — for it is my earnest belief that maternity care, in its best sense, is preventive health care. To work with and help families in the child bearing cycle when most are receptive to and desire assistance, to strengthen self-confidence, to dispel fear, to share accomplishment — that is my *raison d'être* and my joy![44]

This promised a quite different relationship between practitioner and patient, a relationship where the midwife worked *with* the mother and her family, where care extended to the psychic and the social, to before, during and after birth.

Mrs Eileen Goulding, Director of Nursing, 1977–1982 *RWHA*

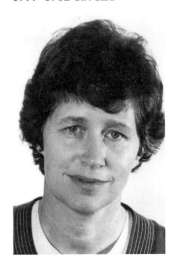

The new director of nursing, Mrs Eileen Goulding, was receptive to change, despite the deep resistance that continued within some of the older nursing and medical staff. Support now came from the Board of Management, which in 1979 was sharply reformed at the direction of the Victorian Health Commission — streamlined, and more focused on the administration of a complex modern hospital.[45] Mrs Lesley Leckie, herself a nurse, strongly supported the reforming midwives and the small group of obstetricians allied with them. In 1979 the English childbirth reformer Dr Sheila Kitzinger was brought out for a 'Birth and Being' Conference organised by the Childbirth Education Association. Percy Rogers went with John Neil, of the Women's obstetrical staff, and despite the clamour of the Primal Screamers who at that time had captured the Childbirth Education Association, Neil was deeply moved: 'I got the impression that for the first time he was really hearing the subjectivity of women'. Neil and Dr Michael Kloss joined with the reforming mid-

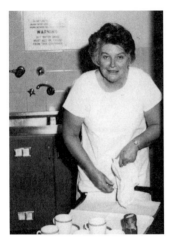

**Mrs Lesley Leckie, past
president, in the Family
Birth Centre** *RWHA*

wives, Mrs Leckie and Percy Rogers to establish the Women's Family
Birth Centre, following in the wake of the more adventurous Queen
Vic. On 17 October 1979 one of Percy Rogers' trained patients was the
first woman to deliver in the Centre:

> She was just terrific. She came into labour and the nursing staff didn't
> know what to do. I came in to see her and she was wearing a pair of
> Richmond footy socks. She apologised, saying she couldn't get the
> Carlton ones. I said it was all right — I'd deliver her anyway.
>
> But the nursing staff were outside, hovering. They'd come in: 'Is it
> all right if we feel your tummy — are we intruding — can I take your
> blood pressure?'
>
> The couple were very affable — a lovely couple. They required
> nothing.
>
> 'Do you feel like an injection?' 'No, I feel happy.'
>
> She pushed the baby out beautifully — breathed and panted it out.
>
> And one of the sisters standing next to me I felt was going to throw
> her arms about me in a most unprofessional way; then said: 'Oh it's just
> like Beethoven's 7th symphony.' And I said, 'If the 9th is an 'Ode to
> Joy', then I guess the 7th is an 'Ode to Life'.

The Family Birth Centre was both a medical success, even though
'the rest of the obstetricians were waiting for the disaster they felt was
inevitable', and an outstanding public relations success for the hospital,
lifting its profile among young middle-class women. (In 1976 the hospital
had suffered damaging public criticism of its midwifery wards from a
prominent woman journalist, Iola Mathews, who had written on her
shock at a sudden transference from a Lilydale hospital after a post-partum
haemorrhage: the noise from the wards, the demand feeding and con-
struction work had robbed her of sleep.[46]) Soon Frances Perry House
began to lose patients, so it too had to modify its birth practices; and
before long the normal public wards relaxed their rules about shaving
and enemas and birth positions and analgesia. The Birth Centre remains
immensely popular nearly twenty years later, a symbol of humane human
birthing, even though its practices are now scarcely distinguishable from
normal deliveries in the public suites of the hospital. The hospital accepted
the Family Birth Centre, and its champions accepted the necessity of
remaining in a large hospital where specialist help was immediately at
hand. The Birth Centre acted, however, as a catalyst for change throughout
the hospital, and as the Royal Women's most successful bid to establish
itself as the maternity hospital for all women, not just the poor, the unfortunate or the unrespectable.

The hospital was, however, prepared to address the areas of women's
reproductive health that were more controversial. Gytha Betheras and
her 'girls' running the Family Planning Clinic had become increasingly
aware of women's needs for sexual counselling, and that the hospital had
a special opportunity to reach a section of the population that was outside
the reach of private middle-class sexual counsellors. Again there was resistance from some of the old consultants (one even told Gytha that he had
never had a patient with a sexual problem); again the same group of pro-

gressive doctors, nurses and Board members stood by them. The doctors running it needed special training, but again it more than justified their belief in the need for it. It opened for patients on 17 March 1977, a special date because it was the day the Queen came to visit the hospital. Gytha reflects on the sexual difficulties she has seen over her long medical practice, and how women have asked for help:

> Women might have complained many years ago if intercourse was impossible, and if it was possible, they gritted their teeth. They next complained if it was painful. Now they're brave enough to complain if it's not pleasurable or if they don't have orgasms. So there's been a progression.
>
> In a family planning clinic, most people you're seeing because they *do* have intercourse, so they were complaining of pain, lack of libido or of pleasure, no orgasms and then there were a lot of media writings about orgasm and multiple orgasm.
>
> Then pressure came from the male partner who began to judge himself as a lover not just by how he performed, but by whether he could give his partner an orgasm.
>
> In the earlier days I had a lot who used to come about the stage their second child went to school saying, 'Doctor — I have no interest.

The Family Birth Centre
RWHA

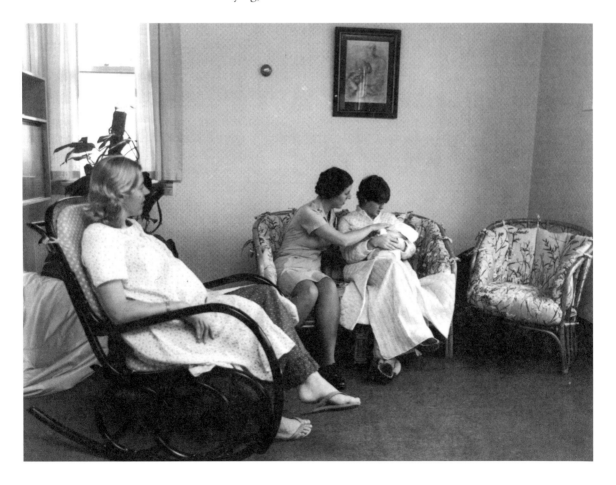

My relationship is going to break up. We never make love.' They had got into the bad habits that get established with babies and young children — fatigue and all those things — and the relationship had just perished.

Nowadays I'm seeing these people much earlier — at the time these bad habits are being established in the months after a child is born. They come in and say, 'I'm not interested. I'm not responsive. I'm too tired.'

So if that means people are taking preventive action much sooner, then that's a good thing.

The sad little group that I see — DINKS (double income, no kids) have been joined by the DINS (double income no sex). These are often young, married or de facto, they're both working like demons and suddenly the fun's gone out of the relationship. All work and no play; all pressure and no relaxation.

But there are also tremendous numbers of younger and older women with non-consummation of their marriages or relationships. Some days every patient I see is at different stages of that. It's a very common problem. They think they're the only ones in the world. And it's just a great relief to have the young ones come almost straight away if they're having difficulty.

Another old concern of the hospital, venereal diseases, benefited from the 'permissive society' in that again the hospital could humanely and rationally devote specialist resources to it. As the Sexually Transmitted Disease Clinic it began in the late 1960s, and as it became better known and young people became more sexually adventurous its case load rose. In 1971 there were four cases of syphilis, in 1973 there were thirty, in 1974, twenty. In the early 1970s it did not seem warranted to keep records of genital herpes or warts, although their incidence was rising. (Perhaps the sexual revolution really lasted only from the Pill to herpes.) The patients were predominantly young, reported the doctor in charge, Michael Kloss in 1977:

The youngsters are usually very brave, to them any Venereal Disease is no worse than a cold or some other illness. They ignore the frightful havoc that is brought about in their later reproductive life by such an illness. Older people in more stable relationships are inevitably horrified, embarrassed and ashamed. Young people on the other hand will rapidly and cheerfully notify all their friends and contacts about their latest acquisition, older patients will go to unbelievable extremes to deceive anyone who might be likely to suspect them. Another noteworthy aspect of the younger patients was their state of personal hygiene, whilst obviously there were exceptions, the vast majority deserved low marks for personal cleanliness and in some patients, one could only be appalled. Multiple venereal diseases were pretty common in most young people and one can understand that, when one looks at their sexual behaviour pattern. Multiple sexual contacts were frequent, some of the younger girls had truly athletic contact records. 5–10 contacts per week were not uncommon and I have no reason to disbelieve them. The only exception to the above patients, namely multiple sexual contacts and cleanliness, were the professional prostitutes. They were as a rule spotlessly clean, and although they made multiple contacts per week, the number for any given girl was usually constant, few of them worked overtime! The many and varied aspects of their profession are quite a separate topic, but their health care demands are very real and pressing and I believe, are inadequately dealt with in our society.[47]

The hospital had come a long way from the punitive attitudes of the past: each patient, however much removed from doctor or nurse in values and way of life, was a person, a woman needing care. Into the 1980s new conditions became the concern of the clinic — chlamydia (rising alarmingly among young women of all classes, threatening them with sterility), hepatitis, and of course HIV. By the 1990s the clinic was called the Communicable Diseases Clinic and half its case load was chlamydia (56 per cent), with herpes next (19 per cent), gonorrhoea, HIV, hepatitis B and C, non-specific vaginitis, and *molloscum contagiosum* all 8 per cent, and genital warts 6 per cent.[48] The hospital still saw young women who were gravely ill and affected for life, and women who exposed themselves to terrible risks of disease.

But most controversial of all, and the most dangerous for the hospital's public standing, was its decision in 1975 to establish the Pregnancy Advisory Service, financially made possible by Medibank. This clinic was to provide legal termination of pregnancy for its public patients. Since the Menhennit ruling, it had largely been private patients who had benefited. The hospital argued its case on the grounds of women's and patients' rights:

> In order to accept abortion we must accept a woman's right to control her reproductive function and concede that termination is part of the female health demand. Opponents have always focussed their attention on the right of the foetus, but they have completely ignored the other rights in this equation. The rights of the patient, the rights of the family, the rights of the husband and they totally ignore the misery, the hardship and psychological damage that ensues as a result of an unwanted pregnancy. They ignore the problem of the pregnancy, the unwanted and impossible pregnancy. The average woman has a negative attitude to termination, but she is faced with a situation if it continues, which will be worse. Most women, in my experience, are unhappy about having a pregnancy terminated, but once having made the decision, they are relieved and show no remorse later on.[49]

The women who came in during the 1970s were ordinary Australian women, half of them married, 35 per cent single, the rest separated or divorced. Most already had children. A quarter had already had an abortion, and 5 per cent had had more than one. Half were born overseas.

The hospital's social work department undertook the counselling, a load of work that in time almost overwhelmed its resources. After her pregnancy was confirmed, the patient would be assessed by a social worker — a psychiatrist was called in only if the patient was 'grossly disturbed', because the idea of a patient being assessed by a panel of experts was too much like an inquisition. As Beth Stevenson recalls:

A major focus of the Social Work interview was to ensure that the woman was fully informed of her options — without anyone being pushed — that is, continue the pregnancy and keep the baby, continue the pregnancy and consider adoption or request a termination of pregnancy. There was always a percentage who decided to continue with the pregnancy.

A report of the patient's 'social and emotional set-up' was prepared, discussed and the patient interviewed again in the weekly clinic: where termination was discussed, she was medically examined and, what the hospital considered was essential, advised on contraception: 'We are adamant about contraceptive measures to be taken after termination and we do this not from a punitive point of view but because we genuinely believe that contraception is preferable to termination'. 'Gytha's girls' provided much of the medical workforce. Gytha again:

> I believe that the follow-up appointment is *the* moment to make
> an on-going relationship with that woman, to offer her on-going
> contraception. And for the hospital: I believe it brings her back when
> she is ready to have her children, so it's constructive for the hospital,
> not just to do the termination, but to make a relationship with her to
> help her achieve what she wants. Most of the young women who have
> terminations, later want to have families. And if we've made a positive
> impact, if we're looked upon as competent and caring, and ready to
> meet their needs if possible, they'll come back. And the better we treat
> them, the less traumatised they'll be — that's good therapy. They're not
> lesser mortals because they had a termination.

But those opposed to abortion were not prepared to permit the hospital to openly provide terminations for public patients. The hospital's Tracy-Maund lecturer for 1976 was Dr Kelvin Churches, a member of the honorary staff from 1948 until 1974, and formerly chief of the cancer unit. He had had enough of Victoria's hypocrisy over contraception and abortion and gave a history of '120 Years of Abortion in Melbourne', naming a number of qualified and unqualified abortionists of the past, telling the tragic story of post-abortal sepsis, especially of gas gangrene. He applauded the fact that abortion had finally come out of the shadows and that the Royal Women's Hospital, after decades of avoiding the issues, had accepted that it had a responsibility to the community in family planning and safe, legal terminations for public patients. An edited version of the lecture was published in the *Age* on 24 April 1976, just three days after Iola Mathews had criticised the hospital for its noisy wards. The Churches article included dramatic graphs of the rise in terminations performed at the Women's Hospital since 1965 — a rise from a handful to over 1300. And the publicity made the hospital the focus of the Pro-Life movement. On 26 June Nancy Dexter reported in her column in the *Age* some intelligence released by the ever-vigilant Protestant Federation, which maintained its surveillance of the Catholic press. It had noticed a small advertisement from the Australian Pro-Life Youth Alliance, asking readers to enrol as contributors to the Royal Women's Hospital before 30 June. The cost was only $2 and the reward was the right to vote in the coming Board of Management elections. No elections had been held for seventy-five years, but this time there would be, as the Pro-Life Alliance intended contesting five of the seven seats to gain anti-abortion representation on the board. The hospital and its pro-abortion supporters were galvanised into action. Five hundred alliance support-ers had become contributors; three hundred pro-abortion contributors signed up from the University of Melbourne Student Union alone, plus many others from the Royal Melbourne Institute of Technology and the Melbourne Teachers' College. The Women's Electoral Lobby supplied many, so that when the elections came, the hospital had 3000 member subscribers and 5000 others. At the election, the Right to Life polled only 500 votes; the sitting members over 2000.[50]

This was only the beginning of years of confrontation with the Right to Life Association, whose unshakeable conviction that termination of pregnancy was wilful murder drove them to take extreme measures. A huge banner was strung across its front declaring 'THIS HOSPITAL KILLS BABIES', distressing not only staff, many of whom found abortion distasteful also, but especially parents with tiny babies in the neo-natal intensive care unit. On the footpath a priest prayed; inside they harassed staff and patients. Gytha Betheras:

> They came on our premises. They challenged the patients going in, they challenged staff. Staff might have strong beliefs and not approve of termination of pregnancy, but would not stand in the way of someone else coming to the hospital for treatment.
> And some were coming into the wards and reading theatre lists to find out patients' names.
> There were big letter writing campaigns to staff.
> I found it distressing because it went so against my belief. I respect their beliefs and respect their right not to have an abortion and their right to counsel their child or their partner not to have an abortion. But they don't have the right to stand between the practice of medicine and another person who has different beliefs.

Senior staff were harassed at home; the Chief Executive Officer had his front door daubed. The hospital had them charged with trespass and finally they were found guilty.[51] The last recourse was a court injunction granted on 5 June 1986, still in force, which forbids Right to Life demonstrators from coming any closer to the hospital than the southern side of Grattan Street.

Every burst of publicity for the Pregnancy Advisory Service, good or bad, brought desperate women flocking to the hospital for terminations of pregnancy. The Queen Victoria Medical Centre also provided the service, but after its amalgamation into the Monash Medical Centre its role as a provider declined until it stopped altogether. By 1997 the Royal Women's Hospital struggled, as the only public provider in the state, to serve the thousands of Victorian women who still were seeking the termination of an unwanted pregnancy.

The manner in which these new services were being conducted exemplified a profound change that had overtaken the hospital since the early 1960s. There was a new respect for the personhood of the patient; she had rights and so did her family; no matter who she was and no matter what she had done. The spirit of Medibank lived on in its Coalition form of Medicare, so that gradually the difference between public and private patient diminished: not that private patients did worse, but that public patients were entitled to care and conditions as good as the private. They had paid for them also, as taxpayers. Perhaps post-war prosperity had removed some of the stigma of being a charity patient because the working class now earned enough to pay tax. Taxpayers had rights to things they had paid for. But the psychic changes were more complex and human, and they were revealed in no more dramatic a way than in multiculturalism. Multiculturalism was born and nurtured in schools and hospitals, and it was the hospitals' migrant employees who perhaps achieved most on behalf of their fellow migrants. Margaret Peters acknowledges that it was the migrant staff who made them understand migrant needs:

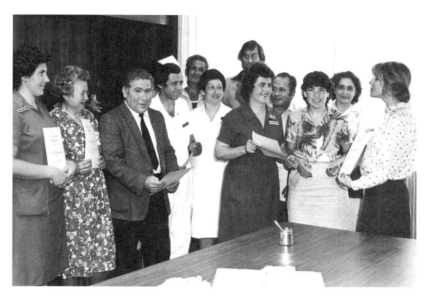

Staff who completed the hospital's migrant English course in 1982 receiving their certificates from their teacher, Jill Tucker. From left: Anka Najari, Elizabeth Bolyos, Luigi Corbisiero, Frank Naskopoulos, Paolo Musmeci, Rosie Ursmando, Clive Ansell (Education Department supervisor), Stephani Sanartizi, Frank de Clemente, Vicki Simanovska, Dragica Perduv. Hidden from view, Michelle Desira. *RWHA*

Some of those men and women worked here for all their post-arrival lives and there was always a great family spirit. You may not have always understood what drove them to come to Australia, but you certainly understood what drove them to work here and educate their kids. You'd work here with men and women whose English was rudimentary and who were doing essential but basic work around the place, whose kids were graduating as God-only-knows-what from Melbourne University across the road. And it was a great joy to watch that evolution. I always enjoyed working with those people because they did work hard and with great commitment to this place. We had our odd strikes from time to time, but fundamentally they'd do anything for patient care around here. It's a great spirit.

In 1978 Liliana Ferrara returned to work at the Women's after raising five children, and could not believe the 'beautiful changes':

At lunches the sisters knew more about the Italian sauces than me. And wines! In fifteen years, 1964 to 1978, it was a big change.

Their neighbours were Italian and they understood. They saw that they were ordinary people, nice people. They'd say, 'I have this lovely Greek neighbour, or Italian neighbour, who gives me food. Such a good cook.'

They started to trust them.

And they grew up too, the migrants. They opened restaurants.

Within the hospital, the treatment of the patients was unrecognisable:

I met a different kind of patient — Arabic speaking. By then the Italians I'd interpreted for were coming in for gynaecological problems — hysterectomy, some unfortunately had cancer. Now in midwifery it was the Lebanese, the Egyptians, Syrians and Palestinians.

And everyone was trying to accommodate them. 'Bring your own food.' They even had a microwave — they can heat their soup, their food, they can do anything they want.

Pamphlets by the thousand in every language — which in the past, I did everything myself.

But they were still missing a bit of the act because a lot of them could not read or write. So in actual fact, 'Italian?' 'Yes' 'Oh, I'll give you this', in an Italian she could not understand. They would say 'yes' but they were too embarrassed to tell the doctor they could not read or write very well.

Or they would say, 'How long have you been in Australia?'

'Twenty-seven years.'

'Oh you speak English then.'

They presumed that because you can do your shopping and can say 'I'll have this or that in English', that you understand little things like 'hysterectomy'.

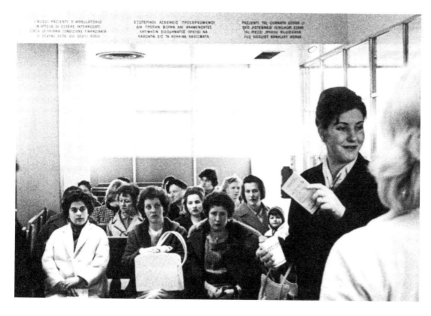

Multilingual Outpatients department
Mark Strizic, RWHA

The labour ward was different in every way:

> They knew the customs. With my Arabic speaking patients they had
> the freedom of the labour ward. The mother-in-law or mother would
> come and sit on the floor. The husband would be there. (Actually he
> didn't want to be there.) They encouraged them in every way to have
> supportive people around them. If you want to lie on the floor to have
> a baby, do what you want.
>   It took me a year before I could find myself—am I in the same
> place?

The expanding role and profile of the Social Work department was
vital in the transformation of the relationship between hospital and
patient. The social workers under Isobel Strahan and later Kath Lancaster,
developed a high skill in the adoption service, but as a professional department within the hospital, they lacked the authority they deserved. They
were always understaffed, but they also suffered from the (one-sided)
special relationship with the ladies of the 'old' Board, who while giving
the social workers essential moral support, also sought to use the department to satisfy their need for a more traditional 'hands-on' philanthropy.[52]
The workload with the single mothers was immense — by 1974 around
1000 were delivered in the hospital every year, half of them being under
eighteen years of age. But here also changing social values affected the
hospital's work: as sexual mores became more tolerant, the 'shame' of
unmarried motherhood diminished and more women felt confident
enough to keep their babies: in 1968 more than 40 per cent did so and
by 1972 the proportion had risen to 60 per cent. The federal Labor
government's expansion of social benefits for single mothers saw 80 per
cent keep their babies by just 1975.[53] Social workers themselves, including
Kath Lancaster, by now had serious reservations about the desirability of
adoption on the large scale it had been practised in the 1960s. Evidence
was mounting that some adopting families did not bond adequately and
the child welfare community was shocked by cases of abuse of adopted
children in 'nice' middle-class homes which were presenting at the Royal
Children's Hospital. More commonly, adopted adults were increasingly
curious about their biological mothers, and some were quite distressed
by their lack of biological identity. The protocols of adoption were under
question, while among the childless the expectation had been planted
that they too could have a family. As the number of babies relinquished
for adoption fell, the waiting lists of couples wanting to adopt continued
to rise, creating in part a captive market for the growing new technologies of assisted reproduction.

The decline in adoptions and the decision not to see all single or separated women automatically — that is, they were no longer, by definition,
a 'social work problem' — released the social workers for other duties.
Their work expanded into specialised counselling in the neo-natal
intensive care unit, the new Pregnancy Advisory Service, oncology and
the artificial insemination by donor programme. In the 1960s the acute
shortage of staff had been relieved by bursaries for traineeships from the
Hospitals and Charities Commission and by the 1970s the department

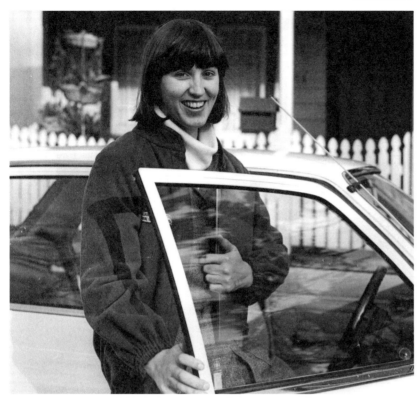

Domiciliary nurse
RWHA

had a special student unit. In the 1980s, under Bethia Stevenson, the Social Work department developed more grief counselling — for families who had lost a baby, for women with cancer.

But some of the new work with patients was, in the next decade, to move to other professionals, in particular midwives. Eileen Goulding died in 1982 after a long and tragic illness which had prevented her from implementing many of her reforms, and she was succeeded as Director of Nursing by Mrs Netta McArthur, a Scot coming from a tradition where midwives enjoyed greater professional autonomy and standing. She was an instinctual reformer and found a powerful ally in Gary Henry who rose to be the first non-medical Chief Executive Officer in July 1984. Both were committed to a public hospital system where the public patient was deserving of the same care and respect as the private patient. Many visiting doctors, pupil midwives and medical students had been revolted by the conduct of the Outpatients Clinic, while those who worked there every day were soon oblivious of the patients' embarrassment, humiliation and outrage. But few critics were ever as eloquent as the new Director of Nursing:

> Outpatients was like a cattlerun. I've never seen anything like it in my entire life. The patients came in at one end like a factory and got weighed and urine tested and something else — blood taken and then GIVEN A NUMBER — not even a name, just a number. Then they'd sit in a great big barn of a place on these old recovered seats and their number would be called. And I asked why they were given a number

and I was told that it was because the names were too difficult to say!

Then they were taken into cubicles—like two cells—get undressed, put a gown on and sit there and wait until somebody came to get them and sat them on top of a wooden box. There was little conversation—just wobbled their belly, listened to their foetal heart, and their backsides were facing the curtains that were hardly ever drawn and with people walking up and down this back corridor.

Women were considered available for medical training—they shouldn't be given any options. And they had medical students examining them—doing pelvics on them without permission. It was unbelievable. Because you were a public patient, that's how you were going to be treated—you can't afford to go private, so you're lucky we're looking after you. The doctors and the midwives really cared about the women's health, but there was a dichotomy—it was the pregnancy they cared about rather than the person.

I just used to find that really shocking. I'd not seen anything like that before—not even in the worst parts of Britain.

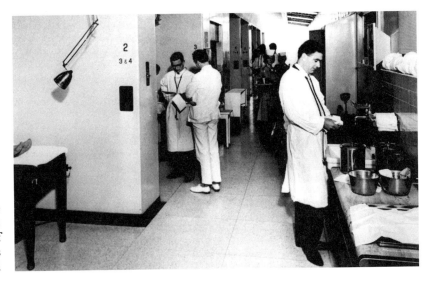

Long corridor outside cubicles in Outpatients: note the absence of screens for patients
RWHA

The nursing division had been slowly adjusting to change and seeking it, but now in the 1980s the climate was ready for profound change. Netta McArthur had come first to the Women's in 1979 on an appointment to integrate Frances Perry House with the rest of the hospital, now that funding arrangements and policies for private hospitals had changed. She found the 'old culture' of the Women's 'controlling', even oppressive and she was determined to liberate both patients and nurses and midwives. She wanted to put the decision-making back into the workplace, giving the charge sisters, who were now called unit managers, control over their workforce and their budgets: 'Even today some of them have the fear of making a decision and being crucified for not making the right decision'. The loosening up was difficult for many, but in fact there was no reason why patients should not have visitors at any time, and that if a patient had a visitor when a nurse needed to get sutures out, then perhaps it was the patient's, not the nurse's decision as to whether the visitor could stay: 'Nursing still hasn't lost that need to control and the need to know all'. She was to call all this the 'transformational model of nursing' which is 'based on values, on people taking risks and making decisions and being able to communicate with each other and with patients, and to be able to create an atmosphere of change'. The goal of nursing and midwifery is to work in partnership with women, their families and the medical staff:

> We still think we know best, and we've still got a long way to go until we're in true partnership with women. As I keep saying, 'When was the last time we asked that woman — what is it that you want us to do for you while you're here? What is the most important thing for you to accomplish and achieve? And work with them to achieve that before they go.

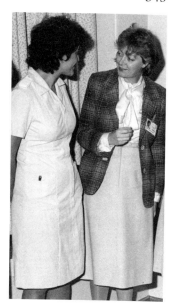

Mrs Netta McArthur, director of nursing, 1982–1997 *RWHA*

High on Netta McArthur's reform list was changing the method of midwifery and neo-natal nurse education and the transference of midwifery education to the university. She succeeded in reducing the annual intakes of students from four times to three and then to twice a year. She had been very critical of the way pupil midwives were sent first to the post-natal wards where their complete lack of experience could have baleful effects on new mothers struggling to breast feed or fighting post-natal depression or simply getting to know their babies. Younger nurses welcomed the enhanced status university degrees would give them; other nurses often had doubts that you could learn to be a good nurse in a lecture theatre. In 1994 the Royal Women's Hospital nursing school closed, and while the beginning of a new era for midwifery, it was also the end of an era for the hospital which had been the first in Australia to train nurses.

A new receptiveness to change pervaded the hospital, and while it was often the same key medical staff, backed by the reformed board, the new ethos in nursing and the opening of the hospital to new ideas made the 1980s the most creative decade in the hospital's history. While its stature as a research and teaching hospital grew both nationally and internationally, given public prominence by its advanced work in reproductive biology, it now emerged as the most innovative women's hospital in social medicine and women's health. Many of its services now became pace setters in the hospital world: its catering, for so long stodgy and culturally insensitive, became both imaginative and palatable. Nurses and the catering department worked together to serve meals to patients so that they could leave their beds, use the ward like a living room, sit at a table, entertain visitors — and if Netta McArthur had had her way, not even wear bed clothes but ordinary clothes, if they wanted, as maternity patients. Rooms with double beds were provided for public patients who had complications or a loss and needed their partner with them. Wards were renovated and made to look like home, spa baths installed for oncology patients in chronic pain, pre-admission clinics prepared women for childbirth and surgery, and those who came in for day surgery had their transport home planned before admission. As hospital stay time for both

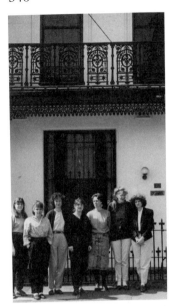

CASA House and staff, Kate Gilmore on far right
RWHA

midwifery and gynaecology dramatically shortened, more care had to be taken in Outpatients to follow up care. A Breastfeeding Assessment Centre assisted women at home with their babies; parentcraft classes prepared them in advance; a Young Mothers Clinic dealt specifically with teenage pregnancies; a Chemical Dependency Unit served drug- and alcohol-abusing patients (by the 1990s the most vulnerable group of the Victorian population to maternal death). The hospital also did more outside its walls: ante-natal clinics for Turkish and Vietnamese women in first North Melbourne then Flemington, collaborative work with community health centres, shared care with general practitioners and a clinic in Broadmeadows, bringing the hospital's services into the outer western suburbs of Melbourne. It also took responsibility for non-clinical outreach to the community: with a 'Women's Health Line', the Women's Health Information Centre in a shop in Carlton, a Well Women's Clinic, and perhaps its most radical venture, CASA, the Centre Against Sexual Assault.

When the Queen Victoria Medical Centre moved into the Monash Medical Centre at Clayton, there was a need for a rape crisis service in the centre of Melbourne. The Women's won the contract and appointed a feminist social worker, Kate Gilmore, as co-ordinator. From the beginning the hospital working group, under the leadership of Dr Les Reti, knew that the counselling and advocacy side must not be accommodated within the hospital and that the medical model was no longer appropriate. Wendy Weeks, as a social work academic, was invited on to the planning committee:

> Some of the original design had a lot of hierarchy which people thought wasn't feminist — high paid psychologist, low paid clerical worker. It was a standard package. Therefore it was reworked through this committee (that Les Reti chaired) so that it was much more consistent with what we understood internationally to be feminist theory and practice.
>
> So in the first six months on the committee we talked out the philosophy of the centre. And the key issue was — what was the problem? who were the audience? who were the participants? who was it for? what was it going to do? We had to grapple with what rape was, what sexual assault was; where did it come from; whose problem was it: what did you have to change if you wanted to abolish it?[54]

CASA House opened in June 1987 in a terrace in Cardigan Street. It operated twenty-four hours a day, seven days a week on the 'rights advocacy' model of service provision, seeking to empower survivors of sexual assault — to be their advocates rather than agents of the legal/medical system, and seek 'to ensure the safety and security of the victim/survivor' and promote 'their right to gain control over their experience'.[55] It was not merely a success as a sexual assault crisis service; it offered an ideological challenge to the rest of the hospital, providing an intellectual shape to the shift in practice which had its roots in the 1970s. Many people — doctors, nurses and always social workers — had been moving towards what Wendy Weeks would call 'women centred practice':

> You can't talk about the shift to women centred practice at the

Women's Hospital without talking of the contribution Kate Gilmore made. Apart from the fact that she is very committed and very talented, she also has a wonderful analytical mind. She was able to look around, listen and learn and talk to a range of people, and say, OK, what is sexual assault? what is rape? who are the women who are being affected and what are they saying? So Kate pushed the agenda, but always openly and with a strong educative stance and she kept true to the analysis of the women — Why call women 'patients', they're women? What's wrong with the word 'woman'? And now we're saying — why can't women be citizens?

It was a seed that fell on already fertile ground: the 'enormous clinical material' had graduated to being 'patients'; the next step was 'citizens'.

Again political change impelled institutional change. A state Labor government was elected for the first time in twenty-seven years in 1982 and, federally, Labor returned to power in 1983. But the preceding coalition governments had funded significant growth in the public hospital system so that by 1982–83 Margaret Mabbitt, now Associate Director of Midwifery, could feel for the first time in her long association with the hospital that staffing levels were where they should be. The federal Labor government brought in a new Medicare scheme, and the hospital was now so accustomed to major changes, that it took them in its stride. But these Labor governments of the 1980s were of a new breed, desperate not to be tarred with the brush of big-spending and reckless management

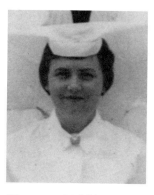

Margaret Mabbitt *RWHA*

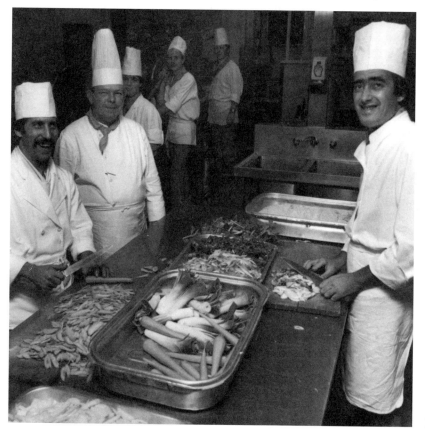

Kitchen staff *RWHA*

of the Whitlam years. And there was a longer term trend that by 1984 was becoming clear. Medical carers had significantly expanded the range of their care: full care required a range of interventions, supports and structures from many different professionals. Medicine had not become just more technologically complex, it had become sociologically so. Illness and natural functions like reproduction were social as well as biological phenomena. In every way, it had become more expensive, but governments could not, or would not, underwrite a perpetual expansion of services. In 1983 the state government imposed major budget cuts, and it would seem to those inside hospitals, that from then on they would lurch from crisis to crisis, cut to cut, change to change to the end of the millennium and beyond. At the same time, hospital workers of all kinds were demanding long overdue improvements in pay and conditions. Middle-class professionals no longer considered themselves above going on strike. In 1984 the hospital experienced its first major industrial dispute with doctors; in 1985 the first actual nursing strike; in 1986 its staff joined a shattering nursing strike that lasted fifty days, culminating in even the midwives walking off the job. In 1984 the Director of Medical Services, Dr Cliff Flower, commented prophetically:

> Looking back over annual reports of the past decade it becomes very obvious that there has been a marked change in the climate within which hospitals operate. Perhaps the expectation of the community today in relation to hospital and health services is higher than this same community is able or willing to pay. Perhaps we are about to look at quite new, and possibly less expensive patterns of health care delivery. We may even recognise belatedly that greater funding for and attention to health maintenance and preventive medicine could lead to a reduction in demand for some therapeutic services. It is also likely that the near future will see more shared-care programs being developed between hospitals and community-based resources.[56]

The 1980s was a decade of social planning, strategic management, corporate plans, mission statements — a whole vocabulary of structured power which sometimes gave the appearance of social concern rather than the performance. Hospital management had become an academic discipline driven by new theories of organisation which sought to transform the power structures within these vast and complex institutions. Within the Women's Hospital major structural reform was instituted to break down divisions between departments, devolve day-to-day decision making to the workers at the 'coal face', remove hierarchies and administer from a small top executive. Services would be co-ordinated into large aggregates for better interdisciplinary work and the reduction of professional boundaries and privileges. Most dramatically, the power of doctors was reduced. They became members of teams rather than the ruling class. While some welcomed it, others were deeply disorientated. Much of this reform was driven not only by the new theories of hospital management, but also by the continuing budget cuts under both the Labor government and the new Liberal government elected in 1992; and with each crisis, the new style of management endeavoured to

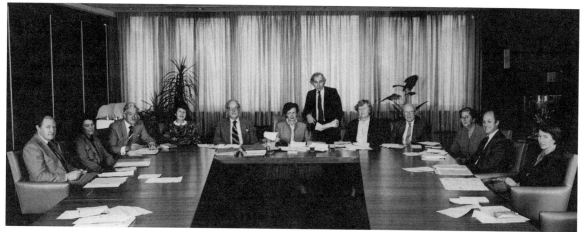

empower staff in the decision making. If it was more democratic and often more creative, it none the less marked a further loss of power for medical staff. Unwittingly, the way was prepared for the entry of accountants into medical practice. Doctors one day would have to be financially accountable for every clinical decision they took.

But the most dramatic reform in the hospital's history was reserved for the state Liberal government. Inheriting a public hospital system which was over-concentrated in the older sections of the metropolitan area, rationalisation was clearly necessary. A strategic review recommended the amalgamating of the Royal Women's and Royal Children's Hospital into a Women's and Children's Healthcare Network which shared administrative resources but retained separate campuses. The state government had also introduced a radical new form of hospital funding called Casemix (an extension of the clinical funding mechanisms instituted by the state Labor government), which funded hospitals according to the procedures and rewarded the most efficient in business terms: the more patients treated for the least expenditure of resources. Casemix had many supporters among the health industry (as it had now become), but few were happy at the financial cuts which came simultaneously. Hospitals were expected to do more with less: be less wasteful with staff, time and materials, and the culture of business managerialism which had crept into the world of administration now entered the door of the clinic. The Royal Women's entered this new era in a stronger position than most, having benefited from sound financial management in the 1980s and early 1990s, but within the network it felt somewhat shabby and tainted by its work for the poor and the delinquent compared with its partner the Royal Children's which had thrown off its pauper past, and glowed with goodness and the innocence of childhood in the public mind. The Royal Women's had worked very hard to establish itself as the hospital for all women, but it refused to abandon its duty to those for whom it had been founded.

In July 1995 the Board of Management, the direct descendant of the committee of godly women who had sought out Dr Tracy and Dr Maund to found a lying-in hospital for poor women, met for the last time. Only two of its number — a professor and one lay woman — were to be trans-

Board of Management, 1983. Left to right: Mr A. S. McLaughlan, Mrs Mary Murdoch, Mr John Lewis, Mrs Alison Leslie, Mr Gordon Leckie OBE, Mrs Judith Adam (president), Dr William Chanen, Lady Woodward, Mr Harry Wexler OBE, Dr Gytha Betheras, Professor Roger Pepperell, Mrs Dorothy Heeley.

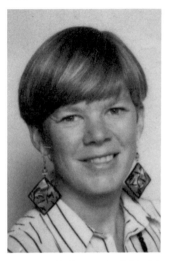

Dr Chris Bayly *RWHA*

lated on to the board of the new network. In that sense the Royal Women's Hospital was no more. However, the network promised that it would retain the hospital's individual identity and its focus. The restructuring also brought new challenges. Now it was to be the hub of services to women, with spokes extending into the community, not just through community health centres and satellite clinics, but even through private general practitioners and other community providers. Dr Chris Bayly is Director of the Division of Community Health Services which now includes around twenty departments, from sexual counselling to social work to breast screening to health education and the organisation of outpatients. The division works with a consciously feminist model of health care as well as the biomedical model: 'My vision for the future is for the biomedical and social models of health working with more mutuality. There'll always be some conflict and that can be constructive, but perhaps a questioning, slightly uneasy peace'.[57]

Chances 16

By the early 1970s the Royal Women's Hospital was firmly established in the forefront of medical practice in women's reproductive health and of neo-natal care; and it projected itself to the community as a leader in medical science and technology.[58] Fittingly in 1970 Professor Lance Townsend was knighted and Dr Kate Campbell was made a Dame of the British Empire. (The president of the Board, Mabel Coles, was also made a Dame.) Kate Campbell had been retired five years, but Professor Townsend had another seven years ahead of him. His strategic planning of the hospital's research work was now bearing fruit, and the research culture pervaded all clinics and units of the institution. Everyone was expected to be doing some sort of research in addition to their clinical work. The Pathology Department had a staff of a hundred (twenty of them part-timers associated with the twenty-four-hour transfusion service). The hospital assumed a responsibility for state-wide epidemiology, especially statistics on stillbirth and neo-natal deaths and congenital defects, and Townsend continued to publish annual clinical reports, which if lacking in analysis of quality and recommendations for improvement, did establish benchmarks of practice for both the Royal Women's itself and for women's health services throughout Australia. Many individual clinics, from Family Planning to Oncology, had research projects. The hospital continued to make use of its 'marvellous clinical material' — the large numbers of both normal and high-risk pregnancies that passed through its wards and clinics. The sheer volume of patients made it easy to mount major investigations, and the security of tenure for the senior staff, especially the university appointments in the Professorial Unit, made it possible to plan for the very long term. The hospital also benefited from the 'university precinct': the university was next door, the Royal Melbourne Hospital ten minutes walk away, as were the two Catholic hospitals, St Vincent's and the Mercy Hospital for Women which were both now teaching hospitals for the university. Further down Swanston Street was the Queen Victoria Medical Centre, occupying the site of the

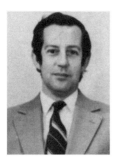 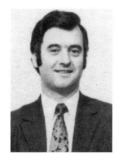 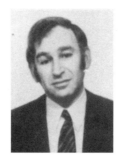 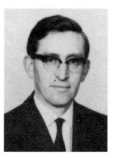 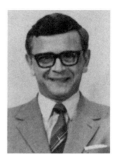

Left to right: Drs Douglas Adey, Donald Byrne, William Chanen, Denys Fortune and Michael Kloss in 1972

original Melbourne Hospital. If the Queen Victoria was more adventurous in social medicine, the Royal Women's had other research strengths, and groups from the two collaborated on special projects. The international medical world was also closer, as cheaper air travel abolished the tyranny of distance and Australian researchers could attend single conferences or take short study trips more often. Australian medical science was now firmly part of the international scientific community. The hospital had the intellectual critical mass to be an exciting place to work, for young researchers, for clinicians coming in from general practice and for senior staff alike. Townsend protected his younger researchers from the scepticism and interference of the older honoraries and bore the brunt of the inevitable feuding that erupted. It was by necessity a volatile mix of minds and (largely male) egos.

Two of his special initiatives were now bringing their rewards both to patients and to the hospital itself. In 1965 W. H. Kitchen had been appointed as paediatric first assistant (a university appointment) in the Professorial Unit to oversee the introduction of the newly evolving practice of neo-natal intensive care. He was sent on three-months study tour to Europe and North America, but Kitchen was concerned with the long-term outcomes for the babies, not merely their short-term survival and progress in intensive care. He read an Edinburgh study of the outcome of infants weighing less that $3\frac{1}{4}$ lbs born in the late 1950s and early 1960s:

> The findings really were to me devastating. Less than a third went to normal school and normal school meant you weren't more than two grades behind your peers. Another third were educable in schools for the blind or physically handicapped. And a third were just ineducable in any form.
>
> And with the intensive care that was coming out, it looked as though things should be better, but so many of the previously used techniques which had seemed a good idea at the time, had proved devastating — Streptomycin or its precursor, a lot of the kids were deaf; Vitamin K analogue produced a type of cerebral palsy. So it seemed terribly important when we introduced new techniques here, that there was a surveillance of what went on. They call that 'Quality Assurance' or something now.[59]

There was a group in San Francisco and another in the United Kingdom who were following up very low birth weight babies, but their results were all 'up on bookshelves' and not processed. Kitchen and this team took advantage of the new computer technology and the results were entered on a data base. The other advantage they had was the stability of the Victorian population compared especially to the USA, and when they assessed their first cohort at the age of eight, they were able to find 90 per cent of them. A few had returned to Italy or Greece with their families, but even many of these were found. The assessments were medical, psychological and educational, and the first cohort was drawn entirely from the Women's own patients, consisting of babies born between 1966 and 1970.

That first cohort was a dreadful disappointment. How you define disability depends on how you view it. Some follow-up people make the statement that if you exclude those who are severely disabled, the rest are the same as the normal population. Which is a nice piece of creative thinking. But our first group was severely socio-economically disadvantaged and about a third were Greek or Italian parentage. There were quite a lot of minor impairments and something like 10 per cent that were severe.

The results on survival were very gratifying however: from 1965 to 1971 the death rate among infants weighing between 1000 and 1500 grams had fallen from 47 per cent to 33 per cent. Over the next twenty-five years the improvement would be spectacular, with well over 90 per cent of babies weighing 1000 to 1500 grams living, and the unit saving babies of 23 and 24 weeks gestation. This was good news not only for premature babies, but also for mothers with life-threatening pre-eclampsia or other conditions where early delivery might be necessary. In the 1990s the greater confidence in neo-natal intensive care makes a caesarean at 27 or 28 weeks an easier decision for all concerned.[60] The Royal Women's, like all large maternity and children's hospitals, widely publicised its success stories, and the 'high tech' imagery reshaped community perceptions of

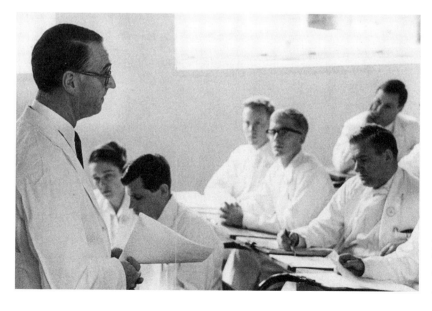

Professor Sir Lance Townsend lecturing to medical students
Mark Strizic

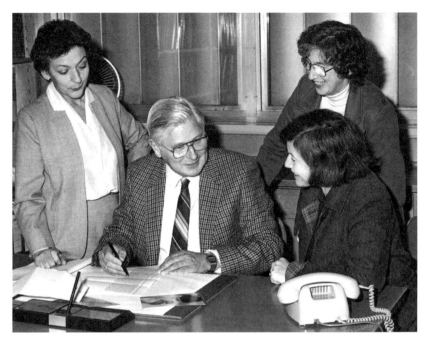

**Dr Margaret Ryan
(research social worker),
Dr W. H. Kitchen,
Dr Anne Rickards
(research psychologist),
Sister Val Lissenden
(nurse/midwife)** *RWHA*

what went on in hospitals. But the neo-natal work which won the Royal
Women's and Bill Kitchen's team international acclaim was the 'Follow-
up of Infants Weighing Under 1500 grams'. Victor Yu from the Queen
Victoria collaborated on the 1979–80 cohort and eventually it became
the outcome for the whole state which reduced the bias of the sample.
The project is still continuing under Associate Professor Lex Doyle.

But the follow-up produced some other startling findings. The social
worker, Maggi Ryan, 'did the very strange thing of actually talking to
the mothers, and not only that, she listened to them':

> And when we got our group back aged two, quite a bit of the
> assessment time was spent with the social worker. And the stories that
> came out of that were heart-rending. The old nursery had a small
> window in the corner where the mothers pressed their noses to the
> glass, although certain of the humane nurses let them in at night.
>
> But they were coming with stories like, 'All I ever saw were his
> feet', and the information for these parents was sparse, usually given by
> nurses who weren't particularly *au fait* with neonates. Doctors rarely
> met them. The whole emphasis was on prevention of infection and
> apparently the worst in the world were parents. We should have
> realised this at the time that really the people who ultimately care for
> these children are not the doctor and the nurse but the parents.
>
> So out of this came a real revolution in the pastoral care of families
> — firstly mothers, then fathers and then perhaps moving on to the
> extended family. And the pastoral care for the parents is extraordinarily
> important, perhaps even more so than the intensive care for the infant.

They found that around 40 per cent of the mothers were still suffering
from depression when their children were two-year-olds, and the unit

which in the 1970s was one of the most sophisticated high-tech activities in the hospital, was also one of the most advanced in the emotional care of patients.

The techniques of intensive care, investigation and diagnosis are enormously satisfying intellectually, and it's easy to make that the sole criterion by which you judge the efficacy of treatment. The counselling of patients just didn't initially go on and the feeling was that if you had a very sick child, you told the mother that it probably wouldn't survive, and then if it did, she was supposed to be pleased about it. The social worker came across one lady who called her baby 'Lozaro', 'Lazarus', coming back from the grave. And this anticipatory

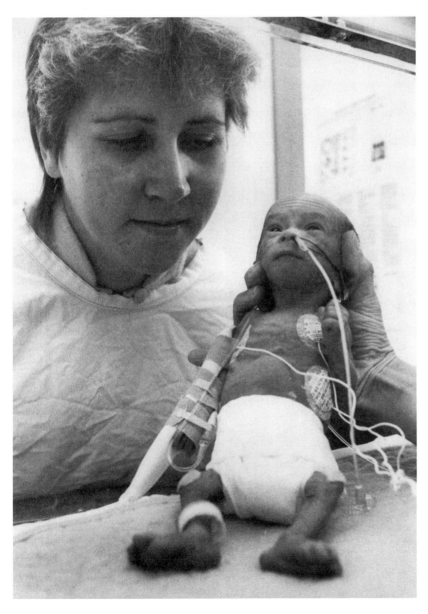

Premature baby and nurse *RWHA*

grief was an area we were very keen to counsel people properly on. If anything it's better to remain optimistic and deal with the death when it happens, rather than anticipate it.

The neo-natal intensive care unit was almost an anomaly. There medical, nursing and social work staff were close, and kept largely to themselves amidst the wider culture of the hospital. They also were realistic about the psychological toll of their own work, about the burn-out that came from working with intense concentration with very sick babies, and the grief when a baby they had nursed for months ultimately died. The medical staff also suffered, trying to decide priorities over levels of treatment when resources were limited. A number scoffed when Bill Kitchen appointed a psychiatrist to the unit: 'was it for the babies or the staff?', but the psychiatrist proved invaluable counselling staff and mediating ethical debates. Kitchen had no illusions about the 'old Women's': 'This place was terrible: the antenatal clinics were like running a veterinary practice — everything was done to stop communication'. But it was not surprising perhaps that it took paediatricians to start the process of humanising the Women's: 'Paediatricians are used to being cut down to size by their patients — someone drags your coat, you look round — "Big April Fool"'.

The second major intellectual investment by the hospital had been in Endocrinology, with the appointments from Scotland of J. B. Brown, and later of James Evans. Townsend, although a cancer specialist, realised that endocrinology had a large place in gynaecology and in Brown he had found an outstanding researcher who would attract others to come to the Royal Women's. Brown was unique in that he had designed the oestrogen assays which made the measurement of oestrogen possible for the

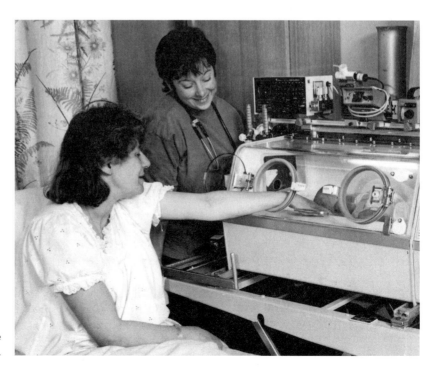

Mother and premature baby *RWHA*

first time, and the unit was to become recognised for knowing more about oestrogen than any other place in the world. With Pincus Taft and James Evans, he pioneered the induction of ovulation, using human pituitary gonadotropins. Brown extracted his own, but tragically a contaminated batch manufactured by the Commonwealth Serum Laboratories was given to a small group of the Royal Women's patients. This contaminated batch was implicated in the 1990s in five women in Australia developing C J disease. Such a tragedy, coming close on other disasters with pituitary extract used by the Royal Children's Hospital to overcome growth abnormalities, aggravated long-held community fears of 'hormone' treatments, masking the immense benefits this growing field of clinical research was bringing. 'Hormone treatments' had long been feared as something which transgressed the boundaries of the natural; medicine, which by definition was an intervention in 'natural' processes of illness and disablement, 'went too far' when it interfered with hormones. Treatments which might incidentally or temporarily change secondary sexual characteristics like facial hair or promote weight gain or stimulate skin eruptions, were psychically threatening in a way quite different from surgery. Fertility treatments which might cause women to hyper-ovulate and conceive quadruplets, or even worse, shocked and disgusted many. It was treating women like breeding animals; it was veterinary medicine rather than human medicine. Therefore just as medical science was beginning to unravel the secrets of the chemical messengers which controlled the reproductive system, deep anxiety was aroused in the non-medical world. Even among many who were medically trained, including obstetricians and gynaecologists, there were some who recoiled from this new, secret, biochemical narrative of human reproduction and experience.

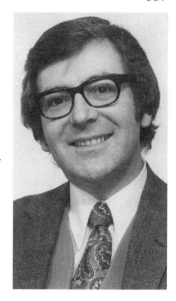

Dr James Evans, endocrinologist and hospital historian *RWHA*

Even the apparently life-affirming task of making the barren fruitful laboured under a taint of 'interfering with the natural', of 'going against Nature'. But there was another stigma which afflicted research and treatment of infertility — the widespread belief that infertility was the wages of sin. The Women's had been only the second hospital in the world to start an infertility clinic. Crown Street, Sydney, had been the first in 1937, and J. W. Johnstone had followed suit at the Women's in 1945. In the absence of significant scientific knowledge, it was assumed that infertility was the fault of women. (Seminal analysis developed by McLeod at Cambridge in 1945 was just beginning to be studied at a community level.) Men rarely volunteered a semen specimen, and they were not required to do so when their wives sought treatment, so little could be studied. If a man could produce an ejaculate, he assumed he was fertile. Women who were infertile were either unfortunate women who could not ovulate, or they were diseased women whose fallopian tubes were too damaged by pelvic inflammatory disease for conception to be possible. The pelvic inflammatory disease was assumed to have arisen from a septic abortion (most likely induced), or a sexually transmitted disease (most likely gonorrhoea). And those pathologies were again assumed to have been the consequences of sexual promiscuity.[61]

In 1968 Ian Johnston, as the most junior member of the consultant gynaecological staff, was told to run the starkly named Sterility Clinic, which he quickly renamed 'Infertility'. He had no previous interest in infertility, but he was fascinated by the new technology of laparoscopy, which offered a radically new way to explore the pelvis. Around a third of the patients the clinic were seeing had a history of PID, but when Johnston began investigating each patient routinely with the laparoscope, he began to learn about the problems the patients really had, and the treatment of infertility was transformed from something of a medical art into a science. They began to get a proper basis for diagnosis, and with that, a launching pad for treatment. They discovered more endometriosis than anyone had expected, and they found more apparent PID than the patients' histories had disclosed. Johnston made a large-scale study, which he never published, of the aetiology of all this PID, and found that around a third had had an acute appendicitis when they were young which had been missed and had turned into peritonitis; another third had no history of anything (although later he would speculate that some may have had chlamydia); the remaining third did have some history which you could relate to their infertility:

> Not always an illegal termination of pregnancy; in fact the bulk of them were in women who'd had a simple pregnancy, a normal delivery and they'd developed a puerperal infection or they were unlucky enough to have had one or two spontaneous miscarriages and they'd get infected afterwards. So the number of whom we could actually say that their past sexual behaviour contributed to infertility problems was probably less than 10 per cent of the whole population.
>
> I could sense the disbelief about everything, so I said, let's look at it. I wasn't unique in looking at it — there was quite a lot in the literature, all giving similar results. But it depends on the community. It was important at that time in that hospital because we had been through the era of 'Bung' Hill and Hildred Butler and all the work they'd done on *Welchii* infections. And I grew up as a student and a resident watching women die of *Welchii* infections.

The immediate response to these damaged women was surgical: opening them up to clear the pelvis of adhesions, and mobilise the uterus, ovaries and tubes. 'But it was heavy handed stuff and we had no idea of the harm we were doing surgically to the tissues in those days, because it's not until you start to do surgery under the microscope that you can actually see the damage you're doing'. Johnston and his colleague Andrew Spiers went to the St Vincent's Hospital's microsurgery school, and those new techniques did have some success in the restoration of tubes which had been tied off for sterilisation. But for those women whose tubes were internally a mass of scar tissue from infection, microsurgery offered no real hope. For Johnston this became the first major indication for in-vitro fertilisation.

In 1971 Johnston met the English embryologist Robert Edwards at a meeting in Japan where he spoke of the work that he and Patrick Steptoe had begun with in-vitro fertilisation (IVF):

> He showed human embryos. Few had ever *seen* a human embryo before, then these incredible slides came up of two-cell and four-cell human embryos. A gasp went round the meeting. He had produced

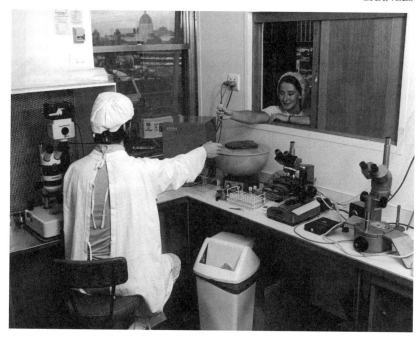

Ova are passed through to an IVF scientist following an ovum pick-up for examination under a microscope prior to fertilisation in the laboratory. *RWHA*

very few of them, but it was very exciting stuff and I came back from that meeting thinking *that's* an area that needs looking at.

The sheep breeders were experimenting in Australia and achieving considerable success, but the essential differences between animals and humans were not appreciated. The sheep breeders were super-ovulating sheep, inseminating them so that they were fertilised *in vivo*, then flushing out the embryos for re-implantation in prepared ewes. The workers on human infertility were attempting to achieve fertilisation *in vitro*, outside the body, and they did not comprehend its immense complexities.

Johnston found little support back in Melbourne, however. Professor Townsend was repelled by the concept and refused to give university funding, then the only source of financial support for laboratory research. Townsend might want the Royal Women's to have an international research profile, but he was only interested in clinical research: 'Jim Brown was the first pure scientist he'd had anything to do with'. The Board did agree to pay the salary of Dr Alex Lopata, but the project could expect nothing else.

Our first laboratory was a cleaner's cupboard in a theatre suite and we put an incubator in there, and the first time we put an embryo into the incubator overnight, the cleaner came along during the night, saw the switch had been left on for the incubator and turned it off.

Then we had a little room that they built for us underneath some stairs. We had a sink in that one, but it had no plumbing—bucket under the sink, water in bottles. But at least it was a room we could lock up and say was ours.

They achieved embryos, but they had no idea if the embryos were genetically normal until they tested them. Convinced of the safety of the embryos, they then had to tackle the problem of implantation. By now, just three clinics in the world were working on IVF, Steptoe and Edwards in England, and two in Melbourne — Professor Carl Wood's Monash University group at the Queen Victoria Medical Centre and Lopata and Johnston at the Royal Women's, and in the race to produce the world's first 'test-tube' baby the English team won. Johnston decided to call a halt until they could find out from Steptoe how they had done it, and the Board, at great expense, paid for Steptoe and his wife to visit Australia. Except that Steptoe didn't tell and hadn't published, convincing Johnston that he would not follow suit. The only thing they found out from Steptoe was that he was doing it with natural cycles, not over-stimulated ones. The Women's team changed tack and in late 1979 achieved their first pregnancy. On 23 June 1980 Candice Reed was born in the Royal Women's Hospital, Australia's first 'test-tube baby'. The Monash team never forgave them for winning the Australian race, and the myth was nourished that Monash had in fact achieved the first.[62] But the Royal Women's had not only produced the first Australian baby, it was the first research team in the world to publish the full report of the procedure, the article appearing in *Fertility and Sterility* of February 1980, four months before Candice was born.

Initially, however, success rates were so low as to make IVF scarcely worth while, so the strategy of implanting multiple embryos was adopted; but while the hospital had successes such as the world's first IVF quadruplets, the rates of pre-term delivery and perinatal mortality were unacceptably high. Rather than throw embryos away, the doctors looked to

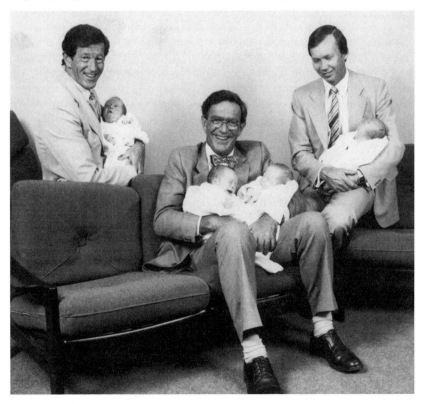

Dr Ken Mountain, Mr Ian Johnston and Dr Andrew Spiers with the first IVF quadruplets
RWHA

freezing them, and in 1985 the French developed a good technique which the Women's put into practice the following year. This conferred much greater control of the process and over the years the clinic has achieved a published perinatal mortality of 8–10 per 1000, lower than that of the general community.

Monash's successes received more publicity, but the Royal Women's Hospital soon became one of the major clinics training people from all around the world — from thirty-two countries at the last count. It brought the hospital more repute and some money, but the administration still expected the clinic to pay its own way in research. The funding now came increasingly from the patients themselves, while Medicare still refused to support treatment. Public patients were treated free; private patients paid and raised funds for equipment. Even government funding for the very successful Donor Insemination programme was kept by the hospital for other purposes and not passed on to the clinic. None the less, the perception grew that IVF was somehow taking millions of dollars away from other, more 'legitimate' areas of medicine, because for all its technological and human triumphs, it was arousing hostility and distrust in influential sections of the community.

There was considerable opposition from within the medical profession itself — that it was somehow 'going too far', putting human life into the laboratory, diverting valuable funds, indulging people who should learn to resolve their grief over their childlessness. When so many vital areas of health care remained neglected and underfunded, none more deserving than Aboriginal health, IVF looked like bourgeois self-indulgence. But there was also ethical anxiety about human interference in the biological mysteries of reproduction which were the realm of God, not man. The Roman Catholic Church was an expected critic and again Right to Life was prominent in its attacks on the hospital, but the critique was wider and the new philosophical discipline of bioethics grew in response to the profound questions that reproductive technologies were raising about both the sanctity of life and the proper place of secular science. While many other areas of medicine and experimental science aroused bioethical concerns, IVF was, in the public mind, the trigger. The later regulation of reproductive biological research in fact was to outlaw many of the procedures which had been essential to its development.

While the opposition from the Catholic Church was expected, that from the women's movement came as a surprise. Feminists deplored the invasion of women's bodies by male, high-tech science — women's reduction into 'living laboratories'.[63] They reported the disappointment and the stress, and they opposed the polarised debate about surrogacy which, to social work academic Wendy Weeks, was essentially 'a repeat of adoption, and we already knew as social workers that there was a problem with adoption'.[64] If the controversy took some of the gloss off the achievements of in-vitro fertilisation and its associated technologies, the growing success rate tempered the disillusionment. Again social workers were part of the team which supported the families in the IVF programme, as the social work department refocused itself away from adoption towards supporting, counselling and advocating for patients in all parts of the hospital. Men were admitted as patients to the hospital for the first time in

1968 and their compulsory attendance with their wives enabled the clinic to begin to understand the extent of male infertility and to develop, in the mid 1970s under Dr Gary Clark, Melbourne's first public Donor Insemination programme. The hospital developed a bank of frozen sperm and Australia's first Natural AID workshop was held at the Women's in 1978. Reproductive biology, as it became known, transformed the pattern of gynaecological admissions from the early 1970s, leading to a new expansion of gynaecological activity in the hospital just as the midwifery declined with the changing demographics of Melbourne. It also extended the hospital's reach into the middle class, as women sought the best science in their quest to have a baby. By the 1990s reproductive biology had retreated from being the hospital's busiest research area as most of the physiological problems infertile couples faced had a technological solution of reasonable efficacy. The most recent addition to this technology is intra-cytoplasmic sperm injection (ICSI) which enables men with very poor sperm production to father children, and this one new device has revolutionised infertility treatment. Roger Pepperell, the Dunbar Hooper Professor of Obstetrics and Gynaecology since 1977, believes that the increasing practice of safe sex and a resultant decline in sexually transmitted diseases will in time reduce some infertility; as would a reversal of the present trend for women to start their childbearing in their mid and late thirties.[65]

In the 1990s the hospital's most active research became perinatal medicine: looking at what makes mothers and babies sick. The Perinatal Medicine Unit's major interest became pre-eclampsia and eclampsia in mothers; with babies it has been the three remaining major killers of babies in Victoria: congenital malformations, pre-term delivery and poor growth within the womb. The unit's research methodologies ranged from a gene sequencer to identify gene defects, to public health programmes to assist women to stop smoking in pregnancy — by now the largest preventable cause of low birth weight in Australia. Research midwives interviewed women and their families to tease out the now recognised genetic component of pre-eclampsia, and worked with the antenatal patients in the anti-smoking programme. Even health policy and economic dimensions are included as part of the unit's work.

Now that infection has been controlled in Australia and embolism preempted by early ambulation and the greater physical activity of pregnant women, pre-eclampsia and eclampsia remain the major medical disorders of human pregnancy, and they are among the top three killers of pregnant women in the world. In Australia they take first or second place in the aetiology of maternal mortality, and the World Health Organisation estimates that 50 000 women die of eclampsia a year. Babies also are imperilled: antenatally because the pre-eclampsia affects the functioning of the placenta and can limit the supply of oxygen and nutrition to the baby. And given that delivery is the ultimate cure for pre-eclampsia, and that it must occur at whatever stage of the pregnancy that the disease strikes, that can mean the baby goes from a difficult life in the womb to the rigours of premature life in a neo-natal unit. Perinatal loss remains around 10 per cent. Pre-eclampsia itself is finally beginning to be understood. Professor Shaun Brennecke:

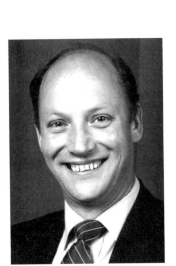

Professor Roger Pepperell
RWHA

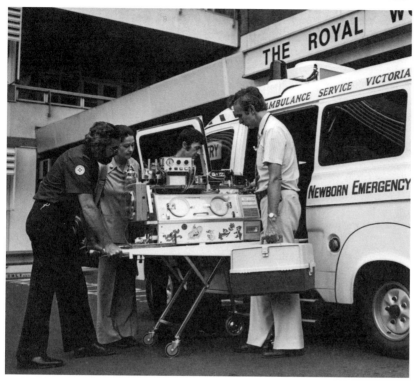

NETS: Newborn
Emergency Transfer
Service, with Dr Neil
Roy, far right *RWHA*

It is thought that in the early weeks the placenta does not attach itself
to the womb as well as it should, so that the mother is never able to
feed the placenta enough blood for the metabolic needs of the
placenta and the baby to be met. The placenta becomes relatively
hypoxic (insufficient oxygen), and eventually, as the placenta grows and
the oxygen needs increase, there comes a time in the second half of
pregnancy where the placenta can't cope and so begins to release
significant quantities of toxins into the maternal circulation. The idea
of a toxin has come back into vogue, although now it's thought to be
an internal toxin that the placenta produces. This toxin damages the
fragile endothelial cells that line the mother's blood vessels. These
endothelial cells make a lot of hormones, in particular a couple of
hormones that are meant to dilate the blood vessels of the body which
keep the blood pressure low. This results in a net preponderance of
hormones left in the woman's body which want to make the blood
vessels constrict and put up the blood pressure. Hence the high blood
pressure which is one of the most important clinical features of the
disease.

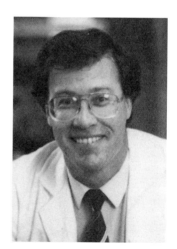

Professor Shaun
Brennecke *RWHA*

And because the blood vessels are constricted, the blood flow
around the body is restricted, so that the brain and the kidneys don't
get as much oxygen and nutrition as they would like — the brain is
hypoxic hence the convulsion, the kidneys can't work as well so they
begin to leak protein. And when the endothelial cells become damaged they become very leaky so that fluid in the mother's bloodstream
leaks out into the extra-vascular spaces which appears as oedema or
swelling.[66]

The cause, or causes, remain unresolved, although it is clear that the condition clusters in families. It is not a simple and predictable inheritance, 'probably because you're not dealing with individuals, but with two individuals — mother and foetus — who are present together'. The Royal Women's is one of the groups around the world seeking the genetic defect that it is hoped will revolutionise the treatment of pre-eclampsia. The hospital has also been one of the pioneers of the prophylactic use of low-dose aspirin for pre-eclampsia.

Causes other than pre-eclampsia of low birth weight are also the concern of the unit. Dr Robin Bell has worked on smoking in pregnancy, and at the end of the twentieth century smoking and social class have become closely allied:

> If you look at pregnancy outcomes in relation to social class, it is thought that smoking is responsible for a lot of what you can show is a relationship between social class and outcome in our community. It may not have always applied and that isn't to say that there isn't anything left, but let's say it's a powerful part of the influence.[67]

Smoking is also the single most preventable cause of low birth weight and of Sudden Infant Death (now that babies' recommended sleeping positions have been changed). And it remains a major health problem for the Royal Women's Hospital where 30 per cent of its antenatal patients are usually smokers before becoming pregnant. While men's smoking rates are falling, the smoking rates in young women and adolescent girls are still far too high. Robin Bell:

> It's interesting talking to the women here. Very many say that they always thought they'd give up when they were pregnant and are very

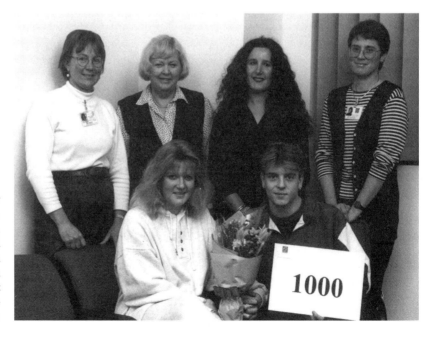

The Smoking Study Research Team. Sue Bishop, Lois Harrop, Mary Panjari and Dr Robin Bell, with Tomina Carr and Darren Lewis, the 1000th patient to participate in the study.

disappointed with themselves when they haven't. They all thought they'd stop at thirty, or some magical time in the future, not realising how very very addictive smoking is. Starting smoking as an adolescent when you're detached from the consequences and believing you can do anything including giving up smoking, then confronting the fact that you can't, is very difficult.

But these days Australian women are very healthy in pregnancy — significantly healthier than they were even thirty years ago. Professor Pepperell:

> Their haemoglobins are better, they're much more aware of what's going on pregnancy. They come to classes. They have iron therapy during the pregnancy and some don't need it because their iron levels are OK. They're seen more frequently. Minor problems are recognised and treated before they become a major disaster.
>
> Rheumatic fever as a childhood illness is now very rare. In the past it was very common and we saw them twenty years later when they were having their babies and were in real trouble. The commonest problem we have now in the cardiac area is congenital heart disease, where the kids who had heart problems at birth, had them corrected either partially or completely. We're now seeing them in difficulty but very rarely do they die.

This general well-being, however, masks the very real dangers of pre-eclampsia for those women at risk. No one wants to talk or know about the 'downside of pregnancy' and the danger with pre-eclampsia is that by the time the clinical symptoms become troublesome, the woman, and possibly her baby, are very sick. Shaun Brennecke again:

> I have always been amazed at how well women feel until their disease is very advanced. I have vivid memories of a woman who had very severe pre-eclampsia who walked from the bus stop because of a taxi strike or something — some kilometres to the hospital where I was working. And then there was a lift breakdown and she walked up five flights of stairs and then presented and said she felt a bit unwell.
>
> It's always very difficult to convince women who are severely pre-eclamptic that they have a disease that needs urgent treatment in hospital and a prompt delivery, because they often feel relatively well. And it comes as a great shock to them to be turned around in this way, to have their expectations of a normal pregnancy stifled and end up in hospital, lots of drips, lots of blood tests, monitoring and possibly early delivery within a day or two of coming into the hospital.

For Dr Chris Bayly, Director of the Community Health Services Division, unrealistic expectations are now one of the major dilemmas in women's health care:

> Because things are so much better now regarding mortality rates and so on, people expect that nothing's going to go wrong and somehow

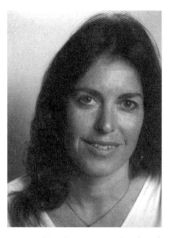

Dr Suzanne Garland
RWHA

Dr Les Reti *RWHA*

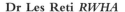

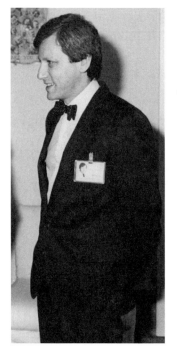

we should prevent everything from going wrong. Every time something does go wrong, it has to be somebody's fault. And providers can be as guilty in placing those expectations on ourselves — we've got to be able to fix everything, we've got to be able to find an answer to everything. Which sometimes means that we intervene in situations which are best left alone, where the real problem is about talking and listening and about adjustment to a situation rather than trying to solve a problem that can't be solved.

Neither do all the childbirth classes guarantee an ecstatic birth experience, and while birthing has been vastly humanised, some women are still unprepared for the levels of pain they experience or the interventions that become inevitable if their babies are to be born well.[68] None the less, now that modern medicine can take most of the suffering out of sex, humanity is left with the political problem of the delivery of that medical relief. Neither can medical intervention overcome poverty and inequality, and the sufferings of gender, class and ethnicity remain for too many. The sicknesses of women seen in the infirmary wards in the nineteenth century still afflict women in developing countries. (In rural Bangladesh, a study has found eight out of ten women to be suffering health problems of some form as a result of pregnancy or delivery.[69]) Class, however, has almost disappeared as a determinant of women's reproductive health in Australia, leaving only Aboriginal women whose health remains that of women in the Third World. The Royal Women's Hospital, through its chief microbiologist, Dr Suzanne Garland, now has outreach both into Mongolia with a World Health Organisation (WHO) programme, into Thailand, and into Aboriginal communities in northern Australia. Her team has pioneered patient self-collected specimens on tampons and uses molecular biology analysis for the detection of sexually transmissible organisms. Compliance is very high (95 per cent in one Aboriginal community), and accuracy far greater than with conventional diagnostic techniques. The project is to diagnose and treat STDs, such as gonorrhoea, which leave their victims more vulnerable to HIV infection. And the assessment of STD/HIV/AIDS diagnosis is the project that WHO asked her to bring to Mongolia. The HIV/AIDS education campaign has made young Australians use condoms more. When Suzanne Garland went to the Royal Women's in 1984, they saw at least one case of gonorrhoea a week, now she might go six months or more before seeing one. The challenge now is to reduce STD/HIV infection in northern Australia and in the Third World.[70]

The biological destiny of women in the developed world has been transformed in the lifetime of this hospital. To Dr Les Reti, it's obvious:

> It was very hard to have a women's movement if a quarter of women were anaemic and two thirds pregnant. And they couldn't have sex after the menopause because it hurt so much. I believe that after contraception, the single biggest advance has been Hormone Replacement Therapy because it's opened the second half of women's lives.[71]

But the wonders of modern medicine are not there for all women around

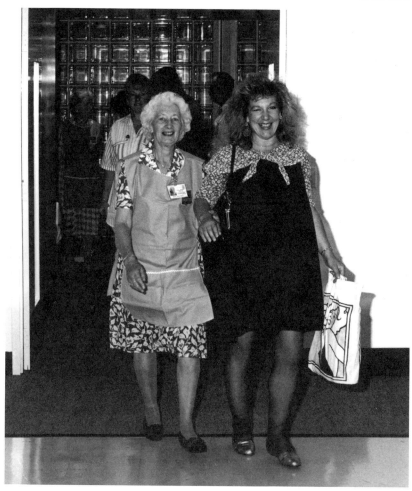

**Modern motherhood:
antenatal patient
accompanied by RWH
volunteer** *RWHA*

the world, because of political and social systems; and perhaps they are
threatened even within developed countries because costs are perceived
to be rising too fast. Les Reti again:

> Even though there have been enormous advances on a scientific level,
> I think there are system problems. Now that the systems are so
> complex, the reasons that patients don't get the best care aren't that the
> doctors are crummy, or the nurses are crummy or the technology's
> crummy — probably all three, and the many other facets of care are
> very good — but because the thing does not come together very well.
> There are system failures.

The answer he sees is the eternal vigilance of auditing, assessing, amend-
ing and re-auditing, a cycle of 'quality assurance' combined with the political and community will to continue to care about women and the
medical conditions peculiar to them. And here remains the single most
compelling reason for the preservation of the single-purpose hospital —
advocacy. The great women's hospitals are disappearing around the world
— in London, in Boston and within Australia, in Sydney, Adelaide and
Perth. The Queen Victoria Hospital was absorbed so well into the Monash

Medical Centre that it is but a memory. While delivering babies can be conducted in a general hospital, the total focus of the Royal Women's Hospital on women's health in all its aspects and stages of life and its advocacy for women, is vital not just for Melbourne, but for the nation and the region. When Richard Tracy and John Maund first talked of a lying-in hospital for the young colony, one which would not only deliver babies but specialise in the diseases peculiar to women and children, they recognised that women and children had specials needs that the general hospital could not meet. Nearly a century and a half later that has not changed.

Appendixes

Appendix I
Confinements 1857–1887

	1857	1858	1859	1860	1861	1862	1863
Confinements	108	181	188	197	230	298	295
Maternal deaths	0	0	3	5	1	2	4
Stillbirths	10	18	8	17	13	17	15
Neo-natal deaths	0	1	13	1	2	3	7
Birthplaces							
Australia	0	1	1	3	7	15	13
England	40	67	84	68	75	90	90
Ireland	61	96	84	106	128	153	155
Scotland	4	12	17	13	18	35	32
Other	3	5	2	7	2	5	5
Single	19	59	47	72	74	104	110
Mother's Age	108	181	184	197	230	298	295
15–20	18	34	25	41	34	56	44
21–25	41	82	69	80	99	102	122
26–30	37	47	60	53	59	88	85
31–35	7	11	21	14	25	38	25
36–40	4	6	8	9	9	11	12
40+	1	1	1	0	4	3	7
Parity	108	181	188	197	229	298	295
1	71	122	115	115	130	164	159
2	19	33	24	35	37	48	57
3	12	8	24	18	19	24	20
4	2	6	11	8	8	25	11
5	0	4	3	10	13	13	14
6	2	1	4	7	5	11	5
7	2	1	1	2	7	5	14
8	0	0	3	1	7	5	5
9	0	1	2	1	6	4	5
10	0	0	0	0	1	1	4
11+	0	3	1	0	1	2	3

Confinements 1857–1887 (continued)

	1864	1865	1866	1867	1868	1869	1870	1871	1872	1873	1874	1875
Confinements	338	392	398	384	371	384	402	445	490	445	446	420
Maternal deaths	4	4	7	6	5	7	5	2	4	16	5	7
Stillbirths	21	41	42	37	40	33	33	29	44	28	28	31
Neo-natal deaths	6	3	0	4	4	7	2	10	2	2	1	0
Birthplaces												
Australia	25	20	34	40	53	68	84	94	122	138	179	163
England	103	106	121	116	124	99	108	137	136	110	110	100
Ireland	144	196	201	185	158	169	172	169	196	167	128	125
Scotland	38	52	34	27	29	37	31	33	28	21	23	23
Other	8	18	8	16	7	11	7	12	8	9	6	9
Single	121	153	145	151	149	161	176	164	185	192	261	216
Mother's Age	338	392	398	384	371	384	401	445	488	445	446	420
15–20	69	72	60	81	84	71	89	89	124	122	120	113
21–25	117	155	156	122	136	123	135	155	156	149	165	127
26–30	105	106	103	106	101	104	109	112	104	79	94	98
31–35	29	39	44	41	32	45	29	58	58	49	40	51
36–40	12	15	26	24	12	27	28	19	28	32	16	24
40+	6	5	9	10	6	14	11	12	18	14	11	7
Parity	336	390	398	384	370	384	400	443	471	419	431	415
1	165	213	198	201	190	187	198	214	243	222	220	194
2	70	81	79	66	76	77	89	87	93	92	100	89
3	33	35	33	37	27	31	28	47	33	23	34	42
4	16	20	13	12	20	19	29	31	25	19	21	27
5	19	15	14	22	15	14	11	19	23	23	16	21
6	12	9	15	16	10	16	16	9	11	9	9	13
7	11	5	21	8	12	12	14	12	9	9	9	13
8	5	6	8	8	14	11	6	8	9	8	8	9
9	2	2	9	10	3	8	6	8	9	3	8	6
10	3	2	4	2	2	4	0	4	8	7	2	1
11+	0	2	4	2	1	5	2	4	8	4	10	5

Confinements 1857–1887 (continued)

	1876	1877	1878	1879	1880	1881	1882	1883	1884	1885	1886	1887
Confinements	397	504	541	594	590	673	571	601	600	358	215	479
Maternal deaths	3	9	5	13	11	27	7	13	38	17	7	5
Stillbirths	37	37	39	43	56	47	40	30	46	25	9	29
Neo-natal deaths	0	1	0	0							3	
Birthplaces										355		478
Australia	194	271	298	359	375	468	416	453	457	265	170	352
England	94	96	103	90	110	102	82	72	80	46	18	62
Ireland	80	112	89	91	92	66	60	62	54	31	15	28
Scotland	0	0	0	0	0	0	0	0	0	0	0	0
Other	29	25	51	54	13	18	12	14	9	3	3	16
Single	225	289	280	331	306	378	334	362	361	221	125	268
Mother's Age	397	504	534	593	590	663	563	595	599	356	215	478
15–20	124	165	162	203	195	219	211	171	202	115	72	139
21–25	122	163	188	217	228	232	208	260	245	150	87	195
26–30	74	98	95	85	91	82	79	90	82	59	30	75
31–35	37	36	45	44	41	50	36	35	37	22	12	45
36–40	25	26	31	25	27	25	21	33	29	6	13	21
40+	15	12	13	19	8	8	8	6	4	4	1	3
Parity	385	498	541	594	589	612	555	595	550	330	213	476
1	208	266	281	315	322	342	333	330	324	206	118	249
2	70	115	107	126	120	155	112	134	130	65	48	120
3	29	31	35	40	47	29	31	39	33	23	16	35
4	22	18	29	32	25	14	22	26	13	10	9	24
5	19	15	24	21	17	16	13	19	13	13	3	16
6	6	10	14	14	18	14	16	16	12	4	6	14
7	4	11	15	15	10	12	9	9	7	1	5	7
8	12	3	13	14	7	10	5	5	6	1	3	5
9	3	12	9	3	6	6	5	5	7	2	1	4
10	6	6	3	6	17	14	12	12	5	5	4	8
11+	6	11	11	8								

Confinements 1857–1887 (continued)

	1857	1858	1859	1860	1861	1862	1863
Pelvic Contraction	4	4	4	8	5	6	4
Version	0	1	0	0	1	0	0
Forceps	4	6	9	12	7	8	13
Inertia	0	0	9	0	4	0	9
Craniotomy	0	1	0	1	2	0	2
Induction of Labour							
Episiotomy							
Torn Perineum	0	1	4	0	5	2	1
Eclampsia	0	0	1	0	0	2	1
Albuminuria							
Placenta Praevia	0	1	0	0	1	0	0
APH	0	1	0	0	1	0	2
PPH	0	0	0	1	0	6	8
Adherent Placenta	0	0	1	0	0	1	0
Mania/Psychosis	0	0	1	1	0	1	0
1 Syphilis	0	1	0	1	1	0	1

2 Gonorrhoea
3 Tuberculosis
4 Alcoholism
5 Diarrhoea/Typhoid
6 Pneumonia
7 Heart Disease
8 Infectious Diseases
9 Cancer
10 Scarlet Fever/Scarlatina
11 Tonsilitis
12 To Infirmary ?sepsis
13 Septicaemia
14 Salpingitis
15 Hydramnios
16 Renal Disease

Confinements 1857–1887 (continued)

	1864	1865	1866	1867	1868	1869	1870	1871	1872	1873	1874	1875
Pelvic Contraction	8	10	7	18	15	16	8	15	11	0	3	3
Version	2	0	0	1	3	5	3	2	5	2	3	3
Forceps	21	15	9	21	18	12	17	18	41	31	32	23
Inertia	11	3	5	5	1	10	9	10	7	0	0	0
Craniotomy	2	3	2	2	2	2	0	2	3	1	1	1
Induction of Labour						2	2	0	6	0	2	0
Episiotomy												
Torn Perineum	0	0	0	1	0	1	0	4	0	0	1	1
Eclampsia	2	2	0	3	6	5	2	3	2	3	3	2
Albuminuria												
Placenta Praevia	2	1	0	0	1	0	0	0	1	3	1	1
APH	1	1	1	0	0	0	0	1	0	0	0	0
PPH	6	2	4	1	4	5	11	12	3	2	0	1
Adherent Placenta	0	0	0	1	2	1	5	8	9	2	0	0
Mania/Psychosis	0	0	0	0	0	4	2	4	2	1	1	2
1 Syphilis	1	0	0	0	9	5	8	0	0	0	0	1
2 Gonorrhoea					1	0	0	0	0	0	0	0
3 Tuberculosis					1	2	5	2	0	2	1	1
4 Alcoholism					1	3	0	1	0	0	0	0
5 Diarrhoea/Typhoid						1	1	0	0	1	0	1
6 Pneumonia						1	1	0	0	0	0	1
7 Heart Disease							1	1	0	0	0	0
8 Infectious Diseases									1	0	0	0
9 Cancer												0
10 Scarlet Fever/Scarlatina												1
11 Tonsilitis												1
12 To Infirmary ?sepsis												
13 Septicaemia												
14 Salpingitis												
15 Hydramnios												
16 Renal Disease												

Confinements 1857–1887 (continued)

	1876	1877	1878	1879	1880	1881	1882	1883	1884	1885	1886	1887
Pelvic Contraction	3	1	0	0	0	0	0	0	0	1	4	3
Version	3	2	0	1	0	1	0	0	0	0	0	4
Forceps	28	25	29	29	11	17	12	29	17	11	11	26
Inertia	0	0	0	0	0	0	0	0	0	0	0	4
Craniotomy	0	0	2	0	0	4	0	0	0	0	1	0
Induction of Labour	0	0	0	0	0	1	0	1	0	1	2	2
Episiotomy	0	0	0	0	0	0	0	0	0	0	0	0
Torn Perineum	2	0	0	0	0	1	0	0	0	0	48	25
Eclampsia	2	4	5	0	1	4	2	2	2	2	1	7
Albuminuria	1	0	0	0	0	0	0	0	0	0	10	10
Placenta Praevia	1	2	0	2	1	2	1	0	0	0	1	1
APH	0	1	0	0	0	1	1	0	0	0	0	0
PPH	0	0	3	6	1	1	0	0	0	0	3	4
Adherent Placenta	1	1	0	1	1	2	0	0	0	0	0	6
Mania/Psychosis	2	0	1	0	1	6	1	0	0	0	0	0
1 Syphilis	0	0	0	0	1	3	1	0	1	0	2	5
2 Gonorrhoea	0	0	0	0	0	0	0	0	0	0	0	0
3 Tuberculosis	0	1	0	0	1	1	0	1	0	1	1	4
4 Alcoholism	0	0	0	0	0	0	0	0	0	0	0	0
5 Diarrhoea/Typhoid	1	1	9	3	1	4	3	2	9	9	1	1
6 Pneumonia	0	1	0	0	0	3	3	0	2	1	1	3
7 Heart Disease	0	0	0	0	0	0	0	0	0	0	0	4
8 Infectious Diseases	0	2	0	0	0	0	0	0	0	0	0	0
9 Cancer	0	0	0	0	0	1	0	0	0	0	0	0
10 Scarlet Fever/Scarlatina	0	0	0	0	0	2	0	0	0	0	0	0
11 Tonsilitis	0	0	0	3	0	0	0	0	0	0	0	0
12 To Infirmary ?sepsis						5	8	0?	1	0	3	6
13 Septicaemia											5	2
14 Salpingitis											1	0
15 Hydramnios											1	0
16 Renal Disease												1

Appendix II

Obstetrical Deaths, 1939–1940

Clinical Report, 1939–1940,
pp. 26–32

TABLE XIX.—OBSTETRICAL DEATHS.
Admitted Before Delivery.

No.	History No.	A. or E.	Age	Para	Cause	Notes.
1	H/369 (1939)	E	18	1	Pre-eclamptic Toxaemia. Post-partum Haemorrhage.	Admitted at full time in labour—history of oedema of legs for two months, and spots before the eyes for twenty-four hours. Urine contained much albumen, and blood pressure 170/130. Given eliminative treatment and sedatives. Baby born eight hours after admission. Fairly severe post-partum haemorrhage occurred—Crede's expression of placenta. Patient in condition of shock afterwards, improved with treatment, but collapsed and died two hours later. Post-mortem performed.
2	E/22 (1939)	E	22	2	Eclampsia. Pulmonary Oedema.	Admitted when thirty-four weeks pregnant, in semi-conscious condition with history of one eclamptic fit. One fit occurred in hospital. Baby delivered normally fourteen hours afterwards, but condition of patient gradually deteriorated till death, thirty hours after admission. Post-mortem performed.
3	E/28 (1939)	E	30	4	Eclampsia. Pulmonary and Cerebral Oedema.	Admitted when thirty-six weeks pregnant with history of two eclamptic fits before admission. Was comatose on admission. Improved slightly with elimination and sedatives. Stillborn baby delivered naturally ten hours after admission. Patient collapsed and died twenty minutes later. Post-mortem performed.
4	E/34 (1939)	E	25	1	Eclampsia.	Admitted unconscious at full time with history of several eclamptic fits before admission. Several fits occurred before death five hours later, despite treatment. Post-mortem Caesarean section—stillborn baby. Post-mortem performed.
5	E/12 (1940)	E	18	1	Post-partum Eclampsia. Bronchopneumonia.	Admitted in strong labour at full time and was rapidly delivered. An eclamptic fit occurred seven hours later, and was followed by nine others in the next eight hours. Treatment by elimination and sedatives was carried out, but bronchopneumonia developed and the patient died 36 hours after admission. Post-mortem performed.
6	E/20 (1939)	A	24	3	Eclampsia. Chronic Nephritis.	Admitted when thirty-two weeks pregnant with history of five eclamptic fits. Past history—first pregnancy terminated for severe pyelitis at five months, second pregnancy resulted in stillborn baby at full time. Despite eliminative treatment and morphia had eight fits before delivery of stillborn baby by forceps four hours after admission. There was gross peripheral circulatory failure after delivery and patient died in four hours. Post-mortem performed.
7	E/37 (1939)	A	19	1	Eclampsia. Gangrene of Lungs.	Admitted when thirty-two weeks pregnant in early labour. Urine contained no albumen. Blood pressure 170/130. An eclamptic fit occurred twenty-four hours later, followed by other fits before delivery by forceps under nitrous oxide and oxygen anaesthesia of living male child three hours later. Blood pressure fell rapidly, patient became cyanosed within a few hours and temperature rose to 103 deg. Death occurred forty-eight hours after delivery. Post-mortem performed.
8	E/8 (1940)	A	24	1	Eclampsia. Sub-arachnoid Haemorrhage.	Attended ante-natal six times, last attendance one month before admission when one week post-mature. Had an eclamptic fit shortly before admission and remained unconscious until death 7½ hours afterwards. Lumbar puncture yielded pure blood. Died undelivered. Post-mortem performed.
9	E/11 (1940)	A	42	11	Eclampsia. Bronchopneumonia.	Admitted to hospital when thirty-four weeks pregnant with mild albuminuria and hypertension (blood pressure 190/140). Quickly improved, and was discharged. Re-admitted one week before due date with history of one eclamptic fit. Blood pressure 240/140 and urine contained 1/3 albumen. Four fits occurred before delivery twelve hours later, despite eliminative treatment, morphia, and venesection. One fit occurred after delivery. On the following day blood pressure fell to 75 mms. Hg. and patient was very cyanosed. Blood pressure gradually rose again, but bronchopneumonia developed, and the patient died on the fifth day. Post-mortem performed.
10	D/60 (1939)	E	28	4	Accidental Haemorrhage. (Revealed and Concealed).	Admitted when twenty-eight weeks pregnant with history of severe vaginal haemorrhage, and abdominal pains for a few hours. Uterus enlarged, tense, and tender. Treated by morphia, followed by packing of vagina, and blood transfusions. Stillborn baby delivered normally nineteen hours after admission, followed immediately by placenta and much retro-placental clot. Patient suddenly collapsed and died two hours later. Post-mortem revealed polycystic kidneys.

375

OBSTETRICAL DEATHS (Continued).
Admitted Before Delivery.

No.	History No.	A. or P.	Age	Para	Cause	Notes.
11	D/2 (1940)	E	33	9	Accidental Haemorrhage. (Revealed and Concealed). Severe Anaemia. Oedema of the Lungs.	Admitted in thirty-sixth week of pregnancy on account of sudden profuse painless loss of blood. One hour after admission the os was found to be dilated to two fingers, membranes intact, vertex presentation, no placenta felt. Vagina packed with cotton wool. Packing was removed thirty-three hours later, as no pains or bleeding had occurred. For the next three days there was slight bleeding. Medicinal stimulation given without effect. Six days after admission the patient suddenly collapsed, and complained of continuous abdominal pain. Some dark fluid was lost P.V. Under general anaesthesia the os was found to be 2/3rds. dilated and membranes bulging. Babe hydrocephalic. Head perforated and child extracted. Placenta was manually removed—much dark blood clot followed. An intravenous saline with glucose 5% was commenced, followed by blood transfusion. Condition improved only slightly, and patient died three hours after delivery.
12	D/13 (1940)	E	31	9	Concealed Accidental Haemorrhage.	Admitted when thirty-eight weeks pregnant with history of severe vaginal haemorrhage four hours before admission, and pains in back and lower abdomen. Considerable shock on admission. Urine contained some albumen, uterus large and tense. Condition gradually became worse and the patient died seven hours after admission. Blood transfusion was attempted. Died undelivered. Post-mortem performed.
13	D/15 (1940)	E	40	8	Accidental Haemorrhage. Pyelonephritis. Chronic Nephritis.	Admitted when thirty-two weeks pregnant with history of oedema for four weeks, abdominal pain for two weeks, and severe vaginal hemorrhage a few hours before admission. Patient in state of severe shock. Urine contained much albumen. Uterus enlarged, tense and tender, and there was generalised oedema. An immediate blood transfusion given, also morphia and pituitrin. Thirty-six hours later macerated foetus born. There had been no urinary output. Blood urea was 104 mgms. per 100 c.cs. blood. Intravenous normal saline was continued, later intravenous sodium sulphate, also hypertonic saline and glucose, but there was no urinary output for five days. Blood urea rose to 446 mgms. and condition gradually became worse till death on 12th day. Post-mortem performed.
14	H/459 (1939)	E	45	10	Pyelonephritis. Coronary Sclerosis. Myocardial Degeneration.	Admitted when thirty-six weeks pregnant with history of pain in loin, frequency and scalding micturition. Temperature elevated and pulse very rapid. Pus and bacilli in urine. Treated by alkalies, sulphanilamide and morphia with very little improvement in general condition. Labour commenced on fifth day, and child was delivered normally in 40 minutes. Fifteen hours later became very cyanosed and restless, and died in three hours. Post-mortem performed.
15	J/213 (1939)	E	42	6	Chronic Myocarditis. Congestive Cardiac Failure.	Admitted when thirty-six weeks pregnant in moribund condition. Died five minutes after admission to hospital. Post-mortem performed.
16	J/42 (1939)	A	22	1	Mitral Stenosis. Cardiac Failure.	Admitted when thirty-six weeks pregnant with considerable degree of cardiac insufficiency. Labour commenced thirty-six hours later and lasted twelve hours, being terminated by forceps delivery because of maternal distress. Nitrous oxide and oxygen anaesthesia used. Patient died of acute pulmonary oedema within five minutes of delivery. Baby stillborn. Post-mortem performed.
17	C/5 (1940)	E	40	4	Obstructed Labour. Lower Uterine Segment Caesarean Section. General Peritonitis.	Admitted in labour when six to eight weeks post-mature. Membranes ruptured prematurely before admission. Labour pains good, but head did not advance. Lower uterine segment Caesarean section thirty hours after membranes ruptured. Foetus stillborn—weighed 7 lbs. 10 ozs. (previous largest baby—8 lbs.). The patient rapidly developed signs of a general peritonitis, and later a faecal fistula. Became markedly jaundiced, and developed bronchopneumonia and an empyema. Died on 18th day.
18	J/46 (1940)	E	36	1	Intestinal Obstruction. Perforation of Bowel. General Peritonitis.	Admitted one month before due date with history of onset of abdominal pain and vomiting seven days previously. Vomiting severe and persistent for twelve hours before admission. An enema yielded a poor result. An intravenous saline was given and classical Caesarean section performed under spinal anaesthesia. A band was found constricting the lower ileum, which was gangrenous and perforated. The area was excised, bowel anastomosed, and abdominal cavity drained. Death occurred thirty-six hours later.
19	J/56 (1940)	E	22	1	Acute Intestinal Obstruction.	Admitted when fourteen weeks pregnant with history of vomiting for three weeks—copious for four days. Some abdominal pain and distension. Treated by rectal saline and sedatives, but died suddenly forty-eight hours after admission. Died undelivered. Post-mortem performed.
No.	History No.	A. or P.	Age	Para	Cause	Notes.
20	J/94 (1940)	E	32	6	Torsion of Ovarian Cyst. General Peritonitis.	Admitted when a few weeks post-mature. Normal delivery following medicinal stimulation without any interference. On sixth day suddenly collapsed and complained of abdominal pain. Abdomen tender and rigid—examination under general anaesthesia revealed no mass. Thought to be general peritonitis—treated by continuous intravenous saline and gastric drainage until death on fourteenth day. Post-mortem revealed torsion of ovarian cyst.
21	H 201 (1939)	A	28	2	Puerperal Peritonitis. Bronchopneumonia.	Admitted at full time in early labour—one pelvic examination—normal delivery in six hours. Temperature became elevated on fifth day, and remained elevated with only slight remissions until death six weeks later. On fourteenth day a tubo-ovarian mass was palpable vaginally. Abdomen was distended throughout illness, but never rigid, and only slightly tender. Condition was treated by sedatives and repeated blood transfusions. Bronchopneumonia developed about the 28th day. Pus discharged from the right inguinal region on the 46th day without much improvement in general condition. Patient died on 50th day. No post-mortem.

OBSTETRICAL DEATHS (Continued).
Admitted Before Delivery.

	History No.		Age	Para	Cause	Notes.
22	H/55 (1940)	A	24	2	Anaemia of Pregnancy. Puerperal Sepsis. Empyema.	In first pregnancy two years previously had severe puerperal infection with gross anaemia. In this pregnancy at eight months found to have macrocytic anaemia—treated by Campolon, liver, and iron. Admitted at full time in labour—forceps delivery for foetal distress—normal blood loss. Temperature elevated from first day of puerperium. Given a massive blood transfusion on tenth day. Two days later fluid detected in chest, and empyema drained on following day by closed method. Further blood transfusion two days later. Died on 16th day.
23	C/19 (1939)	A	25	3	Ruptured Uterus.	Admitted when thirty-eight weeks pregnant in early labour. Membrane ruptured ten hours later. Three hours afterwards the os was fully dilated. Pains continued for fifteen hours, then patient collapsed and died rapidly. Post-mortem revealed ruptured uterus and massive haemorrhage. Baby weighed 12½ lbs.
24	F/48 (1940)	A	22	1	Hydramnios. Obstetrical Shock.	Admitted when one week post-mature in early labour with ruptured membranes. Labour progressed steadily, but the foetus died after 24 hours. Six hours later, because of maternal distress, the baby was delivered by forceps after a manual rotation of the head. The shoulders became impacted and were delivered with difficulty. An immediate post-partum haemorrhage followed, placenta was expressed by Crede' method. Haemorrhage persisted, so the uterus was manually explored and a hot intrauterine douche given. General condition was poor. A intravenous saline was given, but patient died two hours after delivery. Post-mortem performed.
25	H/156 (1940)	A	27	3	Hyperemesis Gravidarum.	Admitted when eight weeks pregnant with history of vomiting for five weeks, persistent for five days. Rapidly improved with sedatives, and was discharged in five days. Re-admitted three weeks later with history of vague ill-health since discharge from hospital, rapidly becoming worse in preceding three days. Patient was semi-conscious, markedly dehydrated and showed signs of acidosis. Slightly improved with intravenous saline, but became jaundiced, and condition gradually became worse until death on fourth day after admission. Died undelivered. Post-mortem performed.
26	J/118 (1940)	E	46	4	Carcinoma of Thyroid. Bronchopneumonia.	Admitted when 24 weeks pregnant. Subtotal thyroidectomy in general hospital ten weeks previously—section revealed carcinoma. Treated by deep X-ray therapy. Progressive shortness of breath since then. In hospital for eight days with increasing cardiac failure and terminal bronchopneumonia. Died undelivered. No post-mortem.

Admitted After Delivery.

	History No.		Age	Para	Cause	Notes.
27	16/15 (1940)	E	20	1	Late Hyperemesis. Acute Yellow Atrophy of Liver.	Admitted on day following delivery of full-time macerated foetus—history of persistent vomiting for two weeks. Was semi-conscious on admission with gross jaundice. Improved slightly following continuous intravenous saline with 10 per cent. glucose, but died about 18 hours after admission. Post-mortem performed.
28	13/40 (1939)	E	33	2	Puerperal Peritonitis. Subphrenic Abscess. Bronchopneumonia.	Admitted three weeks after birth of full-time living child with history fever and abdominal pains since ninth day of puerperium. Vomiting 24 hours. Signs of general peritonitis on admission. Treated with sedatives and M. and B. 693. Six days later developed pleural effusion. Two weeks later pus withdrawn from chest—three days later intercostal drainage through tenth intercostal space. Patient died six hours later. Post-mortem performed.
29	13/22 (1939)	E	26	1	Puerperal Sepsis. Pelvic Venous Thrombosis. Pulmonary Emboli.	Admitted three weeks after delivery of normal full-time child with history of development of cough three days previously and sudden onset pleural pain 24 hours before admission. Temperature elevated—signs consolidation at base of both lungs when admitted. Sudden attack dyspnoea and cyanosis six days after admission, death occurring a few hours later. Post-mortem performed.

TABLE XXI.—DEATHS FROM SEPTIC ABORTION.

No.	History No.	Age	Para	Cause	Notes.
1	12/165 (1939)	34	3	Streptococcus Haemolyticus. Group A. Septicaemia. Infective Endocarditis. Bronchopneumonia.	Miscarriage at 6½ months during an attack of influenza. Foetus macerated. Admitted 37 hours after miscarriage with high fever and marked icterus and cyanosis. Given intravenous saline and glucose, and 80,000 units anti gas gangrene serum by intramuscular and intravenous routes. On following day there were signs of right basal pneumonia, and vaginal culture grew haemolytic streptococci, group A—given Proseptasine in massive dosage. Condition gradually became worse, and death occurred on seventh day. Blood culture, streptococcus haemolyticus, group A.
2	12/261 (1939)	34	7	Streptococcus Haemolyticus. Group A. Septicaemia.	Admitted with history of irregular bleeding for three months—no history of interference. Temp. 104 deg. on admission. Uterus slightly enlarged. No masses palpable. Blood culture grew haemolytic streptococci, group A. Given sulphanilamide in fairly large dosage, but condition gradually became worse. Developed a streptococcal empyema on 20th day and died on 21st day.
3	12/176 (1940)	42	10	Streptococcus Haemolyticus. Group A. Septicaemia.	History of abortion of foetus the day before admission following fall downstairs when 3½ months pregnant. Hyperpyrexia on admission, but no localising signs. Given M. and B. 693 in massive dosage. Condition became gradually worse till death, on fourth day. Blood culture, streptococcus haemolyticus, group A.

4	12/201 (1940)	25	4	Streptococcus Haemolyticus. Group A. Septicaemia.	No history of amenorrhoea—continuous bleeding per vaginam for one month. Ran high swinging temperature with rigors from time of admission despite treatment with M. and B. 693 and blood transfusion. Gradually became jaundiced and cyanosed, and died on 22nd day. Blood culture, streptococcus haemolyticus, group A.
5	12/211 (1940)	46	10	Streptococcus Haemolyticus. Group A. Septicaemia. Femoral Thrombosis.	Admitted with history of 2½ months' amenorrhoea and history of rigors for 24 hours. No interference. Found to have positive blood culture, but pregnancy continued for six weeks. Septicaemia improved with M. and B. 693, but developed femoral thrombosis one month after admission, and later aborted foetus. Died 6½ weeks after admission. Blood culture, streptococcus haemolyticus, group A.
6	12/215 (1940)	23	1	Streptococcus Haemolyticus. Group A. Septicaemia.	History of abortion five days before admission at three-four months following insertion of tube into uterus. Developed pains, vomiting and rigors on day of admission. Blood culture grew streptococcus haemolyticus, group A. Treated by M. and B. 693 and blood transfusions with no improvement. Died on 30th day.
7	12/215 (1939)	40	9	Anaerobic Streptococcal Septicaemia. Pulmonary Abscess.	Admitted with history of miscarriage four days previously when three months pregnant—denied interference. Uterus contained offensive placenta. Curage performed two days after admission. Frequent rigors followed. Blood culture grew anaerobic streptococci. Despite frequent blood transfusions rigors continued and general condition deteriorated. Bronchopneumonia developed ten days after admission. Gradually became worse, and died on 34th day. Post-mortem revealed pulmonary abscess.
8	12/224 (1940)	35	5	Anaerobic Streptococcal Septicaemia.	Admitted with history of four months' amenorrhoea, and profuse bleeding per vaginam for four days. No interference. Feverish on admission. No localising signs. Frequent rigors occurred, despite M. and B. 693 and blood transfusion, till death on 24th day after admission. Blood culture—anaerobic streptococci.
9	12/95 (1940)	21	1	Anaerobic Streptococcal Septicaemia. General Peritonitis.	One week before admission when three months pregnant passed a catheter into uterus. Aborted foetus five days later. Twenty-four hours after admission abdomen became rigid and distended. Abdomen drained through paramedian incision. Treated by intravenous saline and glucose, and sulphanilamide. Gradually became worse, and died on sixth day after admission. Blood culture—anaerobic streptococci.
10	12/233 (1939)	23	3	Anaerobic Streptococcal Infection. Thrombo-phlebitis Pyaemia.	History of miscarriage at two months, two days before admission. Curettage performed in hospital—discharged well. Re-admitted five days later with pelvic cellulitis. Frequent rigors followed, and condition gradually became worse, despite several transfusions. Blood culture grew an anaerobic streptococci and an anaerobic gram negative bacillus. Died on 21st day after curettage. Post-mortem revealed thrombo-phlebitis of uterine veins, pyaemia and pulmonary abscesses.
11	12/260 (1939)	28	5	Clostridium Welchii Septicaemia.	Induced miscarriage at three months by syringing herself. Indefinite signs of pelvic peritonitis on admission. Eighteen hours later was grossly jaundiced. Given 100,000 units anti gas gangrene serum by intramuscular and intravenous routes and continuous intravenous saline, and alkaline drinks. Total hysterectomy performed. Condition gradually became worse till death, ten hours after operation. Urine culture, and culture from uterus grew bacillus' Welchii. Immediate cause of death was post-operative haemorrhage.
12	12/307 (1939)	31	2	Clostridium Welchii Septicaemia.	History of seven weeks' amenorrhoea, then bleeding for two weeks. No interference known. Became jaundiced 24 hours before admission in semi-comatose condition. Marked peripheral circulatory failure—skin bronzed with purple blebs in some areas. Continuous intravenous saline and anti gas gangrene serum given, but died in three-quarters of an hour. Blood culture grew Clostridium Welchii.
13	12/325 (1939)	32	6	Clostridium Welchii Infection.	History of two months' amenorrhoea, then bleeding for two days and severe abdominal pains. Jaundice marked on admission. Given continuous intravenous saline and anti gas gangrene serum intravenously. Total hysterectomy performed, but patient died shortly afterwards. Cultures of urine and uterine contents grew Clostridium Welchii.
14	12/374 (1939)	34	8	Clostridium Welchii Septicaemia.	History of three months' amenorrhoea. Induced abortion by syringing. Jaundiced twelve hours after admission. Treated by continuous intravenous saline, sulphanilamide, and anti gas gangrene serum by intravenous and intramuscular routes, but rapidly became worse, and died 15½ hours after admission. Blood culture grew Clostridium Welchii.
15	12/15 (1940)	43	5	Clostridium Welchii Septicaemia.	Two days before admission catheter inserted into uterus when seven weeks pregnant, followed by labour pains in 24 hours and development of jaundice. On admission skin bronzed, early peripheral circulatory failure. Uterus size of 8-10 weeks pregnancy, os open. Given 90,000 units anti gas gangrene serum by intramuscular and intravenous routes and continuous intravenous saline and glucose, and alkaline drinks. Five hours later taken to theatre, but patient vomited copiously and died as anaesthesia was commenced. Blood culture—Clostridium Welchii.
16	12/8 (1940)	26	2	Clostridium Welchii Septicaemia.	Twenty-four hours before admission said to have fallen downstairs. Was 18 weeks pregnant. Aborted foetus four hours before admission. Patient in fairly good condition. Twelve hours later slight jaundice noticed—treated by continuous intravenous saline and glucose with 60,000 units anti gas gangrene serum by intravenous and intramuscular routes, followed by blood transfusion. Condition improved. Total hysterectomy performed seven hours after jaundice first noted. Given soluseptasine intramuscularly four-hourly and 100,000 units of anti gas gangrene serum daily and seemed to be improving until fifth day, when patient suddenly died. Post-mortem performed. Blood culture—Clostridium Welchii.

17	12/106 (1940)	28	2	Clostridium Welchii Infection.	Syringed herself when three months pregnant. Aborted foetus 24 hours before admission. On examination somewhat shocked, slight jaundice, severe abdominal pain. Given 40,000 anti gas gangrene serum intramuscularly and intravenous saline commenced. Panhysterectomy two hours after admission. Large perforation found. Further 60,000 units anti gas gangrene serum intravenously. Died 12 hours after admission. Blood culture grew Clostridium Welchii.
18	12/107 (1940)	24	3	Clostridium Welchii Septicaemia.	History of taking some pills when two months pregnant. Bleeding per vaginam for eight hours before admission. Deeply jaundiced on admission. Given 160,000 units anti gas gangrene serum and intravenous saline. Died two days after admission. Blood culture—Clostridium Welchii.
19	12/206 (1940)	31	3	Clostridium Welchii Septicaemia.	Admitted when 2½ months pregnant with history of bleeding per vaginam with vomiting and fever. No interference. Six hours after admission jaundice noted, which gradually increased, also signs of peripheral circulatory failure. Given 40,000 units anti gas gangrene serum intramuscularly and continuous intravenous saline and later a further 100,000 units anti gas gangrene serum. Jaundice gradually increased till death 22 hours after admission. Blood culture—Clostridium Welchii.
20	12/233 (1940)	27	2	Clostridium Welchii Septicaemia.	History of interference with pregnancy at 3½ months. Patient admitted in comatose state with signs of peripheral circulatory failure. Treated by M. and B. 693, continuous intravenous saline, 40,000 units of anti gas gangrene serum intramuscularly as cervical smear showed virulent Clostridium Welchii, and deep X-ray therapy to uterus for 32 minutes, followed by 60,000 units anti gas gangrene serum intravenously. Patient died 18 hours after admission. Blood culture—Clostridium Welchii.
21	12/365 (1939)	21	2	Staphylococcus Aureus Septicaemia. Pulmonary Abscesses.	History of five months' amenorrhoea. Aborted foetus. Bleeding freely per vaginam on admission. Temperature elevated. Placenta had to be removed by curage on fourth day because of free haemorrhage. Ran swinging temperature from seventh day onwards. Blood culture grew staphylococcus aureus repeatedly. Developed abscess over sacrum and few signs in chest. Treated by repeated blood transfusions and sulphanilamide. Died on 40th day after admission.
22	12/91 (1940)	32	1	Staphylococcus Aureus Septicaemia. Abscess in Lungs.	When two months pregnant procured abortion by syringing herself two weeks before admission. Feverish for three days before admission. Frequent rigors after admission—treated with M. and B. 693 and blood transfusion without improvement. Died on 11th day. Blood culture—staphylococcus aureus.
23	12/97 (1940)	47	9	Staphylococcus Aureus Septicaemia. Multiple Abscesses.	Admitted with history of abdominal pain and bleeding for one week. Was five weeks pregnant. Denied interference. Later in day aborted foetus and placenta. Very frequent rigors in next three days—treated with intravenous saline and glucose, and sulphanilamide. Died three days after admission. Blood culture—staphylococcus aureus.
24	12/207 (1940)	4	4	Staphylococcus Aureus Septicaemia. General Peritonitis.	Aborted foetus when three months pregnant without interference. Bleeding freely. Admitted. Temperature elevated immediately afterwards—first signs of peritonitis, later developed pleural friction rub. Condition gradually became worse despite M. and B. 693, and death occurred after eight weeks. Blood culture—staphylococcus aureus.
25	12/358 (1939)	25	3	Vibrion Septique Septicaemia.	Admitted with history of miscarriage when five months pregnant. Jaundice and cyanosis noticed 18 hours later, and death occurred one hour afterwards. Blood culture grew Vibrion Septique.
26	12/84 (1940)	24	1	Vibrion Septique Septicaemia.	Three days before admission when 3½ months pregnant, vagina was packed. Packing removed in 48 hours. On admission was shocked and complaining of severe pains in legs. Treated by intravenous saline and glucose, and soluseptasine. Twelve hours after admission developed crepitus in muscles of thighs, and was given 150,000 units of anti gas gangrene serum. Died 18 hours after admission. Blood culture—Vibrion Septique. Post-mortem performed.
27	12/303 (1939)	35	3	Bacillus Tetanus Infection.	Admitted with history of 3½ months' amenorrhoea. Curettage performed 36 hours before admission—uterus packed afterwards. Aborted foetus at time of admission. On second day developed inflammation in left thigh, gradually going on to abscess formation. On fifth day developed stiffness of jaw and neck—regarded as tetanus, and given anti tetanus serum. Generalised rigidity developed. Twenty-four hours after first symptoms had first tetanic spasm despite intensive treatment with sedatives and much anti tetanus serum. In following 18 hours had six further spasms, finally dying in a spasm seventh day after admission. Given in all 103,000 units of anti tetanus serum, large doses of barbiturate and paraldehyde.
28	12/173 (1940)	20	2	Lead Poisoning.	History of two months' amenorrhoea—two days before admission syringed herself and took lead pills. Admitted with signs of pelvic peritonitis. On sixth day became jaundiced, next day blue line noticed on gums, and stippling of red blood cells discovered. Condition gradually became worse, despite continuous intravenous saline and blood transfusion, and patient died on 14th day.

29	12/363 (1939)	42	7	Septicaemia.	History of miscarriage at stage of five months' pregnancy, followed by repeated vomiting. Marked dehydration and anaemia on admission. Treated by continuous intravenous saline and blood transfusion, but gradually became worse, and died on sixth day. No blood culture taken. Post-mortem appearances those of a septicaemia.
30	12/114 (1940)	34	6	Septicaemia. Septic Pneumonia. Uraemia.	History of syringing herself three days before admission when two months pregnant. Admitted in condition of shock, jaundiced, and complaining of abdominal pain. Given intravenous saline and 150,000 units of anti gas gangrene serum. Cervical culture—non haemolytic streptococci and bacillus coli. Developed complete anuria, also laryngeal obstruction. Died on seventh day in an anaemic state. Post-mortem findings—Abortion. Septic Pneumonia and Nephritis. Septicaemia and Uraemia.
31	12/190 (1940)	27	5	Septicaemia. Pelvic Cellulitis.	History of abortion of 4½ months' foetus one week before admission. Temperature normal on admission. No blood culture taken. Curettage. Low-grade temperature followed, and pelvic cellulitis developed. Suddenly collapsed and died three weeks after admission. Post-mortem diagnosis—Septicaemia.
32	12/193 (1939)	34	9	Pelvic Peritonitis. Pneumonia. Empyema.	Aborted twin foetuses at 2½ months following a fall one week before admission. Frequent vomiting and lower abdominal pain since then. Developed extraperitoneal collection of pus in R. loin, which was drained on 19th day. On 25th day developed R. basal pneumonia, but gradually became worse, despite M. and B. 693, and died on 33rd day. Vaginal culture—no growth.
33	12/174 (1939)	39	5	Acute General Peritonitis.	Admitted with history of miscarriage four days previously when two months pregnant following insertion of knitting needle into uterus. On examination feverish and toxic, with signs of pelvic peritonitis. Abdomen gradually became more distended, vomiting occurred intermittently, until collapse on fifth day, following which condition gradually became worse, till death on seventh day, despite continuous intravenous saline and glucose, and drainage of peritoneal cavity under local anaesthesia. Blood culture—no growth.
34	12/230 (1939)	21	4	General Peritonitis.	Admitted with history of miscarriage two days previously when 2½ months' pregnant. No interference. Uterus size of 4-5 months' pregnancy when admitted—abdomen distended and tender. Collapsed and died suddenly 36 hours after admission. Post-mortem revealed general peritonitis. Vaginal culture—Cl. Welchii, non-lactose fermenting gram negative bacilli.
35	12/248 (1939)	23	4	Tubo-ovarian Abscess. General Peritonitis.	Induced miscarriage at two months—curettage in hospital afterwards, and discharged in 11 days. Re-admitted five days later with history of abdominal pain and vomiting for 24 hours. Had a large left tubo-ovarian mass. No cultures taken. Four days after admission vomited copious amounts of brown fluid, collapsed and died.
36	12/275 (1939)	30	4	General Peritonitis.	Admitted with history of fall three days previously when two months' pregnant—a good deal of bleeding since—denied interference. On examination generalised abdominal tenderness and slight rigidity. Vaginal cultures showed—Clostridium Welchii and Bacillus Coli. Suddenly collapsed 24 hours after admission and died in 12 hours.
37	12/277 (1939)	19	1	Laceration of Vagina. General Peritonitis.	Admitted with history of interference four hours before admission when two months' pregnant. Rather shocked on admission—considerable abdominal pain. Marked generalised abdominal rigidity. Irregular laceration in posterior fornix leading into peritoneal cavity. Treated by continuous intravenous saline and blood transfusion. Aborted foetus on second day. No cultures taken. Died on eighth day after admission.
38	12/309 (1939)	35	3	Perforation of Uterus. General Peritonitis.	History of 3½ months' amenorrhoea—abortion two days before admission. Abdominal pain and vomiting since abortion. Abdomen tender and distended. Vaginal culture—many clostridium welchii, few bacillus coli and non-haemolytic streptococci. Treated by sedatives and continuous intravenous saline. Death on fourth day. Post-mortem revealed perforation of uterus.
39	12/366 (1939)	27	1	Pelvic Peritonitis. Pyaemia.	Admitted complaining of abdominal pain for one week—no definite history of amenorrhoea. Abdomen distended, tender and rigid, especially over lower quadrants. Vaginal culture—bacillus coli, non-haemolytic streptococci. Treated by continuous intravenous saline and glucose, sulphanilamide, and gastric lavage without improvement. Died on third day. Post-mortem performed.
40	12/149 (1940)	25	1	General Peritonitis.	A few hours before admission abortion induced when four months' pregnant by passing catheter into uterus. On admission was bleeding freely, and on following afternoon curage was performed. Vaginal culture—non-haemolytic streptococci and bacillus coli. The following day developed signs of general peritonitis—treated by intravenous saline. Died on fourth day.
41	12/175 (1940)	19	1	General Peritonitis.	Admitted with history of four months' amenorrhoea. Bleeding for one month following miscarriage—curettage. Discharged well on fourth day. Re-admitted five days later with history of sudden onset of generalised abdominal pain two days previously, frequent vomiting and diarrhoea. Clinical signs of general peritonitis—treated by sedatives and intravenous saline. Blood cultures—negative. Vaginal cultures—streptococcus haemolyticus group A, bacillus coli. Peritoneal cavity drained on sixth day.
42	12/192 (1939)	22	1	Septicaemia. Bronchopneumonia.	Admitted with history of three months' abortion three days ago. Denied interference. Signs of bronchopneumonia present and died the following day. Post-mortem fluid in both pleural cavities, small abscesses in lower lobes of lungs.
43	H/400 (1939)	30	8	Hyperemesis. Incomplete Abortion. Syncope.	History of three months' amenorrhoea. Hyperemesis. Treated by outside doctor, who replaced retroverted uterus and inserted pessary. Removed three weeks later, when patient began to haemorrhage. On admission ovum and membranes presenting at vulva. Died when given anaesthetic for curettage. Post-mortem—uterine haemorrhage, syncope. Anaesthetic only a minor factor.

Appendix III

Nursing Notes, 1914–1916

<u>Diagnosis:</u> **Salpingitis**

23 June 1914

Miss J. S.

<u>Age:</u> 27

<u>Occupation:</u> waitress

<u>Present Address:</u> no fixed

<u>Family History:</u> Father healthy. Mother, 50+— not healthy.
2 sisters healthy, 3 brothers healthy, 1 br died as baby.

<u>Previous Health:</u> Health prior to parturition good

<u>Obstetric History:</u> 1 child 4 yrs ago. Healthy. No miscarriages

<u>Menstrual History:</u> onset at 14 years, every month for 6 days

Quantity normal. No pain previous to condition.

<u>Intermenstrual Discharge:</u> for 12 mos after birth of child, then ceased & now returned.

<u>Intermenstrual Pain:</u> none

<u>Present attack.</u> The patient complains that for the last 12 mos she has been losing very freely at the time of her period, gradually getting worse. Last period lasted 3 weeks, now has ceased but has discharge bloodstained and yellow. Period comes on at the night time. In W.H. 5 mos ago, curetted but no relief (worse). No pain. Not getting thin.

<u>General Condition:</u> good

Both tubes and R ovary removed.
Patient made uninterrupted recovery.

WOMEN'S HOSPITAL.		POST OPERATIVE CHAR
Date 25- 6 14 Name ▮▮▮▮▮▮		Surgeon Dr Morton

Time Received from Theatre	12 30. M. 10.
Condition	Unconscious
Colour	Good
Respirations	22
Pulse	80
Temperature	
Extremities	Warm.
Regained Consciousness	1·30.

Time	Temp.	Pulse	Resp.	Urine	Bowels	TREATMENT.	Ozs.	REMARKS.
	96	80	20					
4.30						Face & hands sponged & hot water bottle refilled		

381

6 pm	98⁴	72	20			Catheterized U. D. O 3 v		
6.30								

Summary

Patient has slept during the afternoon Face & hands sponged. & hot water bottle refilled. Catheterized U D O 3 v Is losing P.v. Is comp of Abdominal pain A : P. m. otherwise is comfortable

T 98⁶ P 72. R 20

10	96⁸	80	20			Drink of Soda water
						Dr Embleton visited
						ordered Morphia gr ½
12.30						Morphia gr ½ given
3				3 viii		Catheterized U. O. O 3 viii
2	99⁸	80	24			Drink of Soda water given
6	99⁸	80	24			

Patient has had a fair night, did not complain. Catheterized U. O. O 3 viii T. 99⁶ P. 80. R. 24

J. Higgins

Date 26. 6. 111 _____ Name ███████ Surgeon Dr Morton.

Time	Temp.	Pulse	Resp.	Urine	Bowels	TREATMENT.	Ozs.	REMARKS.
7.						Patient Sponged. Back rubbed c̄ Spirits & powder. Bed made Hot water bottle refilled Cup of tea.		Is losing p. v.
10	99⁶	88	18			Dr Embleton visited Beef tea. 1 bt gauze removed.		
10. 30								
11.				3 viii		Catheterized U. D. O 3 viii cup of Barley broth Dr Morton visited		
2	100⁶	98	20			Face & hands Sponged Back rubbed c̄ Spirits & powder		

Time	Temp.	Pulse	Resp.	Urine	Bowels	TREATMENT.	Ozs.	REMARKS.
2.20						Cup of Tea.		
4						Calomel gr ⅛ given		
5						Calomel gr ⅛ given		
6	100°	96	20			„ gr ⅛ „		
6.45						Orange juice taken.		
						Hot water bottle refilled		
7 p.m						Cal gr ⅛ given		Not complaining
8 p.m.						P.R. ℥ vij		Is losing a little p.r
						Cup of Coffee given		
						Patient has had comfortable day Cal. gr iv given in hourly doses last 7 p.m. Passed urine 8 p.m. Is losing a little p.r.		
10								Sleeping
2								Sleeping
5						Mag Sulph ℥ ij given		
6	99	80	20					

Date 27. 6. 14   Name ████   Surgeon N.T Morton

Time	Temp.	Pulse	Resp.	Urine	Bowels	TREATMENT.	Ozs.	REMARKS.
6.15						Cup of black Tea		
						Patient had a fair night. Comp of right arm feeling sore. Had Mag Sulph Passed urine. T. 99. P.80. R.20		

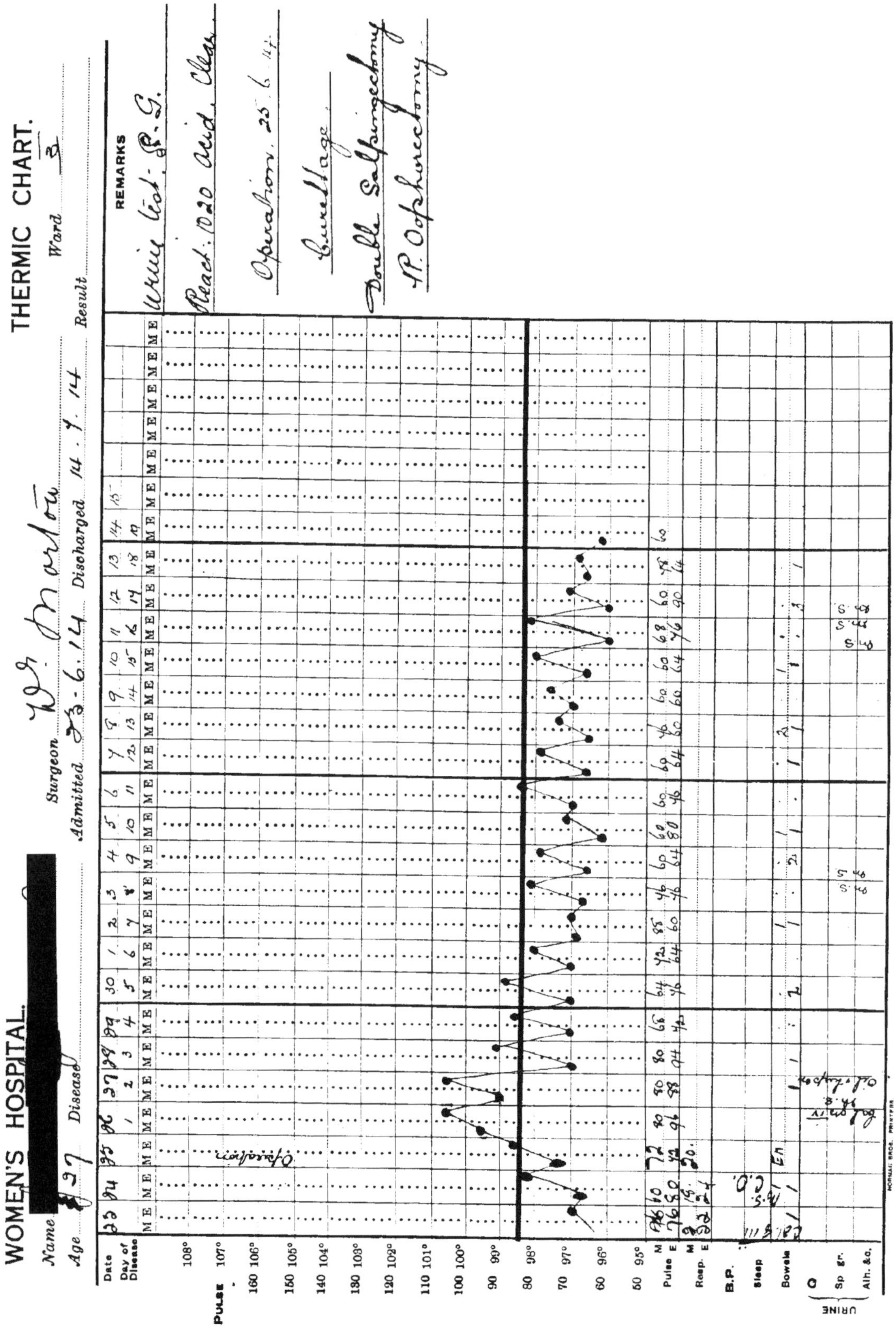

Dr. Morton

Name [redacted] **Age** 27

OPERATION Curettage
Double Salingectomy
R. Oophorectomy.

GAUZES 1 UA

SUTURES C. G. S. W. G. H. H.

Date	25	26	26	27	28	29	30
Day after Operation		1	2	3	4	5	6
Time	A.M. / P.M.	A.M. / P.M.	A.M. / P.M.	A.M. / P.M.	A.M. / P.M.	A.M. / P.M.	A.M. / P.M.
Temp.	2 6 10 / 2 6 10	2 6 10 / 2 6 10	2 6 10 / 2 6 10	2 6 10 / 2 6 10	2 6 10 / 2 6 10	2 6 10 / 2 6 10	2 6 10 / 2 6 10

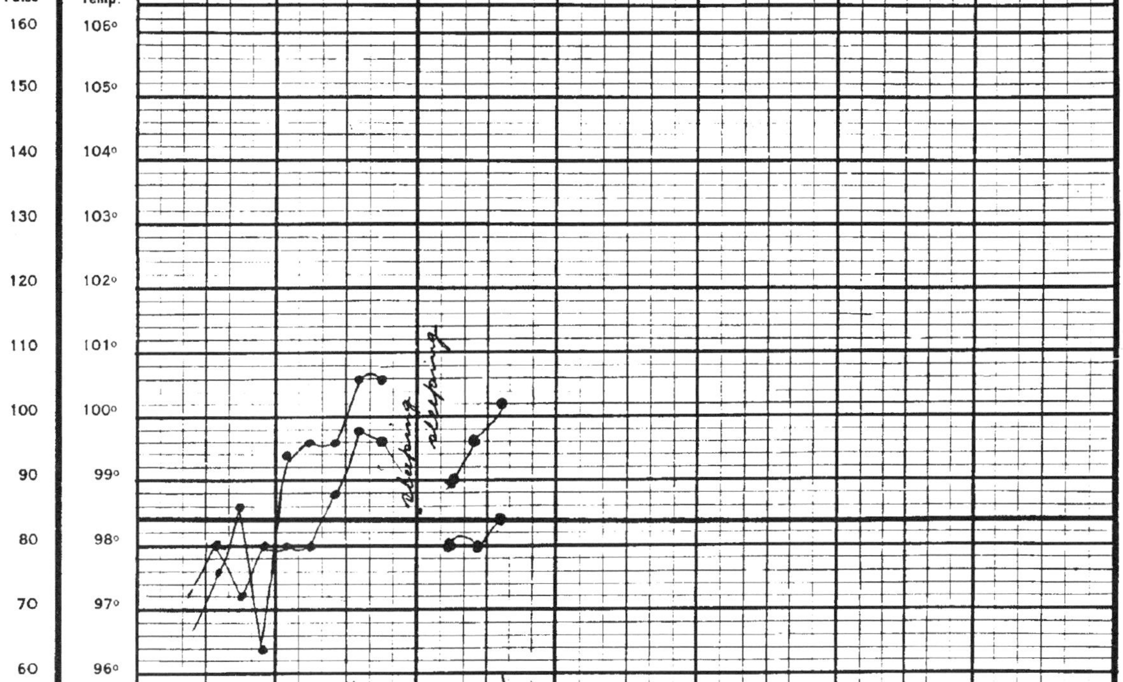

	25	26	26
Pulse	80, 72, 80	80, 80, 88, 96, 96	80, 80, 84
Respr.	20, 20, 20	24, 24, 18, 20, 20	20, 20, 20
Bowels			
Urine			
REMARKS	Catheterized U.D.O. ʒv	Catheterized 3 am U.D.O ʒvii; Catheterized 11 am U.D.O ʒviii	Oil & Turp Enema

Norman Bros., Printers, Melbourne

Diagnosis: **Mild Puerperal Insanity**
18 November 1916
Mrs M. O.

Age: 31

Conjugal State: married 6 years

Present Address: Collingwood

Previous Health: good

Obstetric History: 3rd pregnancy, none living, no history of miscarriage
1st lived 6 mths. 2nd premature. 3rd stillborn.

Menstrual History: irregular. Onset at 15 years, every 6 weeks, lasting 3 days.
last—February. Quantity—scanty. Pain—occasionally in head and back.

Bowels: regular with medicine.

Urine: Some albumen. Sp. gr. 1020. B.P. 150.

Present attack. The patient complains that Transferred from midwifery side in mental condition, refuses to speak, had stillborn child 14 days ago.
Account from Midwifery side: Normal delivery ROA.
Stillborn child on 4/11/16. Patient being eclamptic but no fits recorded; 2 days after delivery showed some mental signs 'wandering' in speech. On fourth day symptoms more acute and got out of bed several times; this continued daily until day of transfer when refused to take any notice of anyone.
About 4th 5th day meningitis was suspected; there being a general rigidity of musculature but no definite signs. Lumbar Puncture gave negative result on 3 occasions.
19/11/16 Some albumen in urine. ?∂ xxx passed. no signs of oedema.
Refuses to notice anybody
Not taking nourishment
20/11/16 General condition much better; talks rationally but wants to go home as would be better looked after there.
Taking some nourishment.
21/11/16 Mental condition not so good again. Says she knows where she is and yet doesn't. Thinks people are laughing at her. Wants to go home away from these people. Taking nourishment well. Some albumen still in urine.

Says she and her husband want a living child, no heart left to go on working without one.
Dr Beattie Smith [psychiatrist] visited 5 pm.
22/11/16 Much the same.
23/11/16 Much the same. Worrying because she hasn't got her false teeth and wedding ring. Latter to be obtained if possible.
Wants to go home. Thinks people are having the loan of her. Not taking nourishment well.
6/12/16 Discharged to mother's home after consultation between Dr Tate Sutherland and Dr Beattie Smith; the latter explaining to her mother that patient was well except for mental condition and that as far as that went the patient was going out at parents' risk, with them understanding the mental condition.
Patient's mental condition much improved.

27 · 11 · 16   Name ███████████   Surgeon Dr Sats Sutherland

Time Received from Theatre	-				
Condition	-	-	-	Urine. 1022 Acid Clear. 26 · 11 · 17	
Colour	-	-	-		
Respirations	-	-	℥XXX.+		
Pulse	-	-	-		
Temperature	-	-	-		
Extremities	-	-	-		
Regained Consciousness		-			

Time	Temp.	Pulse	Resp.	Urine	Bowels	TREATMENT.	Ozs.	REMARKS.
	·					25 · 11 · 16. Taking now well, will have we are all plotting against her, & that her husband has sold her marriage lines, appears to have taken a dislike to him says no one is true to her Patients are jeering at her, she wants to get up & help with work, does not like us to wait on her, when she is quite well Had restless night Sat. trying to get out of bed, did not sleep well 26 · 11 · 16 Very quiet all day, seems very depressed, tried to get out of bed several times. Slept better Sun. night. P.U. B.O.+ 27 · 11 · 16. Still has we are all plotting against her, feels quite well enough to get out & walk about, is reading book & will have it is her own life they are writing about.		

9 · 11 · 16   Name ████████████████████   Surgeon *** Sutherland

Time Received from Theatre	-	Urine
Condition	- - -	S. G. 1000 Acid. Clear.
Colour	- - -	
Respirations	- -	
Pulse	- - -	
Temperature	- -	
Extremities	- -	
Regained Consciousness	-	

Time	Temp.	Pulse	Resp.	Urine	Bowels	TREATMENT.	Ozs.	REMARKS.
						28 · 11 · 16.		

28 · 11 · 16.

Slept much better, not attempting to get out of bed. Husband & friend came to see her Monday evening but Tues morning she did not remember them being here. Her one desire is to get up & walk about, Has not said we were plotting against her since Monday afternoon. Passing about xxxx 3. urine. B.W.O. aperient given Has talked to other patients more & seems much brighter in her self.

29·11·16 Slept very well last night, has been very quiet all the morning, except that she still wants to get up. Taking nour very well. Sat out of bed this afternoon for about 1 hour, was quite satisfied.

30 11 16. Did not sleep very well, & is very depressed this morning crying several times, & p will have people are plotting against her, also her husband, says she is very reserved person & does not make friends, & that is why people are talking & plotting against her says she is being misjudged

Name _____   Surgeon _Tate Sutherland_

Time Received from Theatre -
Condition   -   .   .   .
Colour   -   ..   ..   .
Respirations   -   -   ..   ..
Pulse   -   . .   .   .
Temperature   -   .   .   ..
Extremities   -   -   ..   ..
Regained Consciousness   ..   .

Time	Temp.	Pulse	Resp.	Urine	Bowels	TREATMENT.	Ozs.	REMARKS.
	.					for some wrong she has never done. She has a feeling she has been drugged or got in here without her knowing it, & that she will never leave here. Taking nour. well 2·12·18 Taking nour well quite sensibly.		B.O. P. Urine talking

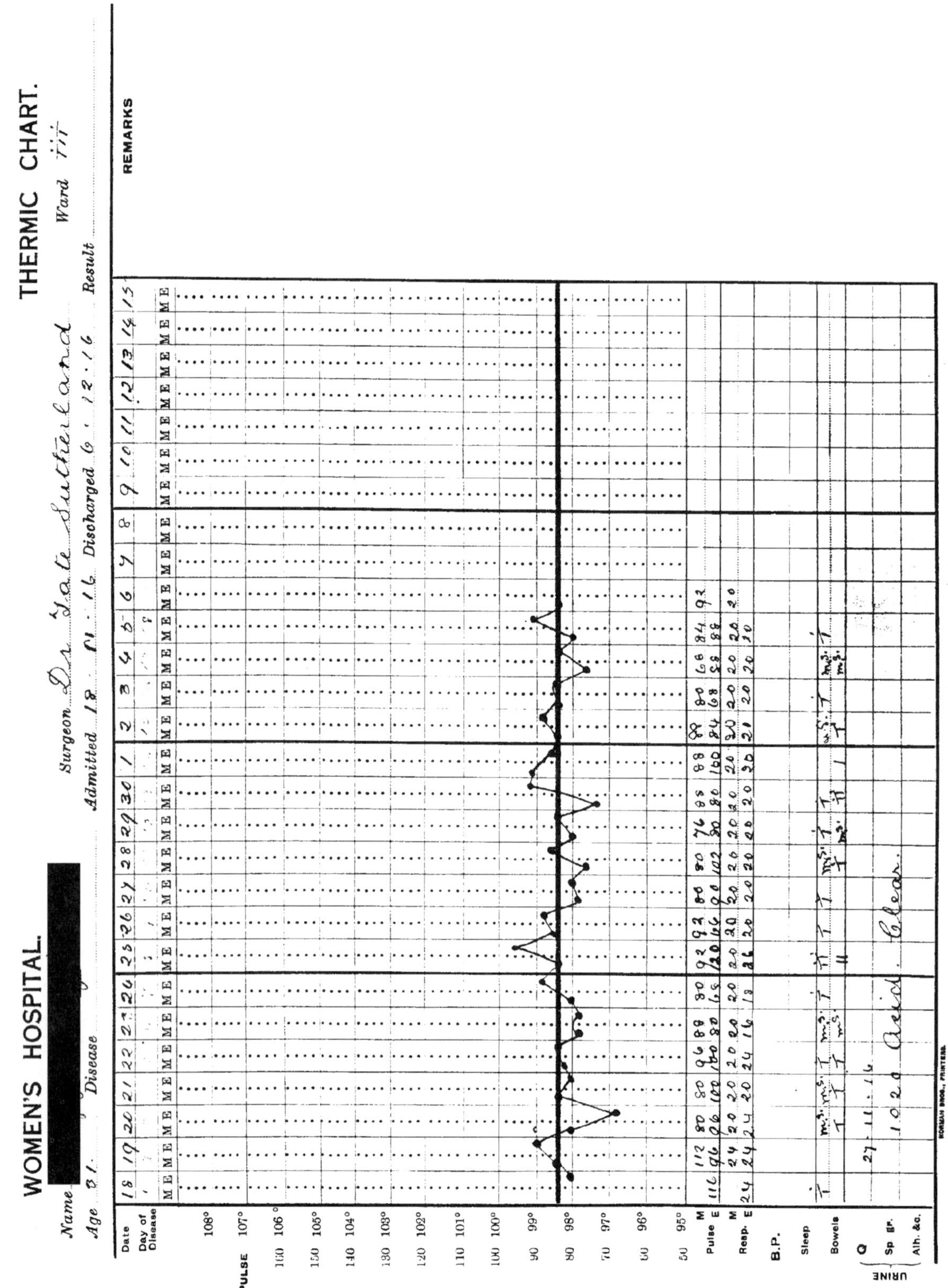

THERMIC CHART.

WOMEN'S HOSPITAL.

Name _____

Age _31.___   Disease _____

Surgeon _Dr. Mc Sutherland_   Ward _iii_

Admitted _18 . 11 . 16_   Discharged _6 . 12 . 16_   Result _____

REMARKS

| Date | 18 | 19 | 20 | 21 | 22 | 23 | 24 | 25 | 26 | 27 | 28 | 29 | 30 | 1 | 2 | 3 | 4 | 5 | 6 | 7 | 8 | 9 | 10 | 11 | 12 | 13 | 14 | 15 |

Richmond Sth
Nov. 29th '16

Mrs K. is very ill. She had a mishap about 2
mos a week ago. When I saw her she had lost a
great deal of blood. I curetted her, but she has
been feverish ever since. She has been in delicate health and has albumen in urine. As she is
much worse this last 24 hours and cannot get
proper care at home she should be admitted to
the Women's Hospital.
Signed. —————
MB BS.

29 November 1916
Mrs E. K.
<u>Aged:</u> 35
[Too sick for further history to be taken]

---

29 · 11 · 16   Name ███████████   Surgeon *Felix Meyer*

Time Received from Theatre	-		
Condition	-	-	-
Colour -	-	-	-
Respirations	=	-	-
Pulse -	-	=	-
Temperature	=	-	=
Extremities	=	-	-
Regained Consciousness		-	

Time	Temp.	Pulse	Resp.	Urine	Bowels	TREATMENT.	Ozs.	REMARKS.
3 45	104²	136	24			Admitted 3·45: Dr ordered Bowel wash-out & Rectal Salines x z to be given. Bowel wash out given ē very slight result		Salines x z to
4·45						Saline x z P. R. given Dr O'Sullivan ordered Salines P.R. to be given 4 hrly.		Not retained Ph. S. O.
5						mouth & tongue v. dirty cleaned.		
5 30						Dr O'Sullivan visited Vaginal smear & Blood culture taken		Off. dis. P.V.
6·	103	12				Head of bed raised n blocks.		Comp of Pain in R. leg.

4.
7.25

Milk & water $\frac{3}{8}$ VI

Rectal Saline $\frac{3}{8}$ X given.

Summary.

Patient is very sick.
Treatment as charted. Rectal Saline
last given 8.25. Comp of pain in R. leg.
was offensive which discharged P.V.
T. 102 P. 112 R. 28.

E. M. Brooks.

le 29—11—16   Name ████████████   Surgeon W.S Meyer

Time Received from Theatre -
Condition   -   -   -
Colour -   -   -   -
Respirations -   -   -
Pulse -   -   -   -
Temperature -   -   -
Extremities -   -   -
Regained Consciousness   -

Time	Temp.	Pulse	Resp.	Urine	Bowels	TREATMENT.	Ozs.	REMARKS.
9								Fairly comf.
10		Sleeping						Sleeping
10.30								Returned saline given at 8.25. P.M. C. Hg. B. action (green stool)
11								Sleeping
12								"
12.30						Rectal Saline 3X given Mouth cleansed.		Saline returned immediatly
2	101⁸	112	24					
3						Cup of Coffee taken		
3								B. O. (Liquid black stool)
3.30						Patient sponged & bed made comfortable		
4.30						Rectal saline 3X given		Saline returned immediatly
5						Cathet. U. K. O 3XXX		

5.30					

Cup of bread & milk taken
Mouth cleansed

| 6 | 103 | 120 | 24 | | |

Summary.
Patient is about the same.
Salines not retained. Cathet. Ut. 16. O₃ xxx
at 5. a. m. no aperient given.

T. 103 P. 120 R. 24   S. Eyre.

.... ·0 · 11 · 16 Name ███████████   Surgeon Dr. Meyer

Time Received from Theatre	-		
Condition	-	-	-
Colour -		-	-
Respirations	-	-	-
Pulse · ·	-	-	-
Temperature	-	-	-
Extremities	-	-	· ·
Regained Consciousness		· ·	

Time	Temp.	Pulse	Resp.	Urine	Bowels	TREATMENT.	Ozs.	REMARKS.
9.						Rectal Saline ʒ v. given		
						Mouth & tongue cleaned		
9.30	2					Milk coffee given	IV	
10	113	108	26					
10.30						Milk bovril	IV	Saline returned
								c̄ slight Bowel
11.15						Milk & water	VI	action (green stool
								R buttock looking
								red same rubbed
								c̄ spirits & powder
								B.W.C. into bed
12.						Dr. Meyer & Dr. O'Sullivan visited		
12.30						Milk & water	V	
2.	104	120	32			Rectal saline v ʒ given		not retained
						Dr. O'Sullivan ordered Salines to be		
						discontinued for 24 hrs.		
4						Water	VI	

4						Water vi
						R leg elevated on Pillows dr--a.a.cr.
						Milk & water iv
4·45						Catheterized U.D.C. xivz.
5·15						Milk & water ii
6.	103	120	32			Sponged all over back. Passed urine into bed
						attended to same looking red.
						air cushion placed under back.
7.						Milk coffee iv

. Summary. Patient about the same, appears very weak
nour taken very well, treatment as charted.

T 103. P 120 R 32 E. Nicholson.

---

e **20 – 11 – 16**   Name ▅▅▅▅▅▅▅▅▅▅▅   Surgeon *Dr Meyer.*

Time Received from Theatre	-
Condition	- - -
Colour	- - - -
Respirations	- - -
Pulse	- - - -
Temperature	- - -
Extremities	- - -
Regained Consciousness	-

Time	Temp.	Pulse	Resp.	Urine	Bowels	TREATMENT.	Ozs.	REMARKS.
9								Sleeping
10	104⁴	56	28					Skin acting v freely
10·15						Cup of Milk & water	vi	
11								Sleeping
11·45						Cup of milk & water	vi	
12·30						Mouth cleansed		
1.30						.		Sleeping.
2		Sleeping						
3						Patient sponged & made		R. buttock still red
						comfortable. back attended		looking
						to. Mouth cleansed.		
3·30						Cup of milk coffee taken	v	
4·30						Cathet U.N.O. 3xvi		
5·30						Cup of warm milk taken	v	
6	103⁸	132	28			Mouth cleansed		

Summary

Patient much about the same.
had a lot of sleep during the night. nourishment
taken well. B. N. O. aperient not given.
Cathet U. K. O. ℥ XVI at 4.30. a. m.

T 103⁸ P 152 R 2.   S. Eyre.

Date 1. 12. 16.   Name ████████████   Surgeon Dr Meyer.

Time Received from Theatre	-		
Condition	-	-	-
Colour -	-	-	-
Respirations	-	-	-
Pulse -	-	-	-
Temperature	-	-	-
Extremities	-	-	-
Regained Consciousness	-		

Time	Temp.	Pulse	Resp.	Urine	Bowels	TREATMENT.	Ozs.	REMARKS.
4.						Milk & water	VI	
8.						Cocoa	II	
9						Milk & water	VI	
10	102	132	48			Beef tea	I	Mouth cleansed
11.30						Dr. Sullivan visited prac...		same v. daily
						...talin 31 to + kin...		...v in kriy...
11.45						Digitalin gr 100 given		
12.						Bed changed back attended to		B.O. & P.U into bed
12.30								Mouth & tongue clea...
1.						Cup milk + water	IV	
						Cal grs i given		Mouth cleaned,
2	103⁸	140	40			Cal grs i "		
2.45						Digitalin gr 100 given		
3.						Cal grs i		Mouth cleaned
						Rambling a lot in her talk. Cup tea given	ii	
						Skin acting v. freely		

							TREATMENT		

(top portion — handwritten chart)

...... *e e oqu ...tted omdete*
H.d. *Strych ⁴⁄₁₀ gr 4 hrly aft...... & H.I. Liq.*
Milk & water   IV
4·   *Cal grs ⁱ   Back rubbed etc.*
4   XVI   *Catheterized U.D. O ℥ XVI*
5   *Strychnine gr ⁴⁄₁₀ given H.I.*   *Coughing a little*
     Refuses nour.
6.   *Milk & water*   III
7.   *H. Inj Digitalin gr ¹⁄₁₀₀ given*

ate *1 – 12 – 16*   Name ▮▮▮▮▮▮▮   Surgeon ....

Time Received from Theatre -
Condition -
Colour -   *Inj Strych ¹⁄₄₀ gr + w....*
Respirations -   " *Digitalin ¹⁄₁₀₀ gr 4 hrly.*
Pulse -
Temperature -   " *Camphor grs IV 4 hrly.*
Extremities -
Regained Consciousness -

Time	Temp.	Pulse	Resp.	Urine	Bowels	TREATMENT.	Ozs.	REMARKS.
7						*Strych ⁴⁄₁₀ gr H.I. given*		
9.30						*Sips of milk & water*		
						Mouth cleaned		
10	103	32	40					*Skin acting freely*
						Dr..... Sullivan visited ... ordered Hypo ..		
						Camphor grs IV – 4 hrly.		
10.40						*Ll Inj. Camphor gts IV ..*		
11						*Digitalin ¹⁄₁₀₀ gr H.I. given*		
12								*Sleeping*
12.30						*Mouth cleaned*		
						Sips of milk & water		
1						*Strych H.I. ⁴⁄₁₀ given*		*Skin acting & freely*
2								*sleeping*
2.30						*Milk taken*	IV	
2.40						*H.Inj Camphor gr IV given*		
3						*Digitalin ¹⁄₁₀₀ gr H.I. given*		*..... ... into bed.*
3.30						*Cup of milk coffee taken*	V	
4						*Patient sponged & made*		*B. W. O into bed.*
						comfatable. ...... H.H. O ℥ III		

						TREATMENT		REMARKS
5						Strych 40 gr H.S. given		quantity of small was
5.15						Drink of tea taken	IV	blisters on abdomen
6	105	132	58			Mouth cleaned		

Summary.

Patient much the same. wandering at time. Treatment as charted. camphor gr IV due at 6.40 a.m.

J.o.3 Pulse 88

S. Eyre.

Date 2 – 12 – 16   Name ▮▮▮▮▮▮▮▮▮▮▮   Surgeon ▮▮ ▮▮▮▮

Time Received from Theatre -
Condition - - - H.S. Strec 40 gr 4 hrly
Colour - - - " " Digitalin too gr 4 hrly
Respirations - " " Camp IV gr 4 hrl
Pulse - - -
Temperature - -
Extremities - - " " 1cc Pituitrin
Regained Consciousness - -

Time	Temp.	Pulse	Resp.	Urine	Bowels	TREATMENT.	Ozs.	REMARKS.
9						Strych 40 gr H.S. given		
9.15	106	160	52					Pulse vol poor
9.30								Seems unable to swallow any nourishment
10	106	168	54			Camphor gr IV given H.S. Mouth cleaned		
11						Digitalin gr too H.S. given		
11.30						Lips moistened. Sips of milk		
12						Pituitrin 1cc H.S. given Lips moistened		
1						Strych 40 gr H.S. given		
2	105	152	50			Camphor gr IV H.S. given		
3						Digitalin gr too H.S. given Lips moistened		Unable to swallow any nourishment
3.30						Patient sponged all over & back attended to		Bowels run into bed

4			

[handwritten medical chart entries, largely illegible]

... , O. 3 × × ĪĪ
Pituitrin 1 cc H. I. given
Sips of coffee given
Strych 40 gr H. I. given
Camphor gr iv H. I. given   Pulse ... weaker

5			
6	106	54	
6.30			

Bowels acted in to bed

Summary.   Could not ...

Patient is very low this morning. see above for treatment

... P. R...   S. Eyre.

Date   2. 12. 16   Name ████████   Surgeon D... Mayer

Time Received from Theatre
Condition
Colour
Respirations
Pulse
Temperature
Extremities
Regained Consciousness

H. Inj Strych 40 gr 4 hrly
   "   Digitalin 100 gr 4 hrly
   "   Camphor grs IV 4 hrly
   "   1 cc Pituitrin 4 hrly

Time	Temp.	Pulse	Resp.	Urine	Bowels	TREATMENT.	Ozs.	REMARKS.
6.40						H. I camphor grs IV given		
7						Cup of milk + water taken	II	Pulse very weak
7						H. I. strych Digitalin gr 100 given		
8						1 pint of water		
9						H. I. Strychnine gr 40 given		
9.30						Mouth cleansed. Cocoa IV taken		
10.40						H. I camphor grs IV given		Pulse weaker.
11						H. I. Digitalin gr 100 given		Mind wandering
11.30						Cup of milk + water Taken IV		Temperature 105.4 in axill.
12						Sponged all over, back rubbed etc. (Temp sponge.)		Slight bowel action into bed + P.u.
12.30						Milk + water taken	IV	Pulse slightly improved.
1						H. I Strychnine gr 40 given		Rambling in speech
2	105	128	52					Pulse vol very poor
2.40						H. Inj camphor II IV given Milk & water	III	

9						... *digitalin* ? too
3.35						... *IV* given
3.~						... $\overline{iii}$
4						Sponged all over Back
						attended to
5						4 *Inj Strych* to given
6	6 105 144 58 $\overline{XII}$					*Caffeine* inj *M.D* (1) 3 $\overline{XII}$
6.40						*H.T. Camphor* gr *IV* given
7						*Digitalin* gr 100 given (*H.J*)
8						1 cc *pituitrin* given *H.J.*

Remarks column:
... W.O + P.u
... Saunders
1 cc *pituitrin* 4 hrly
Seems worse

Summary
Treatment as charted.
Temperature keeping very high
D. Jenner

Date........................ Name ▮▮▮▮▮▮ Surgeon........................

Time Received from Theatre -	
Condition - - -	
Colour - - -	
Respirations - -	
Pulse - - -	
Temperature - -	
Extremities - -	
Regained Consciousness -	

Time	Temp.	Pulse	Resp.	Urine	Bowels	TREATMENT.	Ozs.	REMARKS.
						Summary Patient is not so well.		
						as usual. Cal grs IV given		
						give M. Sin a.m. To on Strych 40		
						Digitalin gr 100 4 hrly Digitalin		
						given last 4 P.m. Catheterized		
						M.D.O 3 $\overline{XVI}$ at 4 P.m		
						T. 102 P 144 R 48.		

Dr. *Meyer*

Name ▓▓▓▓▓▓▓▓▓▓   Age *35.*

OPERATION ....

GAUZES ....

SUTURES ....

Date	29				30				1				2				3				4				5			
Day after Operation																											
Time	A.M.		P.M.		A.M.		P.M.		A.M.		P.M.		A.M.		P.M.		A.M.		P.M.		A.M.		P.M.		A.M.		P.M.

Pulse / Temp.

	2	6	10	2	6	10	2	6	10	2	6	10	2	6	10	2	6	10	2	6	10	2	6	10	2	6	10	2	6	10	2	6	10	2	6	10

Pulse scale: 160, 150, 140, 130, 120, 110, 100, 90, 80, 70, 60

Temp. scale: 106°, 105°, 104°, 103°, 102°, 101°, 100°, 99°, 98°, 97°, 96°

Pulse	136		1	136	112	1		112	120	108	120	120	136	132	132	132	132	140	144	132		132	
Respr.	24			24	26			24	24	26	32		36	28	28	28	48	40	44	40		38	
Bowels																							
Urine																							

REMARKS

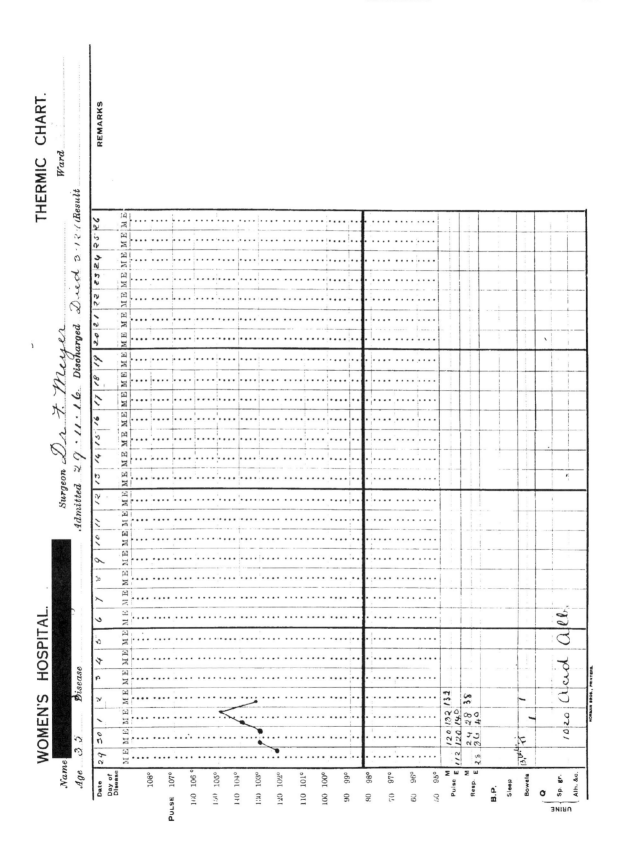

Notes

I: Tracy's Hospital

1 Founding a Hospital

1 Richard Broome, *The Victorians: Arriving* (Sydney, 1984), p. 32.
2 Ibid., pp. 42–68.
3 Paul de Serville, *Port Phillip Gentlemen* (Melbourne, 1980), passim.
4 Brenda Niall, *Georgiana* (Melbourne, 1994), pp. 130–1.
5 K. S. Inglis, *Hospital and Community: A History of the Royal Melbourne Hospital* (Melbourne, 1958), pp. 13–15.
6 R. A. Cage, *Poverty Abounding, Charity Aplenty* (Sydney, 1992), pp. 20–32.
7 Obituary, *AMJ,* December 1874, pp. 364–5.
8 Quoted from a biography of Richard Tracy compiled by the late Dr Colin Macdonald for 'The Book of Remembrance', RWHA.
9 Ibid.
10 Frances Perry, 'The History of Mrs Frances Perry', MSS, Nattrass Collection, RWHA, p. 40.
11 David Fitzpatrick, *Oceans of Consolation: Personal Accounts of Irish Migration to Australia* (Melbourne, 1995), p. 117.
12 *AMJ,* July 1858, p. 229; see Bryan Gandevia, 'William Thomson', *ADB*, vol. 6, pp. 270–2.
13 Inglis, pp. 21–2.
14 RWH Letters, Dean Macartney to the Treasurer of the Colony, 1 August 1856.
15 Mrs Tripp to the Attorney General, 3 December 1856.
16 Dr Motherwell to Dr Tracy, 10 January 1857.
17 From Mr Ham, 20 September 1856.
18 Draft rules for the Management of the Lying-in Hospital, approved 18 September 1856.
19 Letters, 3 and 7 November 1856.
20 Ibid., 1 January 1857.
21 Ibid., 27 February 1857.
22 Ibid., 20 May 1857.
23 Ibid., 13 May 1857.
24 Ibid., October 1857, p. 297; M. Bouchet, *Practical Treatise on the Diseases of Children and Infants at the Breast* (London, 1855), pp. 58–67.
25 *AMJ,* October 1856, pp. 294–5.
26 Ibid., January 1856, pp. 53–7.
27 James Young Simpson, *The Obstetric Memoirs and Contributions of James Y. Simpson* (Edinburgh, 1855), pp. 844–57.
28 See John Harley Warner, 'The History of Science and the Sciences of Medicine', *Osiris,* 1995, 10: 186–7.
29 Royal Women's Hospital Midwifery Book No. I.
30 *AMJ,* October 1857, p. 265.
31 *Argus,* 23 October 1858.
32 *Age,* 23 October 1858.
33 *AMJ,* April 1862, p. 103.
34 Ibid., March 1869, p. 95.
35 Richard Tracy, *Transactions of the Obstetrical Society of London, 1870.*
36 *AMJ,* July 1858, pp. 197–8.
37 RWH Book of Remembrance.

2 Lying-in

38 Judith Walzer Leavitt, *Brought to Bed: Childbearing in America, 1750–1950* (New York, 1986), pp. 87–115; Richard W. Wertz and Dorothy C. Wertz, *Lying-In: A History of Childbirth in America* (New York, 1979), pp. 1–8.
39 B. of M. Minutes, 12 January 1860.
40 Ibid., 29 March 1860.
41 Ibid., 7 June and 2 August 1860.
42 Ibid., 26 January 1860.
43 *Herald,* 6 July 1860; *Argus,* 20 July 1860.
44 *AMJ,* April 1865, p. 119.
45 Ibid., July 1859, pp. 210–13; January 1864, p. 1.
46 Midwifery Book, admitted 29 May 1864.
47 B. of M. Minutes, 25 October 1860
48 F. B. Smith, *The People's Health* (London, 1979), pp. 218–19.
49 Midwifery Book, admitted 5 December 1861.
50 Ibid., 26 April 1860.

51 Ibid., 22 March 1860.

52 Sharon Morgan, 'Irishwomen in Port Phillip' in Oliver MacDonagh and W. F. Mandle, eds, *Irish Australian Studies* (Canberra, 1989), pp. 240–5.

53 Midwifery Book No. 1, 8 December and 20 October 1859.

54 Ibid., 22 November 1860.

55 Royal Women's Hospital, *Centenary of Nurse Training in Australia, 1862–1962,* pp. 1–5; letter to *Argus,* from Nicholas Avent, 8 April 1869.

56 *AMJ,* October 1863, p. 245; J. M. Munro Kerr et al, eds, *Historical Review of British Obstetrics and Gynaecology* (Edinburgh, 1954), p. 14.

57 Herbert Thoms, *Classical Contributions to Obstetrics and Gynaecology* (Baltimore, 1935), pp. 197–291; James Young Simpson, *Memoirs,* 'On the Mode of Application of the Long Forceps', pp. 492–7.

58 Simpson's *Memoirs,* pp. 852–5.

59 Ibid., p. 492.

60 Irvine Loudon, *Death in Childbirth* (OUP, 1992), pp. 135–43.

61 *AMJ,* October 1863, p. 286.

62 Ibid., January 1858, p. 6.

63 Ibid., July 1858, pp. 184–6.

64 Ibid., July 1859, p. 197.

65 loc. cit.

66 Midwifery Book No. 1.

67 *AMJ,* July 1859, p. 197.

68 Charles Rosenberg, 'The Therapeutic Revolution', in *Explaining Epidemics* (Cambridge, 1992), pp. 27–31.

69 Midwifery Book No. 1.

70 *AMJ,* February 1869, p. 63.

71 B. of M. Minutes, 11 October 1860.

72 Dr Suzanne Garland, RWH.

73 These calculations and the commentary are by Dr Robin Bell from a co-authored unpublished paper, 'Birth Weight and the Standard of Living, Royal Women's Hospital, 1857–1997'. This project is still in progress and this 1857–87 series will be disaggregated in a later study.

74 Irving S. Cutter and Henry R. Veits, *A Short History of Midwifery* (Philadelphia, 1964), pp. 110–11.

75 Twelfth Annual Report, for year ending 1868, p. 4.

76 *AMJ,* July 1873, pp. 201–2.

77 Ibid., pp. 206–7.

78 Ibid., January 1868, pp. 20–4; Diana Dyason, 'William Gillbee and Erysipelas at the Melbourne Hospital', *Journal of Australian Studies,* no. 14, May 1984.

3 The Diseases Peculiar to Women

79 I. Baker Brown, *On Surgical Diseases of Women* (London, 1861) p. 233; Michael Mason, *The Making of Victorian Sexuality* (OUP, 1994), pp. 200–3; *AMJ,* February 1873, p. 45; Ornella Moscucci, *The Science of Woman, Gynaecology and Gender in England, 1800–1929* (Cambridge, 1990), p. 105.

80 Dr Rowan's Case Book, no. 4, 14 July 1887.

81 Dr Burke's Case Book, no. 1, 23 October 1883. (Case rediagnosed by Dr James Evans, RWH)

82 Dr Fetherston's Case Book, no. 2, 25 June 1887 (Dr James Evans).

83 Dr Balls-Headley's Case Book, No. 1, 19 July 1885.

84 *AMJ,* October 1863, pp. 284–5.

85 Mason, pp. 181–3.

86 Mary Poovey, ' "Scenes of an Indelicate Character": the Medical "Treatment" of Victorian Women', in Thomas Laqueur and Catherine Gallagher, eds, *The Making of the Modern Body,* (Berkeley, 1987), pp. 83–106.

87 Moscucci, p. 126.

88 *AMJ,* March 1871, pp. 85–7.

89 Quoted in admiration in the *AMJ,* January 1858, p. 74.

90 *AMJ,* October 1863, pp. 284–300; ibid., April 1865, pp. 113–24.

91 F. M. C. Forster, *Progress in Obstetrics and Gynaecology in Australia* (Sydney, 1967), pp. 23–8. Ill health prevented Dr Frank Forster from completing his research for a biography of Tracy, but this short book will remain a classic in Australian medical historiography.

92 *AMJ,* April 1865, p. 113.

93 Ibid., p. 116.

94 Ibid., p. 118.

95 Ibid., July 1862, p. 176.

96 Charles West, *Lectures on the Diseases of Women* (London, 1858) pp. 73–4.

97 James Simpson, 'Dilation and Incision of the Cervix Uteri in Cases of Obstructive Dysmenorrhoea', from *Memoirs,* pp. 288–91.

98 *AMJ,* October 1861, pp. 250–2.

99 F. M. C. Forster, 'The Story of the Hysterotome and Incision of the Cervix', *MJA,* 1967, 2: 887 (11 November).

100 *AMJ,* July 1863, pp. 176–9.

101 Ibid., pp. 11–14.

102 Ibid., December 1871, p. 367.

103 Ibid., February 1866, pp. 33–6.

104 Ibid., April 1865, p. 125.

105 Deborah Kuhn McGregor, *Sexual Surgery and the Origins of Gynaecology* (New York, 1989), passim.

106 *AMJ,* October 1861, pp. 269–72.

107 Dr W. Balls-Headley's Case Book no. 1, 8 September 1885.

108 *AMJ,* January 1861, p. 25.

109 Ibid., April 1859, pp. 107–11.

110 Ibid., June 1864, pp. 167–77; May 1874, pp. 129–32.

111 Ibid., December 1864, pp. 362–5.

112 Ibid., March 1866, pp. 65–71.

113 Ibid., December 1874.

II: Sepsis and Antisepsis

4 Fever House

1 de Serville, *Pounds and Pedigrees: The Upper Class in Victoria 1850–1880* (Melbourne, 1991), pp. 200, 303, 522; *ADB*, vol. 3, p. 83.

2 B. of M. Minutes, 3 December 1880, 22 October 1880.

3 Ibid., 1879: May, pp. 213–22 and 257–59; July, 352–7; August, 408–10.

4 B. of M. Minutes, 22 October 1880.

5 Charles E. Rosenberg, *Explaining Epidemics and other Studies in the History of Medicine* (Cambridge University Press, 1992), p. 76.

6 Dyason, 'William Gillbee and Erysipelas at the Melbourne Hospital: medical theory and social actions', pp. 3–28.

7 W. F. Bynum, *Science and the Practice of Medicine in the Nineteenth Century* (Cambridge, 1994), pp. 132–7. Dyason argues that it was this misunderstanding that reveals Gilbee's incomprehension, but this again was a credible 'approximation' since the Group A streptococcus responsible for the worst wound infections was transmitted by droplets and on dust particles.

8 *AMJ*, January 1879, pp. 1–17.

9 Ibid., 15 December 1880, pp. 555–7.

10 Ibid. 15 February 1881, pp. 93–4.

11 Midwifery Book No. 2; B. of M. Minutes, 17 March 1882.

12 Inglis, Hospital and Community, pp. 56–64; *AMJ*, 15 March 1881, p. 141; 15 May 1881, pp. 237–9.

13 B. of M. Minutes, 27 May 1880.

14 Ibid., 4 July, 23 September 1881.

15 Ibid., 7 June 1881.

16 Ibid.

17 Wertz and Wertz, *Lying-in: A History of Childbirth in America*, p. 126.

18 Annual Report, for Eighteen Months ending 30th June, 1883.

19 *AMG*, July 1882, pp. 129–32; *MJA*, 9 October 1937, pp. 626–7.

20 *AMJ*, 15 January 1882, pp. 25–7.

21 *AMG*, April 1883, p. 149; Balls-Headley's Case Book, no. 2, Case of J. O'C, adm. 26 November 1884.

22 Since 1883 it had also been connected to the telephone system, although when honoraries were out on house calls, they still needed to be pursued by messengers.

23 Visitors' Book, 22 April 1884.

24 Letter to *Argus* by Felix Meyer, 31 May 1884.

25 RWH Correspondence: Felix Meyer to Mrs Puckle, 27 April, and to the Board, 3 May 1884.

26 Dr Burke's Case Book, no.1, p. 21.

27 RWH Correspondence, East Melbourne Refuge to Board, 22 May 1884.

28 *Telegraph*, 22 May 1884.

29 *AMJ*, 15 June 1884, pp. 270–2.

30 Ibid., 15 June 1884, pp. 267–8, 15 July 1884, pp. 321–2.

31 Ibid., 15 June, p. 251.

32 Ibid., 15 November 1884, pp. 511–17, 522–3.

33 *AMG*, July 1884, p. 235; and undated cutting in archives.

34 Visitors' Book, 7 July, 19 August 1884.

35 Dr Burke's Case Book, no.1, p. 78.

36 Ibid., p. 88.

37 Dr Balls-Headley's Case Book, no. 1, Mrs S. G., adm. 22 August 1884, p. 77.

38 Ibid., pp. 89 and 98.

39 Dr Rowan's Case Book, no. 1, 12 November 1884.

40 *AMJ*, 15 October 1885, p. 459.

41 Ibid., 15 August 1885, p. 378.

42 Visitors' Book, 29 April, 4 September 1885.

43 *AMG*, October 1885, p. 25.

44 *Annual Report 1884–1885*. The report since mid 1883 analysed deaths for the financial year from July to June. My tables remain divided into calendar years.

45 *AMJ*, July 1886, pp. 306–9.

46 Dr Balls-Headley's Case Book, no. 2, adm. 1 September 1886, p. 246.

47 *AMG*, February 1888, p. 117.

48 Dr Burke's Case Book, no. 2, adm. 18 August 1886.

49 Dr Rowan's Case Book, no. 2, 25 October 1887, p. 120.

50 *AMJ*, 15 July 1887, pp. 294–301.

51 *Annual Report 1887–88*, p. 6.

52 Ibid., 15 May 1888, pp. 211–12.

53 B. of M. Minutes, 6 April 1888.

5 'Servants in the Temple of Purity'

54 B. of M. Minutes, 15 March 1889, 21 September 1894.

55 Dr Balls-Headley's Case Book, no. 2, 8 June 1890, pp. 195–6, 202.

56 Alfred Lewis Galabin, *A Manual of Midwifery* (London, 1886), pp. 265–74.

57 Richard Evans, *Death in Hamburg* (London, 1990), pp. 340–6.

58 Susan M. Reverby, *Ordered to Care: the Dilemma of American Nursing, 1850–1945* (Cambridge, 1987).

59 Alison Bashford, 'Female Bodies at Work: Gender and the Re-Forming of Colonial Hospitals', in *Australian Cultural History*, no. 13, 1994, pp. 65–81.

60 Royal Commission on Charitable Institutions, *VPP*, 1892–3, v. 4, Q. 2093.

61 Ibid., Qq. 3211–12.

62 Ibid., Q. 2451.

63 Ibid., Qq. 4702–5.

64 Ibid. Q. 7133.

65 B. of M. Minutes, 12 June 1896.

66 Ibid., 9 April 1897.

67 R. C. on Charitable Institutions, op. cit., Qq. 4662, 4703.

68 B. of M. Minutes, 7 August 1891.

69 Ibid., 4 January 1889; 31 January and 7 February 1896.

70 Ibid., 2 and 9 March 1894.

71 Ibid., 19 June 1891.

72 *Thirty-fourth Annual Report, 1890–91*, p. 8.

73 B. of M. Minutes, 20 November and 4 December 1891.

74 Calculations and commentary by Dr Robin Bell, co-author of our unpublished paper, 'Birth Weight and the Standard of Living, Royal Women's Hospital, 1857–1996'.

75 S. L. Swain, The Victorian Charity Network in the 1890s, PhD thesis, University of Melbourne, 1977.

76 B. of M. Minutes, 29 January, 15 July, 14 October 1892, 10 March 1893.

77 Ibid., 29 March, 12 April, 9 June 1893.

78 Ibid., 26 June, 3 July 1896, 16 July, 17 September 1897.

79 Mason, *The Making of Victorian Sexual Attitudes* (OUP, 1994), pp. 220–1.

80 B. of M. Minutes, 8 January 1892, 15 March, 22 and 29 November, 6 December 1895, 12 and 19 June 1896, 11 and 18 June 1897; letter to the Sydney Hospital expressing the medical staff's opinion on women resident surgeons, 15 September 1905.

81 B. of M. Minutes, 29 March, 22 February, 13 December 1889; 7 February, 3 October 1890; 20 and 27 January 1893; 25 April 1895; 26 June, 28 August, 22 October 1896; 17 September 1897; 21 December 1900, 18 January, 19 April 1901.

82 *AMG*, 15 July 1894; *IMJ*, 20 February 1902, pp. 84–5.; B. of M. Minutes, 8 September 1899, 27 June, 25 July 1901.

83 B. of M. Minutes, 31 May, 20 December 1901; 31 January, 21 March 1902.

84 *AMG*, 30 February 1902, p. 102; B. of M. Minutes, January–February passim, 14 March, 16, 23, 30 May, 13, 20 June, 29 August and 24 October 1902.

85 Ibid., 3 May, 7 June, 21 June, 11 October, 6 December 1901, 6 June, 29 August, 19 September 1902; Shurlee Swain, with Renate Howe, *Single Mothers and their Children* (CUP, Melbourne, 1995), pp. 87–8.

86 RWH, *Centenary of Nurse Training in Australia, 1862–1962*, pp. 21–3.

87 *New Idea*, 6 November, 1903, p. 433.

88 Ibid., p. 434.

III: Women and Doctors

6 The Sickness of Women

1 *AMJ*, August 1877, pp. 251–5.

2 Cases from Dr Burke's Case Book no. 1 will hereafter be referred to as Burke 1 with date of admission, as also for Dr Fetherston's cases.

3 Burke 1, 20 June 1884.

4 Eugene Anderson, 'The Menstrual Function',

Intercolonial Medical Congress of Australasia (Melbourne, 1889), pp. 704–8.

5 Burke 1, 7 January 1885, comment by Dr Evans.

6 Burke 1, 7 January 1885, 23 October 1883.

7 Galabin, *A Manual of Midwifery*, p. 471.

8 Dr Rowan's Case Book, no. 2, 1 February 1887.

9 Ibid., 24 November 1886.

10 Dr Balls-Headley's Case Book, no. 2, 10 December 1886.

11 Burke 1, 21 November 1884.

12 Ann Larson, *Growing Up in Melbourne, Family Life in the Late Nineteenth Century* (Canberra, 1994), pp. 145–50.

13 Burke 1, 24 October 1884.

14 Eugene Anderson, 'The Menstrual Function', loc. cit.

15 Burke 1, 24 July 1884.

16 Burke 1, 14 December 1883, 5 March 1884.

17 Burke 1, 7 January 1884, 2 October 1884, 7 November 1883.

18 Thoms, *Classical Contributions to Obstetrics and Gynaecology*, pp. 250–5.

19 Walter Balls-Headley, 'On the treatment of So-called Ulceration with Laceration of the Cervix Uteri, by Emmett's [*sic*] Operation of Closure', *AMJ*, 15 November 1882, p. 487.

20 Burke 1, 9 July 1884.

21 Ibid., 16 July 1884.

22 Ibid., 10 November 1883.

23 Fetherston, 2, 5 June 1887.

24 F. M. C. Forster, 'Caesarean Section and its Early Australian History', *MJA*, 1970, 2: 33, 4 July.

25 Walter Balls-Headley, 'Seven Cases of Laparotomy', *Pamphlets* (Melbourne, 1893), pp. 15–6.

26 Balls-Headley's Case Book, no. 1, 26 November 1884

27 Ibid., 18 June 1885.

28 Dr Rowan's Case Book, no. 2, 24 October 1887.

29 Ibid., passim.

30 M. U. O'Sullivan, *The Proclivity of Civilised Woman to Uterine Displacement: the Antidote* (Melbourne, 1894), p. 28.

31 Moscucci, *The Science of Woman*, pp. 14–15.

32 Walter Balls-Headley, *The Evolution of the Diseases of Women* (London, 1894), p. 29.

33 *AMJ*, April 1887, pp. 157–8.

7 The Natural and the Unnatural

34 *AMJ*, September 1887, p. 423.

35 *Intercolonial Medical Congress 1887*, p. 174.

36 *Intercolonial Medical Congress of Australasia, 1889*, p. 629.

37 Ibid., Felix Meyer, 'The Obligations of Gynaecology to Obstetrics', p. 712.

38 Ibid., p. 714.

39 Rothwell Adam, 'Cancer of the Uterus', *IMJ*, vol. II, 20 April 1897, pp. 167–72; George Horne, 'Early Recognition of Uterine Carcinoma', ibid., vol. XIV, no. 8, 20 August, 1909, pp. 381–5.

40 B. of M., Minutes 17 April 1896, 15 May 1896, 11 November 1898.

41 Ibid., 25 September and 26 June 1896.

42 Dr Hooper's Case Book, 1894–1900, adm. 17 August 1899.

43 B. of M., Minutes, 25 November 1898.

44 Ibid., 18 November 1898.

45 *AMG,* 15 April 1895, p. 173; B. of M. Minutes, 25 November 1898.

46 *AMJ,* May 1890, pp. 214–16; see also Thoms, *Classical Contributions to Obstetrics and Gynaecology,* pp. 245–9.

47 *IMJ,* 20 January 1897, p. 19.

48 Ibid.

49 Dr O'Sullivan's Case Book (previously Balls-Headley's until his retirement), Mrs B. W. of Carlton, adm. 14 September 1899.

50 Dr O'Sullivan's Case Book, no. 3, 1 May 1906 and 12 January 1907, Dr Morton's Case Book, 23 June 1909.

51 Dr O'Sullivan's Case Book, no. 3, 4 March 1907.

52 Dr Adam's Case Book, no. 1, 11 June 1897.

53 Dr O'Sullivan's Case Book, no. 3, 30 December 1906.

54 Dr Meyer's Case Book, 15 December 1908.

55 Dr Morton's Case Book, no. 4, 22 August 1909.

56 Lado T. Ruzika and John C. Caldwell, *The End of Demographic Transition in Australia,* Australian Family Formation Project, Monograph No. 5, Australian National University, 1977, pp. 127–91.

57 *ADB,* vol. 12, p. 1, by Farley Kelly.

58 Interview with Dr Gytha Betheras, 5 May 1997.

59 Patricia Grimshaw, Marilyn Lake, Ann McGrath and Marian Quartly, *Creating a Nation* (Melbourne, 1994), pp. 194–5 (Patricia Grimshaw).

60 Simon Szreter, *Fertility, Class and Gender in Britain, 1860–1940* (Cambridge, 1996), pp. 367–439.

61 *Struggletown,* pp. 18–22; and my 'Respectability and Working-Class Politics in Late-Victorian London', *Historical Studies,* vol. 19, no. 74, April 1980.

62 *ADB,* vol. 3, pp. 124–6; RWH Book of Remembrance.

63 Melbourne City Council Archives, no. 3181, Box 384; *Herald,* 4 February 1896.

64 B. of M. Minutes, 20 April 1894.

65 Dr Balls-Headley's Case Book, no.1, 21 July 1884.

66 Dr Morton's Case Book, no. 4, 4 February 1910.

67 B. of M. Minutes 15 February 1889.

68 Ibid., 26 April 1901.

69 Ibid., 19 November 1909.

70 Dr Meyer's Case Book, 5 October 1909.

71 Ibid., 21 March 1909.

72 *AMG,* 22 June 1897, p. 301; *IMJ,* 20 October 1897, pp. 667–70.

73 *IMJ,* 20 September 1907, pp. 498–500.

74 *AMG,* 14 October 1911, p. 137.

75 Dr Adam's Case Book, no. 1, 16 February 1898 and 24 June 1899.

76 Dr Morton's Case Book, no. 4, 22 September 1909.

77 Dr O'Sullivan's Case Book, no. 3, 15 October 1904

78 *IMJ,* 20 February 1907, pp. 57–74.

79 Ibid., pp. 72–3.

80 Michael Roe, *Nine Australian Progressives: Vitalism in Bourgeois Social Thought, 1890–1960* (Brisbane, 1984), pp. 57–88.

81 *IMJ,* 4 May 1904, pp. 264–70; 20 September 1904, pp. 445–69 and 484–7; 4 October 1904, pp. 501–12.

82 Ibid., 20 March 1909, pp. 113–29.

83 *AMG,* 21 December 1908.

84 *AMJ,* 29 July 1911, 7 December 1912.

85 Ibid., 22 February 1913, pp. 916–17.

86 Ibid., 9 May 1914, p. 1551.

87 *AMG,* 21 September 1912, p. 306, 19 October 1912, p. 424; 1 November 1913, p.411; B. of M. Minutes, 13 September 1912, 7 November and 5 December 1913.

88 *AMJ,* 28 March and 4 April 1914.

89 Ibid., 4 November 1911, p. 175.

IV: Class Relations

8 Improving the Race

1 *Age,* 2 February 1918.

2 Minutes of Honorary Medical Staff, 18 April 1912.

3 Interview with Dr Frank Hayden, 16 February 1996.

4 Brian Egan, *Ways of a Hospital, St Vincent's Melbourne, 1890s–1990s* (Sydney, 1993), pp. 88–110, 140–71.

5 Colin Macdonald, 'RWH Book of Remembrance' (draft), Biography of Sydney Herbert Allen.

6 *IMJ,* 20 October 1908, pp. 522–3; ibid., 20 February 1906, pp. 100–3.

7 Minutes of the Honorary Medical Staff, 18 April 1912.

8 B. of M. Minutes, 25 April 1913, 27 June 1913, Report by Felix Meyer on 'The Working of the Gynaecological Department', 25 September 1913.

9 *MJA,* 23 March 1918, pp. 246–8.

10 B. of M. Minutes, 10 May and 2 June 1916, 15 August, 26 September 1919, 19 March 1920.

11 *Age,* 2 September 1921; see also *Argus,* 2 September 1921.

12 Judith Smart, 'The Great War and the "Scarlet Scourge": Debates about Venereal Diseases in Melbourne during World War I', in Judith Smart and Tony Wood eds, *An Anzac Muster: War and Society in Australia and New Zealand, 1914-18 and 1939–45* (Melbourne, 1992), pp. 58–85.

13 *MJA,* 27 May 1916, p. 429.

14 Ibid., pp. 316–18.

15 *Struggletown*, p. 106.
16 Extern Case Book, 11 November 1926.
17 *MJA*, 8 August 1925, p. 158.
18 Ibid., 24 December 1921, pp. 599–603.
19 *Struggletown*, pp. 143–5.
20 *MJA*, 2 June 1923, p. 611.
21 *Annual Report 1911–1912*, Infirmary Report.
22 *Annual Report 1913–1914*, Infirmary Report.
23 *Annual Report, 1917–1918*, Infirmary Report.
24 *MJA*, 3 August 1918, p. 88.
25 Ibid., 14 December 1918, p. 487.
26 Ibid., 3 August 1918, p. 88.
27 Simon Szreter, *Fertility, Class and Gender*, pp. 305–9.
28 *MJA.*, 15 December 1917, p. 492.
29 James A. Gillespie, *The Price of Health* (Melbourne, 1991), pp. 48–56; Philippa Mein Smith, *Mothers and King Baby* (London, 1997), pp. 31–62.
30 Kereen Reiger, *The Disenchantment of the Home* (Melbourne, 1985).
31 *Argus*, 2 September 1921.
32 *Age*, 2 September 1921.
33 Ibid.
34 *Struggletown*, p. 159.
35 *Argus*, 2 September 1921.
36 Letter to President of the Hospital, 27 May 1914.
37 *Struggletown*, pp. 50–1.
38 *MJA*, 15 July 1922, pp. 53–4.
39 Ibid., 3 February 1923, pp. 113–17.
40 Ibid., 8 August 1925, pp. 157–65.
41 H. Cairns Lloyd, 'Caesarean Section', in ibid., 4 March 1922, p. 232.
42 Ibid., 3 February 1923, p. 115.
43 Ibid., 8 August 1925, pp. 157–65.
44 Ibid., 3 February 1923, p. 114.
45 J. A. G. Hamilton, 'The Symptoms, Prophylaxis and Treatment of Toxaemia of Pregnancy', *MJA*, 24 November 1917, p. 434.
46 *MJA*, 8 December 1923, pp. 610–11.
47 Ibid., 21 January 1922, pp. 59–64. Sherwin's comparative statistics on p. 64 are out by a decimal point, giving the Women's a maternal death rate of 21% and Queen Charlotte 2.6%. I suspect there was a typographical error rather than an arithmetical one by Sherwin.
48 Ibid., pp. 78–81.
49 *Argus*, 2 August 1919.
50 *MJA*, 4 March 1922, p. 231.
51 Ibid., p. 229.
52 D. M. Embleton, 'The Hospital Problem of Melbourne and the Commonwealth', ibid., 3 December 1927, pp. 773–9, 896–7.
53 *Struggletown, Ruby Kane*, p. 207.
54 *Argus*, July 1926, see Cutting Book (RWHA), p. 151.
55 *Struggletown*, p. 131.
56 R. Marshall Allan, *Report on Maternal Mortality and Morbidity in the State of Victoria, Australia* (Melbourne, 1929), p. 16.
57 Extern Case Book, 15 March 1921.

58 C. of M., Minutes, 17 October 1924.
59 W. D. Saltau, 'Summary of Radium Treatment at the Women's Hospital, Melbourne, During the Last Five Years', *MJA*, 19 March 1927.
60 *MJA*, 25 July 1925, p. 105.
61 R. Marshall Allan, op. cit., pp. 11–15.
62 Arthur Wilson, Lecture Notes, University of Melbourne, 1926, Lecture 1.
63 Ibid., Lectures 11 and 14.

9 'An Interesting Introduction to the Family Life of the Proletariat'
64 Little George Street, Fitzroy, 17 October 1927.
65 Adam Street, Burnley, 18 April 1927.
66 Napier Street, Fitzroy, 9 December 1922.
67 Newman Rosenthal, *People–Not Cases, The Royal District Nursing Service* (Melbourne 1974), pp. 23–60.
68 Marlborough Street, Fawkner, 25 January 1924.
69 Coppin Street, Richmond, 5 October 1927.
70 Little Docker Street, Richmond, 12 September 1922.
71 Dwyer Street, Clifton Hill, 7 September 1926.
72 Stephenson Street, Richmond, 20 February 1927.
73 Balaclava, 29 December 1922.
74 Homewood Place, Carlton, 15 March 1921.
75 Liardet Street, Port Melbourne, 29 January 1923.
76 Franklin Street, West Melbourne, 19 September 1927.
77 Seake Street, Coburg, 8 December 1932.
78 Brooks Street, South Melbourne, 3 August 1927.
79 Market Street, South Melbourne, 1 November 1926.
80 Bar[nett] Street, Kensington, 1 November 1926.
81 Kerr Street, South Melbourne, 10 October 1921.
82 Victoria Street, Richmond, 6 June 1927.
83 Madden Grove, Burnley, 28 January 1924.
84 Bridge Road, Richmond, 17 January 1921.
85 September 1926.
86 Perry Street, Collingwood, 16 September 1926.
87 *Struggletown*, pp. 223–6.
88 Ibid., p. 193.
89 Nelson Street, Windsor, 13 October 1930.
90 Station Street, North Carlton, 13 November 1926.
91 Abbotsford Street, North Melbourne, 4 April 1924.
92 Canning Street, Carlton, 16 September 1923; Wood Street, North Melbourne, 16 February 1923.
93 Park Street, East Brunswick, 18 May 1927.
94 Medley Street, South Yarra, 28 November 1926.
95 Gray Street, West Brunswick, 6 May 1927.
96 George Street, East Melbourne, 12 December 1926.
97 14 August 1926.
98 15 December 1928.
99 Gipps Street, Collingwood, 16 April 1932.

100 Cobden Street, South Melbourne, 9 March 1927.
101 Mahoney Street, Fitzroy, 2 April 1924.
102 Park Street, East Brunswick, 18 May 1927.
103 Derby Street, Kew.
104 Rosenthal, op. cit., pp. 108–12.
105 Flevelle Street, North Richmond, 27 September 1923; Ferrars Street, South Melbourne, 26 September 1923.
106 Eades Place, West Melbourne, 4 February 1927.
107 *IMJ,* 2 October 1948, Dr George Simpson.
108 Cromwell Street, Collingwood, 31 May 1927.
109 Connell Street, Hawthorn, 24 December 1922.
110 Duke Street, Richmond, 7 August 1923.
111 George Street, Fitzroy, 6 November 1926.
112 Vere Street, Collingwood, 26 March 1921.
113 *IMJ,* 2 October 1948.
114 Invermay Grove, Hawthorn, 14 September 1921.
115 Newry Street, North Fitzroy, 15 July 1927.
116 Rathdowne Street, North Carlton, 25 February 1927.
117 King Street, Richmond, 26 December 1926.
118 Yarra Street, Abbotsford, 26 November 1927.
119 Kelvin Churches, 'Abortion', *Age,* 24 April 1976.
120 e.g. Clifton Hill, 13 November 1930, Port Melbourne, 24 January 1931.
121 James Street, Windsor, 11 November 1930.

V: 'Enormous Clinical Material'

10 Poverty and Pain

1 Interview with Dr Lorna Lloyd Green, 21 July 1993.
2 *Annual Report, 1930–1931,* p. 5.
3 Arthur M. Hill, transcript of 'Prestige' Lecture, 1973, Nattrass Collection, RWHA, Box 6.
4 Interview with Dr Frank Hayden, 16 February 1996.
5 Interview with Dr Ronald Rome, 24 May 1993.
6 Patricia Grimshaw, Lynne Strahan, eds, *The Half-Open Door* (Sydney, 1982), p. 165.
7 'A Hundred Case Histories': Interview No. 10, born 1905, interviewed by Marlene Kavanagh, 1995.
8 Ibid., Interview No. 27, born 1915, interviewed by Marlene Kavanagh, 1995.
9 Calculations and commentary by Dr Robin Bell from co-authored unpublished paper, 'Birth Weight and the Standard of Living, Royal Women's Hospital, 1857–1996'. This project is still in progress.
10 F. B Smith, 'Australian Public Health during the Depression of the 1930s', unpublished MS.
11 R. Marshall Allan, 'The Control of Maternal Mortality and Morbidity', *MJA,* 26 March 1938, p. 554.
12 Laurie O'Brien and Cynthia Turner, *Establishing Medical Social Work in Victoria* (Dept of Social Studies, University of Melbourne, 1979), pp. 19–29.
13 A 1930s case quoted in Bethia Stevenson, Draft of Lecture for Fiftieth Anniversary of Social Work Department, 11 May 1984, pp. 6–7.
14 Ibid., pp. 4–5.
15 Rosenthal, *People not Cases,* pp. 106–12; *MJA,* 18 July 1936, pp. 99–100.
16 Wendy Lowenstein, *Weevils in the Flour* (Melbourne, 1979), pp. 290–4.
17 Swain, *Single Mothers and Their Children,* p. 46.
18 Quoted in Lyn Finch and Jon Stratton, 'The Australian Working Class and the Practice of Abortion, 1880–1939', *Journal of Australian Studies,* no. 23, November 1988, p. 52.
19 Arthur M. Hill, 'Why be morbid? Paths of Progress in the control of obstetric infection, 1931 to 1960', *MJA,* 25 January 1964, p. 101.
20 *MJA,* 14 April 1923, pp. 393–8; 23 November 1935, pp. 707–14.
21 Ibid., 31 March, pp. 390–5, 30 June, pp. 793–5, 28 July 1928, pp. 102–14.
22 Ibid., 15 September 1928, pp. 322–45.
23 Ibid., 19 December 1936, pp. 843–7; H. D. Attwood, 'Patients, Pathologists and Practice', *Aust. N. Z. Journal of Obstetrics and Gynaecology,* (1982), 22: 11, p. 14; C. of M. Minutes, 18 April 1935, 14 May 1937.
24 *MJA,* 21 April, 1928, pp. 491–5; 2 January, 1932, pp. 1–6.
25 'A Hundred Case Histories', No. 58, born 1908, interviewed by Margaret Mabbitt.
26 Interview with Miss Betty Lawson, 27 May 1993.
27 'A Hundred Case Histories', No. 21, born 1911, interviewed by Madonna Grehan.
28 *MJA,* 24 February 1934, p. 269.
29 Arthur M. Hill, 'Post-Abortal and Puerperal Gas Gangrene: a Report of Thirty Cases', *J. of Obstet. Gynae. British Empire,* April 1936, pp. 201–2.
30 The following narrative is reconstructed from Case N. 292, admitted to Ward 3, 12 November 1934, and the report of the case in Arthur M. Hill, 'Post-Abortal and Puerperal Gas Infection', pp. 212–6.
31 Admitted to Ward 3, 24 November 1934.
32 Admitted to Ward 3, 24 November 1934.
33 Admitted to Ward 3, 24 November 1934.
34 Hill, 'Post-Abortal and Puerperal Gas Gangrene', pp. 201–2.
35 C. of M. Minutes, 25 January 1935.
36 Hill, 'Post-Abortal and Puerperal Gas Gangrene', pp. 208.
37 Admitted to Ward 3, 22 November 1934.
38 Admitted to Ward 3, 24 November 1935.
39 Admitted to Ward 6, 21 November 1934.
40 Admitted to Ward 3, 21 November 1934.
41 Admitted to Ward 6, 14 May 1934.
42 Admitted to Ward 6, 28 November 1934; Lowenstein, op. cit., pp. 292–3.
43 Interview with Mrs Kate Picouleau, 29 July 1996.

44 Arthur M. Hill, 'Why be morbid?', pp. 105, 110–11.
45 *MJA,* 23 October 1937, p. 701
46 Arthur M. Hill, 'Why be morbid?', p. 111.

11 Watersheds
47 Arthur M. Hill, 'Why be morbid?', pp. 104.
48 Ibid., pp. 104–5.
49 Ibid., pp. 105–6.
50 Entry on Hildred Butler by H. D. Attwood, *ADB,* vol. 13, p. 320.
51 Interview with Dr Suzanne Garland, 28 July 1997.
52 C. of M. Minutes, 17 December 1937, 1 April, 29 July, 9 September 1938, 13 January 1939; H. D. Attwood, 'Patients, Pathologists and Practice', *Aust. N.Z. J. Obstet Gynae.,* (1982) 22: 11.
53 Leonard Colebrook, 'Puerperal Fever: its aetiology and prevention', *The British Medical Journal,* 21 October 1933; Lucy M. Bryce and Phyllis Tewsley, 'A Bacteriological and Clinical Study of the Professional Personnel of Maternity Hospitals', *MJA,* 9 April 1938, pp. 653–4.
54 Hill, 'Why be morbid?', p. 107.
55 Gwen Williams, conversation with author.
56 Hill, 'Why be morbid?', p. 107.
57 Arthur M. Hill and Hildred M. Butler, 'The Diagnosis, Prevention and Treatment of Puerperal Infection', *MJA,* 21 February 1948, p. 229.
58 Hill, 'Why be morbid?.', p. 109.
59 Ibid., p. 110.
60 Arthur M. Hill, 'Reduction of Staphylococcal Infection in the Newly Born', *MJA,* 31 October 1959, p. 633.
61 Interview with Peggy Taylor, 19 September 1996.
62 Interview with Marlene Kavanagh, 19 September 1996.
63 C. of M. Minutes, 25 March 1938.
64 *MJA,* March 1938, September 1938.
65 Vera I. Krieger and Ronald McK. Rome, 'Toxaemic Pregnancy', *MJA,* 17 May 1941, pp. 611–12.
66 Ronald McK. Rome, 'The Clinical Importance of Renal Function Tests in Pregnancy', *MJA,* 24 March 1945, p. 289.
67 'A Hundred Case Histories', No. 74, born 1916, interviewed by Margaret Mabbitt.
68 Ibid., No. 75, born 1921, interviewed by Madonna Grehan.
69 Ibid., No. 14, born 1920, interviewed by Helen Johnstone.
70 R. H. J. Hamlin, 'The Prevention of Eclampsia and Pre-Eclampsia', *Lancet,* 12 January, 1952, pp. 64–8.
71 T. Dixon Hughes, 'The Importance of the Relativity of Blood Pressure and Other Signs in the Prevention of Eclampsia', *MJA,* 29 December 1951, pp. 871–4.
72 Hamlin, loc. cit., p. 68.
73 Letter to Medical Staff, from John Laver, 24 March 1952.
74 James Smibert, 'Fifty Years of Obstetrics, 1935–1985', *Newsletter, Association of Monash Medical Graduates Inc.,* vol. 13, no. 2, July 1991, pp. 344–5; Lance Townsend, 'High Blood Pressure in Pregnancy', *MJA,* 22 October 1960, pp. 641–53.
75 W. Ivon Hayes, 'Weight Restriction in Pregnancy', ibid., 20 October 1956, p. 605.
76 Interviewed 4 October 1993.
77 James Smibert, 'The Significance of Weight-gain in Pregnancy as assessed by various authors', *MJA,* 29 April 1967, pp. 878–80.
78 Smibert, 'Fifty Years of Obstetrics', p. 345.
79 C. of M. Minutes, 19 July 1946.
80 M. L. Verso, 'Fifty Years of the Red Cross Blood Transfusion Service in Victoria', *Victorian Historical Journal,* November 1980, pp. 218–36.
81 Interviews with Dr Kevin McCaul, 25 May, 3 and 10 June 1993.
82 'A Hundred Case Histories', No. 34, born *c.* 1920, interviewed by Helen Johnstone.
83 H. D. Attwood, 'Patients, Pathologists and Practice', *Aust. N. Z. J. Obstet. Gynae.,* 1982, 22:11, pp. 11–14.
84 RWH, *Medical and Clinical Report, 1939–41,* p. 31.
85 *MJA,* 1 September 1962, p. 340.
86 'A Hundred Case Histories', No. 19, interviewed by Madonna Grehan.
87 *AMA Gazette,* 1 April 1976, p. 12.
88 *MJA,* 11 February, 1951, p. 48; Hugh Ryan, *American Journal of Ophthalmology,* March 1952, p. 338; personal conversation with Professor H. D. Attwood.
89 W. Ivon Hayes, 'Foetal Losses in Childbirth', *MJA,* 19 March 1949, pp. 369–72.
90 Ibid., pp. 151–2.
91 'Current Comment', ibid., 12 September 1942, p. 244; W. Ivon Hayes, 'Caesarean Section: A Review of 486 consecutive operations at the Women's Hospital, Melbourne', ibid., 22 December 1934, pp. 799–807; J. W. Johnstone, 'The Changing Place of Caesarean Section', ibid., 3 February 1951, pp. 188–92.
92 This was for an MD under the supervision of Dr John Colebatch.
93 W. M. Lemmon, 'Rubella in Pregnancy—the Obstetrician's Dilemma', *MJA,* 9 September 1950, pp. 392–4.
94 *MJA,* 17 September 1960, pp. 474–5.
95 Interview with Dr Kevin McCaul.
96 A. M. Hill, 'Why be morbid?', p. 106.

VI: Human Relations

12 Managing Difference
1 McCalman, *Journeyings,* pp. 85 and 79.
2 'A Hundred Case Histories', Interview No. 66, by Helen Johnstone.
3 Interview No. 70, by Helen Johnstone.
4 Jean Martin, *The Migrant Presence* (Sydney, 1978),

p. 33. I am indebted to Jacqueline Templeton for this reference.

5 *Annual Report, 1948–49.*

6 Ibid., *1952–53*, p. 5.

7 C. of M. Minutes, 11 October 1946, 21 October 1949, 9 August 1951.

8 Ibid., 27 March, 25 August, 2 October 1952.

9 John Lack and Jacqueline Templeton, *Bold Experiment* (OUP, 1995), pp. 6–8, 21–3.

10 Interview No. 2, by Margaret Mabbitt.

11 Interview No 76, by Madonna Grehan.

12 Interview No. 29, by Marlene Kavanagh.

13 Interview No. 81, by Liliana Ferrara and Helen Johnstone.

14 Interview No. 98, by Liliana Ferrara and Helen Johnstone.

15 Interview No. 62, by Madonna Grehan, incident related by interviewee's sister who was a midwife at the Women's.

16 Interview No. 88, by Liliana Ferrara and Helen Johnstone.

17 Interview No. 94, by Liliana Ferrara and Helen Johnstone.

18 Interview No. 63, by Madonna Grehan.

19 Interview No. 89, by Liliana Ferrara and Helen Johnstone.

20 John Powles and Sandra Gifford, 'How Healthy are Australia's Immigrants?' in Janice Reid and Peggy Trompf, eds, *The Health of Immigrant Australia* (Sydney, 1990), pp. 77–107.

21 D. R. Dunt and M. L. Parker, 'A computer data processing system for hospital obstetric records—obstetric complications in non-English speaking migrants', *MJA,* 6 October 1973, pp. 693–8.

22 Interview No. 95, by Liliana Ferrara and Helen Johnstone.

23 *MJA,* 2 December 1961, pp. 902–4.

24 *Annual Report, 1967.*

25 Shurlee Swain, with Renate Howe, *Single Mothers and Their Children* (CUP, 1995), pp. 140–1.

26 Valerie Douglas, 'Hospital as an Adoption Agency', *Birthplace,* June 1969, pp. 10–13.

27 *Annual Report, 1956–57*, p. 33.

28 Ibid., *1959–60.*

29 *MJA,* 30 July 1960, pp. 165–6.

30 Swain and Howe, p. 141. They in turn cite J. Shawyer, *Death by Adoption* (Auckland, 1979).

31 Interview with Val Lissenden, 16 September 1996.

32 Interviewed 21 October 1993.

33 Clinical Report, 1955.

34 Source anonymous at request of family.

35 Swain and Howe, op. cit, pp. 88–9.

36 'Endometriosis' by Dr J. O'D., Nattrass Collection, Box. 7. Undated but probably delivered at the 1948 or 1950 congress.

37 Interviewed 16 September 1996.

13 Nurses

38 Val Lissenden.

39 Peggy Taylor.

40 Interview No. 39 by Margaret Mabbitt.

41 Interview No. 11 by Marlene Kavanagh.

42 Interviewed 16 September 1996.

43 Interviewed 16 September 1996.

44 Interview No. 54 by Helen Johnstone.

45 Interview No. 26 by Marlene Kavanagh.

46 Interview No. 82, by Cathy Dedman.

47 Interview No. 49, by Marlene Kavanagh.

48 Interview No. 62, by Madonna Grehan.

49 Interview No. 16, by Madonna Grehan.

50 Interview No. 69, by Helen Johnstone.

51 Interviewed 15 May 1997.

52 Interview No. 64, by Cathy Dedman.

53 Interview No. 65, by Cathy Dedman.

54 'Peg', Interview No. 54, by Helen Johnstone.

55 Interview No. 81, by Cathy Dedman.

56 *Clinical Reports,* 1958, 1959, 1961, 1970, 1972.

57 E. Gruber, 'Social Study of Patients Admitted for Abortions, Royal Women's Hospital, 1 March–31 May 1956', unpublished report, RWH Archives. pp. 23 and 25.

58 Ibid., p. 23.

59 Ibid., pp. 24–5.

VII: Transformations

14 Values

1 Interview with Dr Percy Rogers, 4 June 1997.

2 See Lance Townsend, 'Still Birth in the State of Victoria, 1953–1961', *MJA,* 15 September 1962, pp. 403–6.

3 S. L. Townsend et al., 'Induction of Ovulation', *Journal of Obstetrics and Gynaecology of the British Commonwealth,* August 1966, pp. 529–43.

4 *Annual Report, 1961–62*, p. 13.

5 *MJA,* 4 August 1962, p. 173.

6 Interview with Margaret Peters, 23 May 1997.

7 N. A. Beischer, 'Severe Pulmonary Distress syndrome in obstetrics', *MJA,* 26 November 1966, pp. 1042–3.

8 Interview with Netta McArthur, 24 May 1997.

9 Anon.: Memo to Hon. Medical Staff, n.d., Nattrass Collection.

10 *Annual Report, 1969–70*, p. 10.

11 C. of M. Minutes, 16 April, 1 October 1964, 12 December 1967.

12 Memo to Hon. Executive Medical Staff, 28 March 1968, p. 3.

13 Royal Women's Hospital, *Clinical Report, 1970,* pp. 6–7; *Clinical Report, 1974,* p. 29.

14 *MJA,* 19 April 1969, p. 826.

15 Interviewed 5 May 1997.

16 e.g. *Time,* 24 January 1964, quoted by J. Smibert in 'The Pill—its Place in History', in *MJA,* 11 September 1965, p. 469.

17 *MJA,* 12 May 1962, pp. 715–17.

18 Ibid., 1 June 1963, pp. 809–12.

19 Ibid., 21 April 1962, p. 617; 18 August 1962, pp. 267–8.

20 Ibid., 16 January, pp. 73–6; 6 February, p. 208; 20 February, p. 288; 27 February, pp. 324–5; 3 April, pp. 522–3; 18 September, p. 511; 9 October, 1965, p. 641.

21 Dora Bialestock, 'Neglected Babies', ibid., 10 December 1966, pp. 1129–31; R. G. Birrell and J. H. W. Birrell, 'The "Maltreatment Syndrome" in Children', pp. 1134–40.

22 Carl Wood, 'Aspects of Population', ibid., 5 April 1969, pp. 748–52.

23 Ibid., 11 June, 1966, pp. 1017–19; Kelvin Churches, '120 Years of Abortion in Melbourne', *Age*, 24 April, 1976; *Clinical Reports, 1970, 1972*.

24 'A Hundred Case Histories', Interview no. 24, by Cathy Dedman.

25 Interview no. 99, by Helen Johnstone and Liliana Ferrara.

26 Interview No. 19, by Madonna Grehan.

27 C. of M. Minutes, 10 February 1966.

28 Carl Wood, N. Shanmugan, E. Meredith, 'The Risk of Pre-marital Conception', *MJA*, 2 August 1969, pp. 228–32.

29 Interview No. 75, by Madonna Grehan.

30 Carl Wood et al., 'Birth Control Survey in a Lower Social Group in Melbourne', *MJA*, 27 March 1971, pp. 691–6.

31 B. of M. Minutes, passim May, June 1968.

32 John Leeton and Janet Paterson, 'Family Planning in Melbourne: a Medical-Social Project', *MJA*, 8 March 1969, pp. 538–40.

33 John Leeton, 'A Study of 2,245 women attending a hospital family planning clinic', ibid., 14 July 1972, pp. 67–70.

34 e.g. ibid., 28 January 1967, pp. 163–5; 11 June 1966, pp. 1036–41.

35 Churches, loc. cit.

36 B. of M. Minutes, 11 September 1969.

37 Ibid., 7 February 1970.

38 *Annual Report, 1972*, p. 3.

39 *MJA*, 26 October 1969, pp. 360–2; 25 July 1970, pp. 169–73.

15 Practices

40 B. of M. Minutes, 12 October 1972; 8 February 1973.

41 *Annual Report, 1976*, p. 4.

42 Ibid., pp. 10–11.

43 See Barbara Katz Rothman, *Women in Labour: Women and Power in the Birthplace* (New York, 1982, 1991), pp. 63–77.

44 Transcripts: 'The Hand that Rocks the Cradle', RWH, 1977, Keynote Address, p. 8.

45 *Annual Report, 1979*, p. 5.

46 *Age*, 21, 27 and 29 April 1976.

47 Dr M. Kloss, 'The Permissive Society and its Influence on Gynaecology', in 'The Hand that Rocks the Cradle', loc. cit., pp. 3–4.

48 Clinical Report, 1992.

49 Kloss, loc. cit., 'The Permissive Society and its Influence on Gynaecology', pp. 7–9.

50 *Age*, 26 June, 21 August, 19 September 1976; *Sun*, 30 June 1976; *Australian*, 18 September 1976.

51 *Annual Report, 1984*, p. 6.

52 Interview with Bethia Stevenson, 16 June 1997.

53 B. of M. Minutes, 28 March 1974; *Annual Report, 1975*. p. 8; *Age*, 19 July 1974; *Herald*, 11 September 1975.

54 Interview with Associate Professor Wendy Weeks, 29 May 1997.

55 CASA House Philosophy.

56 *Annual Report, 1984*, p. 12.

57 Interview with Dr Chris Bayly, 5 June 1997.

16 Chances

58 e.g. *Annual Report, 1969–70*.

59 Interview with Dr W. H. Kitchen, 12 June 1997.

60 Professor Pepperell, loc. cit.

61 Interview with Mr Ian Johnston, 9 July 1997.

62 Emma Russell, *Bricks or Spirits? The Queen Victoria Hospital, Melbourne* (Melbourne, 1997), p. 76.

63 See Robyn Rowland, *Living Laboratories* (Melbourne, 1992).

64 Interview with Associate Professor Wendy Weeks, 29 May 1997.

65 Interview with Professor Roger Pepperell, 26 May 1997.

66 Interview with Professor Shaun Brennecke, 29 May 1997.

67 Interview with Dr Robin Bell, 19 June 1997.

68 Stephanie Brown, Judith Lumley, Rhonda Small, Jill Astbury, *Missing Voices, The Experience of Motherhood* (Melbourne, 1994), pp. 84–99.

69 *Maternal morbidity in rural Bangladesh* (Dhaka and London, 1994). Published by the Bangladesh Rural Advancement Committee in collaboration with the London School of Hygiene and Tropical Medicine.

70 Interview with Dr Suzanne Garland, 28 July 1997.

71 Interview with Dr Les Reti, 28 July 1997.

Bibliography

Archival and Official Sources

Melbourne City Council Archives, VPRO
Royal Commission on Charitable Institutions, *VPP,* 1892–93, vol. 4

Royal Women's Hospital Archives

Nattrass Collection
Letters and letter books
Cuttings Books
Colin Macdonald, 'The Book of Remembance'
Perry, Frances, 'The History of Mrs Frances Perry' (Nattrass Collection)
Midwifery Books 1 and 2, 1856–1887
Labour Ward Case Books, 1883–1904
Infirmary Case Books 1883–1910
Infirmary Case Records, 1910–1935
Extern Case Books 1920–1936
Annual Reports 1857–
Medical and Clinical Reports, 1940–
Board of Management Minutes
Committee of Management Minutes
Vistors' Book
Honorary Medical Staff Minutes
Gruber, E. 'Social Study of Patients Admitted for Abortions, Royal Women's Hospital, 1 March–31 May 1956'
Hill, Arthur M. Transcript of 'Prestige' Lecture, 1973, Nattrass Collection, Box 6
Royal Women's Hospital, 'The Hand that Rocks the Cradle', 1977
Stevenson, Bethia, Draft of Lecture for Fiftieth Anniversary of Social Work Department, 11 May 1984
Tracy, Richard. *Transactions of the Obstetrical Society of London, 1870*
Wilson, Arthur. Lecture Notes, University of Melbourne, 1926

Newspapers and Journals

Age
Argus
Herald
New Idea
Telegraph
AMA Gazette
Australian Medical Gazette
Australian Medical Journal
Intercolonial Medical Congress 1887
Intercolonial Medical Congress of Australasia, 1889
Intercolonial Medical Journal
Medical Journal of Australia

Interviews

'A Hundred Case Histories': of women over sixty-five who have had a delivery in the Royal Women's Hospital, conducted 1995–96.
  Interviewers: Liliana Ferrara, Madonna Grehan, Catherine Dedman (Hallam), Helen Johnstone, Marlene Kavanagh, Margaret Mabbitt; co-ordinator: Jane Beer

Interviews by author

Dr Chris Bayly
Dr Robin Bell
Dr Gytha Betheras
Professor Shaun Brennecke
Lorraine Danson
Helen Ferguson
Dr Frank Forster
Dr Suzanne Garland
Dr Lorna Lloyd Green
Catherine Hallam (Dedman)
Dr Frank Hayden
Mr Ian Johnston
Helen Johnstone
Marlene Kavanagh
Dr W. H. Kitchen
Miss Betty Lawson
Val Lissenden
Mary Logan
Margaret Mabbitt

Netta McArthur
Dr Kevin McCaul
Professor Roger Pepperell
Margaret Peters
Dr Les Reti
Dr George Robinson
Dr Percy Rogers
Dr Ronald Rome
Beryl Shannon
Bethia Stevenson
Peggy Taylor
Associate Professor Wendy Weeks

Published Sources

Allan, R. Marshall. *Report on Maternal Mortality and Morbidity in the State of Victoria, Australia.* Melbourne, 1929.
Attwood, H. D. 'Patients, Pathologists and Practice', *Aust. N. Z. Journal of Obstetrics and Gynaecology* (1982), 22: 11.
Balls-Headley, Walter. *The Evolution of the Diseases of Women.* London, 1894.
—— . *Pamphlets.* Melbourne, 1893.
Bashford, Alison. 'Female Bodies at Work: Gender and the Re-Forming of Colonial Hospitals', in *Australian Cultural History*, no. 13, 1994.
Bouchet, M. *Practical Treatise on the Diseases of Children and Infants at the Breast.* London, 1855.
Broome, Richard. *The Victorians: Arriving.* Sydney, 1984.
Brown, I. Baker. *On Surgical Diseases of Women.* London, 1861.
Brown, Stephanie, et al. *Missing Voices, The Experience of Motherhood.* Melbourne, 1994.
Bynum, W. F. *Science and the Practice of Medicine in the Nineteenth Century.* Cambridge University Press, 1994.
Cage, R. A. *Poverty Abounding, Charity Aplenty.* Sydney, 1992.
Colebrook, Leonard. 'Puerperal Fever:

its aetiology and prevention', *British Medical Journal,* 21 October 1933.

Cutter, Irving S., and Veits, Henry R. *A Short History of Midwifery.* Philadelphia, 1964.

de Serville, Paul. *Port Phillip Gentlemen.* Melbourne, 1980.

—— . *Pounds and Pedigrees: The Upper Class in Victoria 1850–1880.* Melbourne, 1991.

Douglas, Valerie. 'Hospital as an Adoption Agency', *Birthplace,* June 1969.

Dyason, Diana. 'William Gillbee and Erysipelas at the Melbourne Hospital', *Journal of Australian Studies,* no. 14, May 1984.

Egan, Bryan. *Ways of a Hospital, St Vincent's Melbourne, 1890s–1990s.* Sydney, 1993.

Evans, Richard. *Death in Hamburg.* London, 1990.

Finch, Lyn, and Stratton, Jon. 'The Australian Working Class and the Practice of Abortion, 1880–1939', *Journal of Australian Studies,* no. 23, November 1988.

Fitzpatrick, David. *Oceans of Consolation: Personal Accounts of Irish Migration to Australia.* Melbourne, 1995.

Forster, F. M. C. 'Caesarean Section and its Early Australian History', *MJA,* 1970, 2: 33.

—— . *Progress in Obstetrics and Gynaecology in Australia.* Sydney, 1967.

—— . 'The Story of the Hysterotome and Incision of the Cervix', *MJA,* 1967, 2: 887.

Galabin, Alfred Lewis. *A Manual of Midwifery.* London, 1886.

Gillespie, James A. *The Price of Health.* Melbourne, 1991.

Grimshaw, Patricia, et al. *Creating a Nation.* Melbourne, 1994.

Grimshaw, Patricia, and Strahan, Lynne, eds. *The Half-Open Door.* Sydney, 1982.

Hamlin, R. H. J. 'The Prevention of Eclampsia and Pre-Eclampsia', *Lancet,* 12 January, 1952.

Hill, Arthur M. 'Post-Abortal and Puerperal Gas Gangrene: a Report of Thirty Cases', *J. of Obstet. Gynae. British Empire,* April 1936.

Inglis, K. S. *Hospital and Community: A History of the Royal Melbourne Hospital.* Melbourne, 1958.

Lack, John, and Templeton, Jacqueline. *Bold Experiment.* Oxford University Press, 1995.

Larson, Ann. *Growing Up in Melbourne, Family Life in the Late Nineteenth Century.* Canberra, 1994.

Leavitt, Judith Walzer. *Brought to Bed: Childbearing in America, 1750–1950.* New York, 1986.

Loudon, Irvine, *Death in Childbirth.* Oxford University Press, 1992.

Lowenstein, Wendy. *Weevils in the Flour.* Melbourne, 1979.

McCalman, Janet. *Journeyings: the Biography of a Middle-class Generation, 1920–1990.* Melbourne, 1993.

—— . 'Respectability and Working-Class Politics in Late-Victorian London', *Historical Studies,* vol. 19, no. 74, April 1980.

—— . *Struggletown: Public and Private Life in Richmond, 1900–1965.* Melbourne, 1984.

McGregor, Deborah Kuhn. *Sexual Surgery and the Origins of Gynaecology.* New York, 1989.

Martin, Jean. *The Migrant Presence.* Sydney, 1978.

Mason, Michael. *The Making of Victorian Sexual Attitudes.* Oxford University Press, 1994.

—— . *The Making of Victorian Sexuality.* Oxford University Press, 1994.

Maternal morbidity in rural Bangladesh. Dhaka and London, 1994.

Morgan, Sharon. 'Irishwomen in Port Phillip', in Oliver MacDonagh and W. F. Mandle, eds. *Irish Australian Studies.* Canberra, 1989.

Moscucci, Ornella. *The Science of Woman: Gynaecology and Gender in England, 1800–1929.* Cambridge, 1990.

Munro Kerr, J. M., et al. eds. *Historical Review of British Obstetrics and Gynaecology.* Edinburgh, 1954.

Niall, Brenda, *Georgiana.* Melbourne, 1994.

O'Brien, Laurie, and Turner, Cynthia. *Establishing Medical Social Work in Victoria.* Dept of Social Studies, University of Melbourne, 1979.

O'Sullivan, M. U. *The Proclivity of Civilised Woman to Uterine Displacement: the Antidote.* Melbourne, 1894.

Poovey, Mary. ' "Scenes of an Indelicate Character": the Medical "Treatment" of Victorian Women', in Thomas Laqueur and Catherine Gallagher, eds. *The Making of the Modern Body.* Berkeley, 1987.

Powles, John, and Gifford, Sandra. 'How Healthy are Australia's Immigrants?', in Janice Reid and Peggy Trompf, eds. *The Health of Immigrant Australia.* Sydney, 1990.

Reiger, Kereen. *The Disenchantment of the Home.* Melbourne, 1985.

Reverby, Susan M. *Ordered to Care: the Dilemma of American Nursing, 1850–1945.* Cambridge University Press, 1987.

Roe, Michael. *Nine Australian Progressives: Vitalism in Bourgeois Social Thought, 1890–1960.* Brisbane, 1984.

Rosenberg, Charles E. *Explaining Epidemics and other Studies in the History of Medicine.* Cambridge University Press, 1992.

Rosenthal, Newman. *People—Not Cases: The Royal District Nursing Service.* Melbourne, 1974.

Rothman, Barbara Katz. *Women in Labour: Women and Power in the Birthplace.* New York, 1982, 1991.

Rowland, Robyn. *Living Laboratories.* Melbourne, 1992.

Royal Women's Hospital. *Centenary of Nurse Training in Australia, 1862–1962.* Melbourne, 1962.

Russell, Emma. *Bricks or Spirits? The Queen Victoria Hospital, Melbourne.* Melbourne, 1997.

Ruzika, Lado T., and Caldwell, John C. *The End of Demographic Transition in Australia.* Canberra, 1977.

Simpson, James Young. *The Obstetric Memoirs and Contributions of James Y. Simpson.* Edinburgh, 1855.

Smart, Judith. 'The Great War and the "Scarlet Scourge": Debates about Venereal Diseases in Melbourne during World War I', in Judith Smart and Tony Wood, eds. *An Anzac Muster: War and Society in Australia and New Zealand, 1914–18 and 1939–45.* Melbourne, 1992.

Smibert, James. 'Fifty Years of Obstetrics, 1935–1985', *Newsletter, Association of Monash Medical Graduates Inc.,* vol. 13, no. 2, July 1991.

Smith, F. B. *The People's Health.* London, 1979.

Smith, Philippa Mein. *Mothers and King Baby.* London, 1997.

Swain, Shurlee, with Renate Howe. *Single Mothers and their Children.* Melbourne, 1995.

Szreter, Simon. *Fertility, Class and Gender in Britain, 1860–1940.* Cambridge University Press, 1996.

Thoms, Herbert. *Classical Contributions to Obstetrics and Gynaecology.* Baltimore, 1935.

Townsend, Lance. *Gynaecology for Students.* Sydney, 1974.

—— . *Obstetrics for Students.* Sydney, 1978.

Townsend S. L., et al. 'Induction of Ovulation', *Journal of Obstetrics and Gynaecology of the British Commonwealth,* August 1966.

Verso, M. L. 'Fifty Years of the Red Cross Blood Transfusion Service in Victoria', *Victorian Historical Journal,* November 1980.

Warner, John Harley. 'The History of Science and the Sciences of Medicine', *Osiris,* 1995, 10.

Wertz, Richard W., and Wertz, Dorothy C. *Lying-In: A History of Childbirth in America.* New York, 1979.

West, Charles. *Lectures on the Diseases of Women.* London, 1858.

Unpublished Sources

Smith, F. B. 'Australian Public Health during the Depression of the 1930s', MS.

Swain, S. L. The Victorian Charity Network in the 1890s, PhD thesis, University of Melbourne, 1977.

Index

References to illustrations are in italics